MEDICAL SHORT CASES
FOR MEDICAL STUDENTS

Medical Short Cases for Medical Students

R.E.J. Ryder MD, FRCP

Consultant Physician
Department of Diabetes and Endocrinology
City Hospital NHS Trust
Birmingham

M.A. Mir MB BS, FRCP, DCH

Senior Lecturer and Consultant Physician
University Hospital of Wales
Cardiff

E.A. Freeman MB, ChB, FRCP

Consultant Physician
Department of Medicine and Care of the Elderly
Royal Gwent and St Woolos Hospitals
Newport

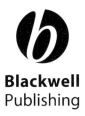

Blackwell
Publishing

© 2000 by
Blackwell Science Ltd
Editorial Offices:
9600 Garsington Road, Oxford OX4 2DQ
23 Ainslie Place, Edinburgh EH3 6AJ
350 Main Street, Malden
    MA 02148 5020, USA
54 University Street, Carlton
    Victoria 3053, Australia

Other Editorial Offices:
Blackwell Wissenschafts-Verlag GmbH
Kurfürstendamm 57
10707 Berlin, Germany

Blackwell Science KK
MG Kodenmacho Building
7–10 Kodenmacho Nihombashi
Chuo-ku, Tokyo 104, Japan

First published 2000
Reprinted 2005, 2006

Set by Best-set Typesetter Ltd,
Hong Kong
Printed and bound in India by
Replika Press Pvt. Ltd

The Blackwell Science logo is a
trade mark of Blackwell Science Ltd,
registered at the United Kingdom
Trade Marks Registry

A catalogue record for this title
is available from the British Library

ISBN-10: 0-632-05729-7
ISBN-13: 978-0-632-05729-0

Library of Congress
Cataloging-in-Publication Data

Ryder, R.E.J. (Robert Elford John)
    Medical short cases for medical
students / R.E.J. Ryder, M.A. Mir, and
E.A. Freeman.
        p.;   cm.
    Includes index.
    ISBN 0-632-05729-7
    1. Diagnosis—Case studies.
    I. Mir, M.A. (Mohammad Afzal)
    II. Freeman, E.A. (Eleanor Anne)
    III. Title.
        [DNLM: 1. Physical
    Examination—Case Report.
    2. Diagnosis, Differential—Case
    Report.   WB 200 R992m 2000]
    RC71.R95 2000
    616.07'5—dc21   00-029741

DISTRIBUTORS

Marston Book Services Ltd
PO Box 269
Abingdon, Oxon OX14 4YN
(*Orders*:   Tel: 01235 465500
                Fax: 01235 465555)

USA
Blackwell Science, Inc.
Commerce Place
350 Main Street
Malden, MA 02148-5020
(*Orders*:   Tel: 800 759 6102
                    781 388 8250
                Fax: 781 388 8255)

Canada
Login Brothers Book Company
324 Saulteaux Crescent
Winnipeg, Manitoba R3J 3T2
(*Orders*:   Tel: 204 837 2987)

Australia
Blackwell Science Pty Ltd
54 University Street
Carlton, Victoria 3053
(*Orders*:   Tel: 3 9347 0300
                Fax: 3 9347 5001)

For further information on
Blackwell Publishing, visit our website:
www.blackwellpublishing.com

Contents

Preface

This book is intended to help medical students with their preparations for medical short case examinations and through this process to enhance the depth and breadth of their knowledge of clinical medicine as well as their clinical skills. Though particularly of use to students sitting their final MB clinical exams, it will also be of interest to more junior students, particularly those who face medical short case clinical exams in their early clinical years. It aims to be useful whether the exam format is of the traditional style or more modern variations such as the Objective Structured Clinical Examination (OSCE).

The book is based unashamedly on its postgraduate predecessor *An Aid to the MRCP Short Cases*. That book, which was first published in 1986, has been purchased by most doctors sitting the MRCP since that time and though this number remains roughly constant, the sales of the book have increased year on year. It became clear that this was because, despite its postgraduate title, medical students were discovering the book and purchasing it themselves to help with their undergraduate short case examinations. Investigations revealed that it was not only students in their final year who were buying it and finding it useful, but also students just starting out in their clinical studies. Thus it seemed appropriate to develop a version of our short cases book specifically for medical students and this is the result. Because the medical students who used the postgraduate version reported to us that they found it exactly what they were looking for, we have retained most of the same style, approach and content in this undergraduate version on the grounds that 'if it ain't broken, don't fix it!'. However, as much basic knowledge is assumed in the main text we have provided a comprehensive glossary in this medical student edition. (Any terms defined in the glossary are indicated with (gl.) at their first mention in each chapter and short case.)

Why should an approach designed for postgraduate doctors sitting the MRCP be found so useful to medical students? The answer, we believe, is that the cases used in the undergraduate medical short case exams are drawn from the same pool as those used in the MRCP examination. Furthermore the examiners are all physicians who are MRCP trained and tend instinctively to use the MRCP style in the examinations that they set and in the approach that they adopt. Though clearly the required standard of performance is lower, there is no question that medical students can benefit by preparing for medical short case exams in a similar way to postgraduates.

In this book, 19 examination *routines* are written around clinical instructions given by examiners to students, with details of the suitable examination steps in response to each command. We have also reduced these *routines* to simple steps (*checklists*) which, if practised, may become spontaneous clinical habits, easy to recall and execute. The bulk of the book presents the examination *routines* for each system and subsystem followed by examples of short cases, both common and rare, and these are illustrated with clinical photographs. The difficult to elicit signs are also illustrated with appropriate clinical pictures. We have individualized 'inspection' to the examination of each subsystem, and have provided a *visual survey* to note the features most likely to be present. The list of 100 short cases chosen for this book is derived from our surveys of various examinations which use the same pool of conditions for both the Membership as well as the final MB examination.

The book sets out initially to be an aid to passing examinations. Nevertheless it is packed with information and there is no doubt that medical students who use it 'to pass their exams', and succeed, will, in the process, have greatly improved their clinical skills and their knowledge of clinical medicine as a result. After all, medical short case exams teach more than they test!

Acknowledgements

We remain grateful to many friends and colleagues who have supported us over the years, a small proportion of whom are listed in the postgraduate book. More than ever we remain grateful to our long-suffering families: to Anne's family, Peter, Lizzie and Jon Williams, to Afzal's family, Lynda, Farooq, Deborah and Joanne Mir and to Bob's family, Anne, Bobby and Anna Ryder. Without their forbearance and help, none of it would ever have happened.

Bob Ryder
Afzal Mir
Anne Freeman

Introduction

The broad aim of medical education is to produce a graduate with an adequate knowledge base who is equipped with the essential skills to understand a patient's complaints, can make a competent clinical assessment, is able to provide a management plan, can explain it to the patient and relatives with sensitivity, and is ready to embark on a further learning experience as a house officer. The final MB examination is designed to test for these qualities, and its colander mesh retains those that are found lacking in one of the three seminal attributes of safety, skills and sensitivity. These attributes and attitudes cannot be pretended or borrowed for the day of the examination, nor is this book a shortcut to bypassing the opportunities for acquiring knowledge, concepts, principles, attitudes and skills during the clinical training. Rather, we hope that you will use this book as a companion to guide you during your learning experiences as you encounter patients on the wards and in clinics.

Medical short case examinations

The structure of medical short case examinations varies not only from country to country but also from medical school to medical school in the same country. For a typical exam, the examiners are divided into pairs and each pair is asked to take a student and test them on a mixture of clinical problems, as many as can be accommodated in 20–25 min. The last few minutes are reserved for the examiners' discussion about an agreed grade. Thus, two examiners will take you for approximately 10 min each to record a separate mark and agree on a combined mark when both of them have completed the examination. This format is used with some minor modifications in many medical schools in the UK. Increasingly, medical schools are introducing the Objective Structured Clinical Examination (OSCE) system, where students are taken to various stations and asked to perform some selected clinical tasks (examine the cranial nerves, chest, legs, etc.).

In most centres, the examiners are encouraged to introduce each patient, for example 'This is Mrs Smith. She is complaining of a cough and breathlessness. Would you please examine her chest and see if you can find a reason for her symptoms.' None the less, the old system often prevails and the examiners may simply ask you, 'Examine this patient's heart, chest or abdomen.' This approach is inevitable when you are asked to make a spot diagnosis, for example 'Have a look at this patient and tell me about your observations', or, when you are asked to examine a subsystem, 'Examine this patient's hands, visual fields, eyes, fundi, etc.' Unlike the Membership examination, the examiners in final MB examinations are usually forthcoming with encouraging remarks or gestures. As you examine a patient and when you give your findings or diagnosis, the examiners will often give you appropriate feedback which should be accepted with good grace and pursued whenever necessary. Remember, they are not misleading or trying to trick you.

The discussion is usually kept to a minimum though they may ask you to give a few causes of an abnormal finding or offer a differential diagnosis. Generally, examiners are discouraged from embarking on a lengthy discussion about the pathophysiology or management plan of a clinical problem in the short cases examination. These aspects are well covered in other examinations.

Survey of the final MB short cases

In 1997, we conducted a survey among the recently qualified medical graduates from 27 medical schools in the UK, and we found that there were 77 short cases which were repeatedly used in these schools (see Appendix 2). We used this survey to guide us in the choice of the 100 short cases chosen for this book from the MRCP/final MB pool which our earlier surveys had shown were commonly used. While diabetic retinopathy is the commonest short case in the Membership examination, examination of the heart (mitral/aortic valve disease), chest (pleural effusion, fibrosis) and abdomen (hepatosplenomegaly, polycystic kidneys, ascites) are the three commonest tasks presented to final MB candidates according to our survey. The examiners are less worried whether you can recognize a polio limb, but they are more concerned whether, after examining apparently normal-looking legs, you can state confidently that there is or is not a neurological lesion. After the examination of an abdomen if you come up with a suggestion that there is splenomegaly, they may quiz you why it is not an enlarged kidney.

They are less likely to let you loose on an unsuspecting public if you cannot decide whether a patient has pneumonia or a smoker's cough!

Preparing for medical short case exams

See patients and learn: The most efficient way of learning clinical medicine is to read up the conditions you meet as you meet them. This applies to all aspects — pathophysiology, aetiology, epidemiology, clinical features, treatment, prognosis, etc. If you talk to and examine a patient and follow through the case — how investigated, how treated, and how the patient progresses — and at the same time read up all aspects of the patient's problem, it will all stay much more easily in your memory than if you only read about the medical condition in a vacuum. With regard to medical short cases there is no substitute to seeing the conditions and clinical signs in real life. Therefore be proactive in seeing as much as you can during your attachments to clinical firms. Seek out and see patients with different conditions. Take their histories and examine them. Whenever you come across a disease, read its features in this book as well as in a textbook of medicine. Use this book to consider the physical signs you might find when you examine the patient. In this way you will remember those signs which are present, by association, and also those that are absent, by dissociation. Remember, during each of your clinical attachments, that you are attached to the hospital and not only to your firm; do not just confine yourself to the patients allocated to you, but look out for all the 'good cases' and 'good signs' passing through the hospital. See as many of these as possible as practice short cases, study their features in this book, and practise presenting them to yourself or to a colleague on a one-to-one basis.

Practise clinical skills: It is not uncommon to see students at the final MB examination who do not correctly hold a tendon hammer, let alone test the ankle jerk. Some students percuss by flexing the middle finger at the metacarpophalangeal joint and some use the force of the whole forearm. Inadequate and clumsy methods look unseemly, are unproductive, and create a bad and unfavourable impression on the examiners. You should practise clinical skills from the very beginning when you first enter into a clinical setting. Watch how your tutors percuss and use the tendon hammer and then practise on a desk and a colleague! As you are taught the examination of each system, practise the clinical skills involved in that examination. Do not take it for granted that you will acquire the correct knack with experience unless you learn the correct method at the outset. Since you will be using clinical skills throughout your practising life it makes good sense to learn the correct methods at the beginning. You may find it useful to use an illustrated book such as *An Atlas of Clinical Skills* (Mir; Saunders) to learn history taking and examination.

Learn examination routines: When an examiner asks you to examine a patient's heart, he expects you to carry out a step by step, integrated examination of that system. It looks bad when you, for example, take the pulse and then appear as if you are in the process of deciding what to do next. Worse still, if you carry out an incomplete series of examination steps in an unorthodox sequence jumping backwards and forwards between parts of the traditional examination sequence — for example, you take the radial pulse and then start to auscultate the heart, then stop to look at the neck to observe the jugular venous pressure, because you had forgotten to do this previously. Similarly, while teaching the examination of the nervous system, tutors have been emphasizing for the last few centuries a particular sequence — bulk, tone, power, coordination, abnormal movements, reflexes, sensations and gait; the examiners may not be amused by your own hybrid if you have not practised this *routine*.

Be aware of the 'downward spiral syndrome': In the postgraduate book this is described as follows:

'The candidate, an otherwise able and experienced doctor, enters the short cases room extremely anxious and lacking in confidence. He is just hovering on the edge of despair and the slightest upset is going to push him over. On one or more of the cases he convinces himself that he is doing badly (whether or not he actually is) and over the edge he goes. The first stage of a rapid 'downward spiral' sets in; the dispirited candidate gets worse and worse and actually gives up before the end in the certainty that he has failed. Months of intensive book work and bedside practice, not to mention the examination fee, go to waste because of inadequate psychological preparation . . .'

This scenario, of course, can also happen to a medical student. The fact that short case exams are practical exams in which you 'perform' in front of examiners can lead to the otherwise able medical student performing poorly simply because of 'stage fright'. If you feel you are particularly prone to performing poorly through lack of confidence and anxiety you may wish to read what we have written on the issue in Section 1 of our postgraduate book. However, it is important to bear in mind that the medical student exam is very different to the postgraduate exam in terms of the examiners' underlying attitude. You should remember that *the final MB examiners would be happy to pass every student*. Even the most hawkish examiners do not wish to fail anyone in their clinical examination. Unless there is anyone who is likely to harm his patients with unwarranted, bubbling overconfidence or demonstrable incompetence no student need fail. A simple statement like, 'I do not know the answer but I would consult a senior or a book before I treat this patient' will often be accepted as reasonable. The examiners are just as happy to pass everyone as they are to fail a few to allow them a few more months experience to get to a level of competence. Doctors are in short supply and there is no compelling reason to fail anyone unless the standard of performance makes it really necessary. It is said that the examiners come with a 100% mark and a student bent on failing nibbles away at it until he fails! In this examination, your good answers get extra credit and the bad ones often pass unnoticed unless they are unsafe. So, go to the examination with the feeling that the examiners are on *your* side and not against you. *Keep thinking and acting positively and put your mistakes behind you.* It is the overall level of competence you show that counts rather than the odd mistake that you make. Remember to think in terms of *the cases are all very easy and you have seen them before.* The vast majority of cases are straightforward and even the rare ones can become well known and recognizable to you. The list of short cases that can be brought to the exam is not limitless and common cases keep recurring in each examination. Further, the examiners' brief is to test your examination technique and how you assemble your findings, and not your diagnostic acumen on rare and weird curiosities. Remember, your best friends are your knowledge and a thorough preparation with short cases and examination *routines*, and your worst enemies are anxiety and overconfidence. You should cultivate the former, discard the latter and prepare yourself psychologically for the examination. If you study the short cases in this book carefully you are unlikely to be surprised in the examination.

The A grade student and the 'belt and braces' student: It is well recognized that the A grade medical student at the final MB (and sometimes even earlier in the clinical years!) can sometimes perform better in their short cases exam than many a postgraduate sitting the MRCP short cases. Such medical students, particularly those who are budding physicians, once they have mastered this book may wish to also study the postgraduate version (*An Aid to the MRCP Short Cases*, 2nd edition), where another 100 short cases can be found. There is more detail on many of the 100 covered in this book, as well as colour photographs of short cases and many accounts of the triumphs and disasters of postgraduates going through their ordeal — accounts full of lessons, and sometimes comedy, and other times tragedy! If the 'belt and braces' student is concerned about any possibility of short cases not covered in this book, he may also wish to dip into the postgraduate version!

Examination *routines*

To help you to satisfy your examiners, we have given comprehensive examination *routines* at the beginning of each subsystem to cover all the tasks necessary for evaluating each short case. These are readily adaptable to your individual methods. We would suggest that you practise each succession of steps repeatedly until you can perform each sequence without having to keep pausing and thinking what to do next, so that you do not miss out important steps. Practise on friends, colleagues and spouses, as well as patients. The *routines* are broken down into numbered constituents to aid memory and *checklists* are given in Appendix 1 which match up to the numbered points in the examination *routine*.

Often you will not need the complete sequence in the examination (for example, it will be rare for you to carry out all the steps in the 'Examine this patient's arms' *routine*; with regard to the 'Examine this patient's chest' *routine*, often the examiner will ask you to only examine 'the back of this patient's chest') but it will certainly increase your confidence if you enter the examination armed with the complete *routines* so that you can adapt them as necessary.

There are some general points that are worth taking on board. You should avoid repeating the examiner's command or echoing the last part of it. Refrain from asking questions like: 'Would you like me to give you a running commentary or give the findings at the end'. Such a response wastes invaluable seconds which could be used running through the *checklist* and completing your *visual survey*. Consider it like a batsman asking a bowler in a cricket match whether he would like his ball hit for a six or played defensively! You should do what you are best at and hope that the examiner does not ask you to do otherwise. A well-rehearsed procedure suited to each subsystem should make it possible for you to start purposefully without delay. Your approach to the patient is of great importance; you should introduce yourself to him and ask his permission to examine him. Permission should also be sought for various manoeuvres, such as adjusting the backrest when examining the heart, or before removing any clothing. Although we encourage you to look for signs peripheral to the examiner's instruction, we would emphasize too that dithering can be counterproductive. In the *visual survey* you should be scanning the patient rapidly and purposefully with a trained eye, not gazing helplessly at him for a prolonged period while you try to decide what to do next. While you are feeling the pulse (heart) or settling the patient lying flat (abdomen), a quick look at the hands should establish whether there are any abnormalities or not. Pondering over normal hands from all angles at great length looks as unprofessional as, indeed, it is. It is of paramount importance to be gentle with the patient and treat him with respect. Make sure that you cover the patient up when you have finished examining him, and thank him.

100 short cases

The 100 short cases dealt with in this book are presented as aides mémoire (clinical descriptions for presentation to the examiner). We have called these aide-mémoire *records*. The style of each *record* imagines you in the examination situation with the patient displaying the typical features of a particular condition; you are 'churning out' these to the examiner along with the answers to anticipated questions. Thus, you play the *record* of the condition to the examiner. Of course the cases in the actual examination will only have some of the features (the *record* tends to describe the 'full house' case), and it is hoped that by becoming familiar with the whole *record* you will be well equipped:
1 to pick up all the features present in the cases you meet on the day by scanning through the *records* in your mind; and
2 to adapt the *record* for the purpose of presenting those features which are present.

To facilitate quick revision, the main points of each short case are highlighted in italics. The smaller print under the rule is a mixed bag of additional features and facts, lists of differential diagnoses and answers to some questions that might be asked. With the lists of differential diagnoses we have tended to put the most important ones (which you should consider first) in large print with longer lists in the small print. The lists are not necessarily meant to be comprehensive.

Next to the diagnoses in these lists we have used brackets to give some of the features of the conditions concerned, or perhaps one or two features you could look for (indicated by ?). The question mark is put there as a cue for you to look for important diagnostic features. We make no apology for repeating some of the features often, in the hope that by constant reinforcement they will become more firmly embedded in your memory. When unilateral signs could affect either side we have not usually specified the side in the *record* but have indicated this by R/L. In these cases, however, each R/L in the *record* refers to the same side. Also . . . is occasionally used for a sign in the lung fields or retina which could occur in any zone or to indicate the size of an organ or sign where the size is unspecified. Words covered in the glossary are indicated with (gl.) at their first mention in each chapter and short case.

Presentation to the examiner

Becoming familiar with the short case *records* will arm you for the examination, though obviously it will not always be necessary, or desirable, for you to use them. Sometimes it may be appropriate just to give the diagnosis—even so it may be still possible to enrich it with some of the well-known features from the *record*. If the examiner's question is 'What is the diagnosis?' you could answer 'mitral stenosis' and await his reaction. On the other hand, if you are certain of your diagnosis, it would be better to say: 'The diagnosis is mitral stenosis because there is a rough, rumbling mid-diastolic murmur localized to the apex of the heart, there is a sharp opening snap and a loud first heart sound, a tapping impulse, an impalpable left ventricular apex, a left parasternal heave and a small volume pulse. Furthermore the chaotic rhythm suggests atrial fibrillation and the patient has a malar flush.'

If you enlarge your response to 'What is the diagnosis?' by giving the features in this way, it is best to give the evidence in the order of its importance to the diagnosis (as shown in the example). However, if the question is: 'What are your findings?' it is best to give them in the order they are elicited: 'The patient has a malar flush and is slightly breathless at rest. The pulse is irregular in rate and volume. The jugular venous pressure is not elevated and the cardiac apex is not palpable but there is a tapping impulse parasternally on the left side and there is a left parasternal heave. The first heart sound is loud and there is an opening snap followed closely by a mid-diastolic rumble which is localized to the apex. These signs suggest that the patient has mitral stenosis.'

Remember, if you are talking in front of the patient, to avoid using words like 'cancer', 'motor neurone disease' and 'multiple sclerosis'. Use euphemisms such as 'neoplastic disease', 'anterior horn cell disease' and 'demyelinating disease'.

Remember also that you can influence any discussion that follows by what you say. For example, the words: 'The diagnosis is aortic incompetence' may produce an interrogation by the examiner, or you may just be moved on to the next case. However, if you say: 'He has aortic incompetence for which there are several causes', this invites the examiner to ask you the causes. It is, therefore, a good answer—as long as you know them!

Chapter 1
Examine this patient's pulse

Possible short cases include

Examination *routine*

As you approach the patient from the right and ask for his permission to examine him* you should $1°$ hypothyroidism

1 look at his **face** for a *malar flush* (mitral stenosis, myxoedema) or for any signs of *hyper-* or *hypothyroidism*. As you take the arm to examine the right radial pulse, continue the *survey* of the patient by looking at

2 the **neck** (Corrigan's sign (gl.)†, raised jugular venous pressure (JVP), thyroidectomy scar, goitre) and then the *chest* (thoracotomy scar). Quickly run your eyes down the body to complete the *survey* (ascites, clubbing, pretibial myxoedema, ankle oedema, etc.) and then concentrate on

3 the **pulse** and note

4 its **rate** (count for at least 15 seconds), **volume** (the upstroke of the pulse wave appreciated by the pulp of the examining finger)‡ and

5 its **rhythm**. A common diagnostic problem is presented by *slow atrial fibrillation* which may be mistaken for a regular pulse. To avoid this concentrate on the *length of the pause* from one beat to another and see if each pause is equal to the succeeding one (see also p. 5). This method will reveal that the pauses are variable from beat to beat in controlled slow atrial fibrillation.

6 Assess whether the **character** (waveform) of the pulse (information to be gained from radial, brachial and carotid) is **normal**, *collapsing, slow rising* or

---

* This may not be necessary if the examiner indicates at the outset that all patients have consented to be examined.

† Any term followed by (gl.) is described in greater detail in the glossary (Appendix 3, pp. 280–294).

‡ A *large volume pulse* suggests diastolic overload (aortic/mitral regurgitation, patent ductus arteriosus, anaemia, thyrotoxicosis, etc.) and a *small volume pulse* suggests low output (mitral/aortic stenosis, low blood pressure).

jerky. To determine whether there is a collapsing quality put the palmar aspect of the four fingers of your left hand on the patient's wrist just below where you can easily feel the radial pulse. Press gently with your palm, lift the patient's hand above his head and then place your right palm over the patient's axillary artery (Fig. 1.1). If the pulse has a *water-hammer* character you will experience a flick (a sharp and tall up-stroke and an abrupt down-stroke) which will *run* across all four fingers and at the same time you may also feel a flick of the axillary artery against your other palm. The pulse does not merely become palpable when the hand is lifted but its character changes and it imparts a sharp knock. This is classic of the pulse that is present in haemodynamically significant aortic incompetence and in patent ductus arteriosus (gl.). If the pulse has a collapsing character but is not of a frank water-hammer type then the flick runs across only two or three fingers (moderate degree of aortic incompetence or patent ductus arteriosus, thyrotoxicosis, fever, pregnancy, moderately severe mitral incompetence, anaemia or atherosclerosis). A *slow*

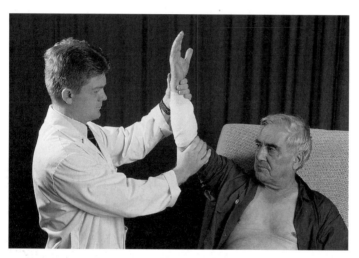

Fig. 1.1 Testing for a collapsing pulse. As you lift the arm the radial artery will impart a flick to your left palm and the brachial to your right palm.

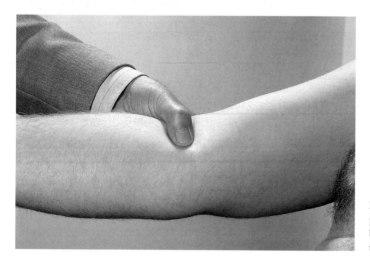

Fig. 1.2 Feeling for an anacrotic pulse. The slow-rising up-stroke can be appreciated in the pulp of the thumb pressing on the artery.

rising pulse (aortic stenosis) can best be assessed by palpating the brachial pulse with your left thumb (Fig. 1.2) and, as you press *gently*, you may feel the anacrotic notch (you will need practise to appreciate this) on the up-stroke against the pulp of your thumb. In mixed aortic valve disease the combination of plateau and collapsing effects can produce a **double-peaked bisferiens pulse**. Whilst feeling the brachial pulse look for any catheterization *scars* (indicating valvular or ischaemic heart disease).

7 Proceed to feel the **carotid** (Fig. 1.3)* where either a slow rising or a collapsing pulse can be confirmed.

8 Feel the **opposite radial pulse** and determine if both radials are the same (e.g. Fallot's tetralogy (gl.) with a Blalock shunt (gl.)), and then feel

9 the **right femoral pulse** checking for any *radiofemoral delay* (Fig. 1.4) (coarctation of the aorta). If you are asked to examine the pulses (as opposed to the pulse) you should continue to examine

10 all the other **peripheral pulses**. It is unlikely that the examiner will allow you to continue beyond what he thinks is a reasonable time to spot the diagnosis that he has in mind. However, should he not interrupt continue to look for

11 **additional diagnostic clues**. Thus, in a patient with atrial fibrillation and features suggestive of thyrotoxicosis you should examine the thyroid and/or eyes. In a patient with atrial fibrillation and hemiplegia or atrial fibrillation and a mitral valvotomy scar, proceed to **examine the heart**.

For *checklist* see p. 275.

Bisferens - 2
Systolic peaks
of aortic pulse
during LV
ejection separated
by midsystolic
dip.

Seen in patients
with mixed
aortic stenosis
and aortic
regurgitation
regurg being
predominant
lesion.

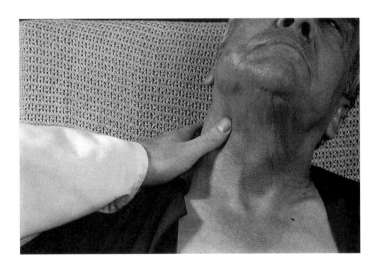

Fig. 1.3 Feeling the carotid pulse.

* Practise feeling the carotid pulse with your thumb and not with all fingers.

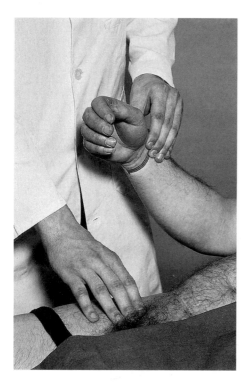

Fig. 1.4 Checking for radiofemoral delay.

1 / Irregular pulse

Record

The pulse is . . . /min and *irregularly irregular* in rate and volume suggesting controlled* (or uncontrolled if rate fast) **atrial fibrillation**. Now look at the *neck* (goitre), *eyes* (exophthalmos), *face* (mitral facies, hypothyroidism† or hemiplegia due to an embolus) and *chest* (thoracotomy scar).‡

Differential diagnosis

The differentiation of an irregular pulse due to controlled atrial fibrillation from that of multiple extrasystoles, will depend upon the observation that only in atrial fibrillation do long pauses occur in groups of two or more (with ectopic beats the compensatory pause follows a short pause because the ectopic is premature). Furthermore, exercise may abolish extrasystoles but worsen the irregularity of atrial fibrillation. Atrial fibrillation can be difficult to distinguish from atrial flutter with variable block, from multiple atrial ectopics due to a shifting pacemaker, and sometimes from paroxysmal atrial tachycardia with block. Only in atrial fibrillation is the rhythm truly *chaotic*.

Causes of atrial fibrillation

Ischaemic heart disease (especially myocardial infarction)
Rheumatic heart disease
Hypertensive heart disease
Thyrotoxicosis
Cardiomyopathy§
Acute infections (especially lung)
Constrictive pericarditis.
Alcohol

---

* Though controlled atrial fibrillation may sometimes feel regular initially, if you concentrate there is a definite irregular variation in beat-to-beat time interval.

† Previously treated Graves' disease now on inadequate thyroxine replacement—pulse rate slow, ankle jerk relaxation slow, etc.

‡ If allowed, follow up any positive findings from this *visual survey* by appropriate examination of the relevant system. If there is no visible abnormality proceed, if allowed, to examine the heart, the neck for a goitre, and thyroid status.

§ Though in most patients with cardiomyopathy no cause can be found ('idiopathic'), sometimes the causal disorder can be identified. Some of the usual causes can be grouped as follows:

1 Toxic (alcohol, adriamycin, cyclophosphamide, emetine, corticosteroids, lithium, phenothiazines, etc.)

2 Metabolic (thiamine deficiency, kwashiorkor, pellagra, obesity, porphyria, uraemia, electrolyte imbalance)

3 Endocrine (thyrotoxicosis, acromegaly, myxoedema, Cushing's, diabetes mellitus)

4 Collagen diseases (systemic lupus erythematosus (SLE), polyarteritis nodosa (gl.), etc.)

5 Infiltrative (amyloidosis (gl.), haemochromatosis (gl.), neoplastic, glycogen storage disease, sarcoidosis (gl.), mucopolysaccharidosis, Gaucher's disease (gl.), Whipple's disease)

6 Infective (viral, rickettsial, mycobacterial)

7 Genetic (hypertrophic obstructive cardiomyopathy (gl.), muscular dystrophies (gl.))

8 Fibroplastic (endomyocardial fibrosis, Löffler's endocarditis, carcinoid (gl.))

9 Miscellaneous (ischaemic heart disease, postpartum).

2 / Slow pulse

Record

The pulse rate is regular at 40/min (irregularly irregular pulse with beat-to-beat variation may be slow atrial fibrillation) and there is *no increase* in the rate on *standing* (complete heart block; mostly in older patients). The JVP is not elevated (unless there is heart failure) but just visible, and there is a complete dissociation of *a* and *v* waves with frequent *cannon waves* (flicking *a* waves occurring during ventricular systole).

This patient has complete heart block.

Other causes of bradycardia

Beta-blocker therapy: about 2% of patients receiving β-blockers have excessive bradycardia (heart rate increases by a few beats on standing and during exercise)

Slow atrial fibrillation: the patient may be on β-blockers and/or digoxin

Hypothyroidism (?facies, ankle jerks, etc. —p. 251)

Sinoatrial disease: bradycardia–tachycardia syndrome

Digitalis overdose.

Cardiac pacing

Most patients with complete heart block will benefit from a demand pacemaker (even asymptomatic patients with a heart rate <40/min).

3 / Peripheral vascular disease

Record

The lower leg(s) are pale (pregangrenous areas may be pink), the toes are bluish-red (there may be digital gangrene) and the *skin is atrophic* (may be stretched and *shiny*) and *hairless*. There are *no pulses** palpable below the femorals (if allowed, listen for a bruit) and the lower legs and feet are *cold* to touch. There is often asymmetry of signs.

These signs suggest peripheral vascular disease (?arcus senilis, ?xanthelasma, ?tendon xanthomata, ?nicotine-stained fingers, ?diabetes†).

Arteriosclerosis obliterans

This, the usual cause of peripheral vascular disease, is due to atheromatous plaques involving the intima of the arteries. As a rule there is superimposed thrombus formation. Degenerative changes occur in the media which frequently calcifies.† The superficial femoral artery is most commonly affected leading to calf claudication. The next most common sites are the popliteal and aortic bifurcation, the latter leading to:

Leriche's syndrome: claudication of low back, buttocks, thigh and calf; limb and buttock atrophy and pallor; impotence, weak or absent femoral pulses, systolic bruits over the lower abdomen and femorals; signs may be asymmetrical; may present as 'sciatica'.

Buerger's postural test

When the legs are lifted to 45° above the horizontal plane, cadaveric pallor develops if the arterial supply is poor. If, while the clinician supports the legs, the patient flexes and extends the ankles to the point of mild fatigue, this enhances the sign. The patient now sits with his feet lowered to the ground for 2–3 min and an impaired arterial supply is indicated by a ruddy, cyanotic hue which spreads over the affected foot (*Buerger's sign*). This sequence indicates occlusion of a major lower limb artery.

The ankle:arm Doppler pressure index

uses a Doppler ultrasonic flow probe to determine the ratio of the peak systolic pressure at the ankle to that in the arm. Symptoms are unlikely to be due to arterial disease if the index is above 0.8. Measurements made immediately after exercise give a good index of disease but are more difficult to perform reliably. In diabetic patients with calcified arteries† the test is unreliable as the pressure in the sphygmomanometer cuff may not reflect that in the artery.

Takayasu's disease

This is an arteritis which affects chiefly, but not exclusively, young women from Japan and the Far East. It involves mainly the aortic arch and the large brachiocephalic arteries. Mononuclear cell infiltrates and fibrous proliferation produce progressive narrowing of the lumen and reduced flow in the upper extremities and to the brain. It develops slowly so that although the pulses gradually vanish (hence the alternative name — *pulseless disease*), collateral circulation opens up allowing it to remain unnoticed for some time. Eventually the patient presents with symptoms such as fainting on turning the head suddenly or rising from supine to sitting, atrophy of the face, headaches, cataracts, optic atrophy, weakness and paraesthesiae of the upper extremities, hemiplegia and convulsions.

---

*The patient with intermittent claudication may have few signs other than reduced or absent pulses in the affected limb. As the atheromatous disease advances, signs of ischaemia appear: low skin temperature, pallor or cyanosis, trophic changes including dry, scaly and shiny skin; the hair may disappear and the toenails can become brittle, ridged and deformed; ischaemic damage may cause persistent reddish or reddish-blue discoloration; ischaemic ulcers and gangrene may develop.

† Peripheral vascular disease in diabetic patients is more progressive, with greater involvement of the more distal vessels which are of smaller calibre; medial calcification is twice as common. See also p. 108.

Buerger's disease (thromboangiitis obliterans)

An obstructive arterial disease with segmental inflammation and proliferative lesions in the medium and small arteries§ and veins of limbs. Mostly affects young males aged 20–40 years, especially in Israel, the Orient and India. Patients are almost always moderate to heavy smokers; there may be an autoimmune mechanism triggered by tobacco products. Clinically the disease is characterized by ischaemia of the extremities§ and *migratory thrombophlebitis*. Raynaud's phenomenen (gl.) is common. If the patient continues to smoke the disease will progress with increasing ischaemia leading to gangrene and amputation of the extremities which is required in a high percentage of patients.

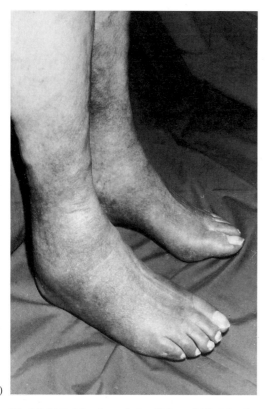

(a)

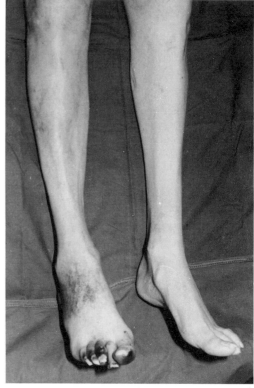

(b)

Fig. 1.5 (a) Peripheral vascular insufficiency. (b) Peripheral vascular disease with gangrenous toes.

§ The features which distinguish this *thromboangiitis obliterans* from the common atheromatous arterial disease (*arteriosclerosis obliterans*), are the younger age of the patient, the relative sparing of larger arteries, the presence of migratory superficial thrombophlebitis, the increased involvement of the upper extremities, and more rapid progression. The diagnosis can be confirmed by biopsy of an early lesion showing a characteristic inflammatory and proliferative lesion on histology.

Chapter 2
Examine this patient's heart

Possible short cases include
Mitral stenosis (lone) (p. 16)
Mixed mitral valve disease (p. 20)
Combinations of mitral and aortic valve disease
Mixed aortic valve disease (p. 26)
Aortic incompetence (lone) (p. 24)
Mitral incompetence (lone) (p. 18)
Aortic stenosis (lone) (p. 22)
Ventricular septal defect (p. 30)
Prosthetic valves (p. 29)
Tricuspid incompetence (p. 28)
Mitral valve prolapse (gl.)
Patent ductus arteriosus (gl.)
Eisenmenger's syndrome (gl.)

Other diagnoses include: atrial septal defect (gl.), coarctation of the aorta, chronic liver disease due to tricuspid incompetence, pulmonary stenosis, cor pulmonale, complete heart block, dextrocardia and left ventricular aneurysm.

Examination *routine*
When asked to 'examine this patient's heart' students are often uncertain as to whether they should start with the pulse or go straight to look at the heart. On the one hand it would be absurd to feel all the pulses in the body and leave the object of the examiner's interest to the last minute, whilst on the other hand it would be impetuous to palpate the praecordium straight away. Repeating the examiner's question in the hope that he might clarify it, or asking for a clarification, does nothing but communicate your dilemma to the examiner. You should not waste any time. Approach the right-hand side of the patient and adjust the backrest so that he reclines at 45° to the mattress. If the patient is wearing a shirt you should ask him to remove it so that the chest and neck are exposed. *Meanwhile*, you should complete a *quick*
 1 *visual survey*. Observe whether the patient is
     (a) breathless,
     (b) *cyanosed*,
     (c) pale, or
     (d) whether she has a *malar flush* (mitral stenosis).

Look briefly at the earlobes for creases* and then at the *neck* for *pulsations*:

(e) forceful carotid pulsations (Corrigan's sign (gl.) in aortic incompetence; vigorous pulsation in coarctation of the aorta), or

(f) tall, sinuous venous pulsations (congestive cardiac failure, tricuspid incompetence, pulmonary hypertension (gl.), etc.).

Run your eyes down onto the chest looking for

(g) a *left thoracotomy scar* (mitral stenosis) or a midline sternal scar (valve replacement†), and then down to the feet looking for

(h) ankle oedema. As you take the arm to feel the pulse complete your *visual survey* by looking at the hands (a quick look; do not be ponderous) for

(i) clubbing of the fingers (cyanotic congenital heart disease (gl.), subacute bacterial endocarditis (SBE)) and splinter haemorrhages (Fig. 2.1) (infective endocarditis).

If the examiner does not want you to feel the pulse he may intervene at this stage—otherwise you should proceed to

2 note the *rate* and *rhythm* of the pulse.

3 Quickly ascertain whether the pulse is collapsing (particularly if it is a large volume pulse) or not (make sure you are seen lifting the arm up).

Next may be an opportune time to look for

4 radiofemoral delay (coarctation of the aorta) (see Fig. 1.4), though this can be left until after auscultation if you prefer and are sure you will not forget it.

5 Feel the brachial pulse followed by the carotid pulses to see if the pulse is a slow rising one (see Fig. 1.2), especially if the volume (the up-stroke) is small.

If the pulsations in the neck present any interesting features you may have already noted these during your initial *visual survey*. You should now proceed

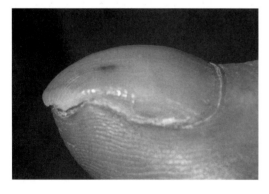

Fig. 2.1 A splinter haemorrhage.

---

*Frank's sign (Fig. 2.2): a diagonal crease in the lobule of the auricle: grade 3 = a deep cleft across the whole earlobe; grade 2A = crease more than halfway across the lobe; grade 2B = crease across the whole lobe, but superficial; grade 1 = lesser degrees of wrinkling. Earlobe creases are associated statistically with coronary artery disease in most population groups.

†Other scars may also be noted during your *visual survey*— those of previous cardiac catheterizations may be visible over the brachial arteries.

to confirm some of these impressions. The Corrigan's sign in the neck (forceful rise and quick fall of the carotid pulsation) may already have been reinforced by the discovery of a collapsing radial pulse. The individual waves of a large venous pulse can now be timed by palpating the opposite carotid. A large *v* wave, which sometimes oscillates the earlobe, suggests tricuspid incompetence and you should later on demonstrate the peripheral oedema and the pulsatile liver using the bimanual technique or, preferably, with your knuckle in the right hypochondrium (Fig. 2.3).* If the venous wave comes before the carotid pulsation it is an *a* wave suggestive of pulmonary hypertension (mitral valve disease, cor pulmonale) or pulmonary stenosis (rare). After

6 assessing the **height of the venous pressure** in centimetres vertically above the sternal angle (Fig. 2.4) you should move to the praecordium† and

7 localize the **apex beat** with respect to the midclavicular line and ribspaces, firstly by inspection for visible pulsation, and secondly by *palpation*. If the apex beat is vigorous you should stand the index finger on it (Fig. 2.5) to localize the point of maximum impulse (PMI) and *assess* the extent of its thrust. The impulse can be graded as just palpable, lifting (diastolic overload, i.e.

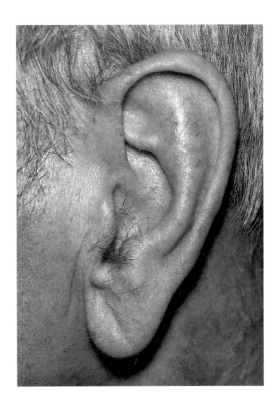

Fig. 2.2 Frank's sign.

* An alternative and useful way of demonstrating a pulsatile liver is to place the knuckles of your closed right fist against the inferior border of the liver in the right hypochondrium (warn the patient beforehand!). Your fist will oscillate with each pulsation of the liver (Fig. 2.3).

† The *visual survey* and examination steps 2–6 should be completed *quickly* and efficiently particularly if you have been asked to examine the *heart*. The objective should be not only to avoid irritating an impatient examiner but also to accommodate as many short cases as possible in the allotted time.

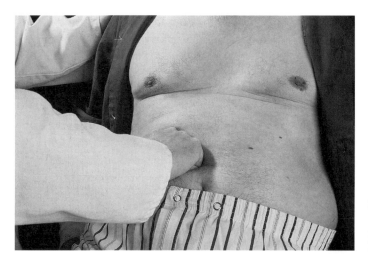

Fig. 2.3 Gently press to feel a pulsatile liver. Warn the patient before you place your knuckle below the right hypochondrium.

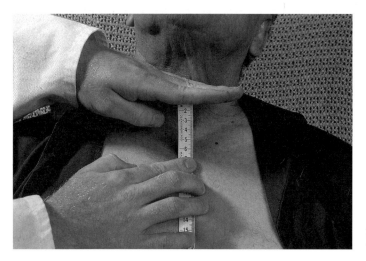

Fig. 2.4 Measuring the height of the venous column.

mitral or aortic incompetence), thrusting (stronger than lifting) or heaving (outflow obstruction).

8 Palpation with your hand placed from the lower left sternal edge to the apex (Fig. 2.6) will detect a **tapping** impulse (left atrial 'knock' in mitral stenosis)* or *thrills* over the mitral area (mitral valve disease), if present.

9 Continue palpation by feeling the **right ventricular lift** (left parasternal heave). To do this place the flat of your right palm parasternally over the right ventricular area and apply *sustained* and gentle pressure. If right ventricular hypertrophy is present you will feel the heel of your hand lifted by its force (pulmonary hypertension (gl.)).

10 Next, you should **palpate** the pulmonary area for a *palpable second sound*

---

* Do not confuse the brief, fleeting and non-localizable tapping impulse with the demonstrably localizable apex beat.

You can avoid this confusion by keeping your fingers in the air while feeling for the parasternal tap with your palm.

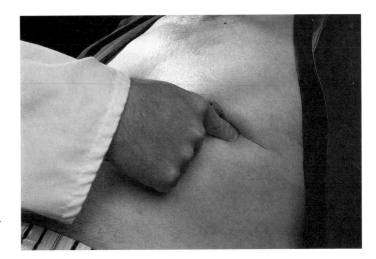

Fig. 2.5 Assessing the apical impulse. Locate the apex beat and stand your finger on it.

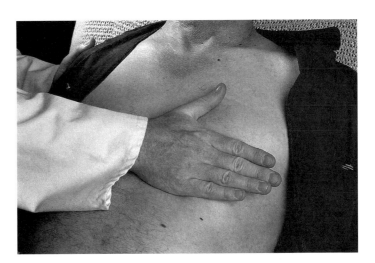

Fig. 2.6 Feeling for a tapping impulse—a fleeting, non-localizable impulse felt parasternally.

(pulmonary hypertension), and the aortic area for a palpable *thrill* (aortic stenosis).*

If you feel a strong right ventricular lift quickly recall, and sometimes recheck, whether there is a giant *a* wave (pulmonary hypertension, pulmonary stenosis) or *v* wave (tricuspid incompetence, congestive cardiac failure) in the neck. A palpable thrill over the mitral area (mitral valve disease), or palpable pulmonary second sound over the pulmonary area (pulmonary hypertension) should make you think of, and check for, the other complementary signs. You should by now have a fair idea of what you will hear on auscultation of the heart but you should keep an open mind for any unexpected discovery.

11 The next step will be **auscultation** and you should only stray away from the heart (examiner's command) if you have a strong expectation of being able

---

*The thrill of aortic stenosis is best felt if the patient leans forwards with his breath held after expiration.

to demonstrate an interesting and relevant sign (such as a pulsatile liver to underpin the diagnosis of tricuspid incompetence). *Time* the first heart sound with either the apex beat, if this is palpable, or by feeling the carotid pulse. It is important to listen to the expected murmurs in the most favourable positions. For example, mitral diastolic murmurs are best heard by turning the patient *onto the left side*, and the early diastolic murmur of aortic incompetence is made more prominent by asking the patient to *lean forwards* with his breath held after expiration.* For low-pitched sounds (mid-diastolic murmur of mitral stenosis, heart sounds) use the bell of your chest-piece but do not press hard, or else you will be listening through a diaphragm formed by the stretched skin! The high-pitched early diastolic murmur of aortic incompetence is very easily missed. Make sure you specifically listen for it.

If the venous pressure is raised you should check for

12 sacral oedema and, if covered, expose the feet to demonstrate any *ankle oedema*.

Auscultation over

13 the lung bases for inspiratory crepitations (left ventricular failure), though an essential part of the routine assessment of the cardiovascular system, is seldom required in the examination. You may make a special effort to do this in certain relevant situations such as a breathless patient, aortic stenosis with displaced PMI or if there are any signs of left heart failure (orthopnoea, pulsus alternans, gallop rhythm, etc.). Similarly, after examination of the heart itself it may (on rare occasions only) be necessary to

14 palpate the liver especially if you have seen a large *v* wave and heard a pansystolic murmur over the tricuspid area. In such cases you may be able to demonstrate a *pulsatile* liver by placing your left palm posteriorly and the right palm anteriorly over the enlarged liver.† Finally, you should offer to

15 measure the blood pressure. This is particularly relevant in patients with aortic stenosis (low systolic and narrow pulse pressure) and aortic incompetence (wide pulse pressure).

For *checklist* see p. 275.

For *checklist* see p. 275.

---

* With the diaphragm of your chest-piece *ready* in position: 'Take a deep breath in; now out; hold it'. Listen intently for the absence of silence in early diastole. Ask the patient to repeat the exercise if necessary.

† See footnote * on p. 11.

4 / Raised jugular venous pressure

Record

The jugular venous pressure (JVP) is elevated (measure) at . . . cm above the sternal angle (look for individual waves and time against the opposite carotid artery). The predominant wave is the systolic v wave which reaches the ear lobes. (If there is no oscillation of the blood column, sit the patient up to find the upper level. Make sure that there is no superior vena cava obstruction (gl.) with congestion of the face and neck, and prominent veins on the upper chest). The carotid pulsation is irregularly irregular and the rhythm is atrial fibrillation (look for the evidence of congestive cardiac failure: ankle and sacral oedema, hepatomegaly, which may be pulsatile in tricuspid incompetence).

The large v wave suggests tricuspid incompetence which is either organic or due to congestive cardiac failure (see also p. 28).

Causes of a raised JVP (if venous obstruction is excluded)

Congestive cardiac failure (ischaemic heart disease, valvular heart disease, hypertensive heart disease, cardiomyopathy)

Cor pulmonale (?signs of chronic small airways obstruction, cyanosis, etc.—p. 45)

Pulmonary hypertension (gl.) (large a wave in the JVP—primary (young females) and secondary to mitral valve disease or thrombo-obliterative disease)

Constrictive pericarditis (abrupt x and y descent, loud early *S3* ('pericardial knock') though heart sounds are often normal, slight 'paradoxical' pulse, *no signs in the lungs*; chest X-ray may show calcified pericardium)

Large pericardial effusion (x descent, pulsus paradoxus, breathlessness, chest X-ray shows cardiomegaly, echocardiogram shows effusion).

5 / Mitral stenosis (lone)

Record

There is a *malar flush* and a *left thoracotomy scar*. The pulse is *irregularly irregu-lar* (give rate) in rate and volume (if sinus rhythm the volume is usually small). The venous pressure is not raised, and there is no ankle or sacral oedema (unless in cardiac failure). The cardiac impulse is *tapping* (palpable first heart sound) and the apex is not displaced. There is a *left parasternal heave*. The *first heart sound is loud*, there is a loud pulmonary second sound and an *opening snap* followed by a *mid-diastolic rumbling murmur* (with *presystolic accentuation* if the patient is in sinus rhythm) *localized* to the apex and heard most loudly with the patient in the *left lateral* position.*

The diagnosis is mitral stenosis. The patient has had a valvotomy in the past. There are signs of pulmonary hypertension (gl.).

Other signs which may be present

Giant *v* waves (tricuspid incompetence—usually sec-ondary; may be primary—see p. 28)

Graham Steell† murmur—rare (secondary pulmonary incompetence; a high-pitched, brief, early diastolic whiff in the presence of marked signs of pulmonary hypertension and a pulse which is not collapsing).

The opening snap soon after the second sound in tight mitral stenosis; longer after the second sound in mild mitral stenosis; absent if the mitral valve is calci-fied (first heart sound soft).

Indications for considering surgery

Significant symptoms which limit normal activity

An episode of pulmonary oedema without a precipitat-ing cause

Recurrent emboli

Pulmonary oedema in pregnancy (emergency valvotomy)

Deterioration due to atrial fibrillation which does not respond to medical treatment

Haemoptysis.

Criteria for valvotomy‡

Mobile valve (loud first heart sound, opening snap, absence of calcium on X-ray screening and thin mobile cusps on echocardiography)

Absence of mitral incompetence.

---

* If unsure about the presence of the murmur, it can be accentuated by exercise—get the patient to touch her toes and then recline 10 times.

† Though associated eponymously with Graham Steell, the original source of the observation was probably George Balfour of Edinburgh, for whom Steell worked as house

physician (*Journal of the Royal College of Physicians* 1991, 25: 66–70).

‡ Should be considered, particularly in the young female who has a desire for pregnancy. Sometimes it can be performed before the development of significant symptoms.

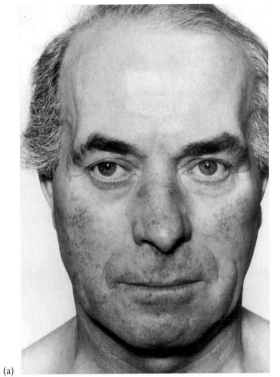 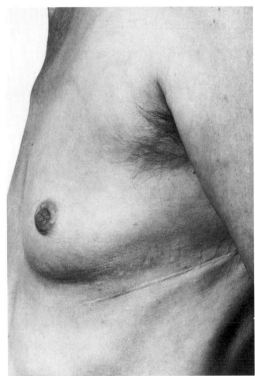

(a)

(b)

Fig. 2.7 (a) Mitral facies. (b) Thoracotomy scar for mitral valvotomy.

6 / Mitral incompetence (lone)

Record

The pulse is regular (give rate). The venous pressure is not raised and there is no ankle or sacral oedema (unless in cardiac failure). The apex beat is *thrusting* in the sixth intercostal space in the anterior axillary line, and there is (may be) a systolic thrill. There is a left *parasternal heave*. The *first heart sound is soft*, and there is a *third heart sound* (both suggest severe mitral incompetence). There is a loud *pansystolic murmur* at the apex, *radiating* to the *axilla*.

The diagnosis is mitral incompetence with signs of pulmonary hypertension (gl.).

Causes of mitral incompetence*

1 Rheumatic heart disease (males more commonly than females; contrast with mitral stenosis which affects females more commonly than males).
2 Previous mitral valvotomy for mitral stenosis (left thoracotomy scar).
3 Papillary muscle dysfunction (ischaemia, infarction or other disease of the papillary muscles or adjacent myocardium).
4 Severe left ventricular dilatation (due to any cause—lateral displacement of the papillary muscles and sometimes possibly dilatation of the mitral annulus† interfere with coaptation of the valve leaflets).
5 Mitral valve prolapse (gl.).

Other physical signs (*which may occur in severe mitral incompetence*)
Mid-diastolic rumbling murmur‡ (brief)
Sharp and abbreviated peripheral pulse (lack of sustained forward stroke volume because of the regurgitant leak)
Wide splitting of the second sound (early closure of the aortic valve because the regurgitant loss shortens the left ventricular ejection time)

Fourth heart sound (acute severe regurgitation with sinus rhythm).

Other causes of mitral incompetence*
Infective endocarditis (fever, splenomegaly, petechiae, splinter haemorrhages, clubbing, Osler's nodes (gl.), Janeway's lesions (gl.), Roth's spots (gl.), etc.)
Annular calcification (especially in the elderly female)
Hypertrophic obstructive cardiomyopathy (gl.)

* Regardless of the aetiology, mitral incompetence is a condition which gradually worsens spontaneously ('mitral incompetence begets mitral incompetence')—enlargement of the left atrium and left ventricle both worsen the incompetence and a vicious circle is set up.
† Left ventricular dilatation is common but the frequency of dilatation of the mitral valve annulus is an uncertain and controversial point. The mitral valve ring is a thick fibrous structure, so that if significant dilatation does occur, it probably indicates severe left ventricular disease.

‡ A short mid-diastolic murmur in the context of mitral incompetence could indicate associated mitral stenosis, or it could represent a flow (left atrium to left ventricle) murmur. The presence of an opening snap in such cases indicates mitral stenosis. In the absence of an opening snap the mid-diastolic murmur has two possible causes: (i) severe mitral incompetence with an increased flow murmur, or (ii) associated mitral stenosis and a calcified mitral valve. In the former there is often a third heart sound. In the latter the murmur is usually longer.

Rupture of the chordae tendinae§ (usually causes acute severe mitral incompetence; causes include infective endocarditis, rheumatic mitral valve disease, mitral valve prolapse, trauma)

Connective tissue disorders:

(a) systemic lupus erythematosus (SLE) (Libman–Sachs endocarditis—p. 182)

(b) rheumatoid arthritis (?hands, ?nodules)

(c) ankylosing spondylitis (?male with fixed kyphosis and stooped posture; aortic valve more commonly affected—p. 268)

Congenital with or without other abnormalities:

(a) ostium primum atrial septal defect (gl.)

(b) Marfan's syndrome (gl.) (?tall with long extremities, arachnodactyly, high-arched palate, etc.)

(c) Ehlers–Danlos syndrome (gl.) (?hyperextensible skin and joints, thin scars, etc.)

(d) pseudoxanthoma elasticum (gl.) (?loose skin or 'chicken skin' appearance in anticubital fossae, inguinal regions, neck, etc.)

(e) osteogenesis imperfecta (gl.) (?blue sclerae, deformity from old fractures, etc.)

Endomyocardial fibrosis (10% of cardiac admissions in East Africa; also occurs in West Africa, southern India and Sri Lanka; the aetiology is unknown).

Indications for surgery

Improvements in surgical techniques and artificial valves, and the reduction in operative mortality have reduced the threshold of physicians for considering surgery in moderately disabled patients (i.e. breathlessness caused by normal activity)—particularly if cardiomegaly and an elevated end-systolic left ventricular volume ($\geqslant 30\,\text{ml}\,\text{m}^{-2}$ body surface area) persists despite medical therapy (digoxin, diuretics, vasodilators). Repair and reconstruction of the valve (annuloplasty), if feasible (mostly in children and young adults), is preferable because of its low perioperative mortality. Asymptomatic patients should not be considered for surgery since the condition progresses slowly;* they may live for many years with little noticeable deterioration in their condition. Acute severe mitral incompetence (e.g. infective endocarditis, ruptured chordae tendinae) may require emergency valve replacement.

§ If the posterior leaflet is predominantly involved the systolic murmur is best heard at the left sternal edge whereas if the anterior leaflet is involved the murmur is best heard over the spine.

7 / Mixed mitral valve disease

Record 1

There is a *malar flush* and a *left thoracotomy scar*. The pulse is irregularly irregular (give rate) in rate and volume and the venous pressure is not raised. The cardiac impulse is *tapping* and the apex beat is *not displaced*. There is a *left parasternal heave*. On auscultation there is a *loud* first heart sound, a *pansystolic murmur** radiating to the axilla, a loud pulmonary second sound, and an *opening snap* followed by a *mid-diastolic rumbling murmur* localized to the apex.

The patient has mixed mitral valve disease. In view of the tapping cardiac impulse, the loud first heart sound and the undisplaced apex, I think this is predominant mitral stenosis. There are signs of pulmonary hypertension (gl.).

Record 2

There is a left thoracotomy scar. The pulse is irregularly irregular (give rate) in rate and volume and the venous pressure is not raised. The apex beat is *thrusting* and *displaced* to the sixth intercostal space in the anterior axillary line and there is a *left parasternal heave*. On auscultation the first heart sound is *soft* and there is a loud *pansystolic murmur* at the left sternal edge and/or apex radiating to the axilla. There is a loud pulmonary second sound and with the patient in the left lateral position I could hear a *mid-diastolic rumbling murmur* following an opening snap.†

The patient has mixed mitral valve disease with pulmonary hypertension. In view of the soft first heart sound and displaced and vigorous apex beat, I think this is predominant mitral incompetence.

It may not be clear clinically which lesion is predominant (e.g. loud first heart sound but enlarged left ventricle)—further investigation with echocardiography and cardiac catheter studies may be required. Table 2.1 shows the factors in favour of a predominance of one lesion or the other.

---

* In the patient with severe pulmonary hypertension when a very large right ventricle displaces the left ventricle posteriorly, the murmur of tricuspid incompetence (p. 28) can mimic that of mitral incompetence. The murmur of tricuspid incompetence is ordinarily heard best at the lower left sternal border, increases with inspiration and is not heard in the axilla or over the spine posteriorly. In tricuspid incompetence giant *v* waves will be present.

† In severe mitral incompetence without mitral stenosis a mid-diastolic flow murmur may be heard without an opening snap. The presence of a third heart sound is incompatible with any significant degree of mitral stenosis.

Table 2.1 Factors pointing to a predominant lesion in mixed mitral valve disease

	Mitral stenosis	Mitral incompetence
Pulse	Small volume	Sharp and abbreviated
Apex	Not displaced; tapping impulse present	Displaced, thrusting
First heart sound	Loud	Soft
Third heart sound	Absent	Present

8 / Aortic stenosis (lone)

Record 1

The *pulse* is regular (give rate), of *small volume* and *slow rising*. The venous pressure is not raised (unless there is cardiac failure). The apex beat is palpable 1 cm to the left of the mid-clavicular line in the fifth intercostal space (the apex position is normal or only slightly displaced in pure aortic stenosis unless the left ventricle is starting to fail) as a forceful *sustained heave*.* There is a *systolic thrill* palpable over the aortic area and the carotids (may be felt over the apex). Auscultation reveals a *harsh ejection systolic murmur* in the aortic area *radiating* into the *neck*, and the *aortic second sound is soft* (or absent). (The blood pressure is usually low normal with a decreased difference between systole and diastole—pulse pressure.)

    The diagnosis is aortic stenosis.

Possible causes

1 Rheumatic heart disease (the mitral valve is usually involved as well and aortic incompetence is often present).

2 Bicuspid aortic valve (commoner in males; typically presents in the sixth decade when the bicuspid valve calcifies).

3 Degenerative calcification (in the elderly; the stenosis is usually relatively mild).

4 Congenital (may worsen during childhood and adolescence due to calcification).

In the late stages of aortic stenosis when cardiac failure with low cardiac output supervenes, the murmur may become markedly diminished in intensity. The murmur of associated mitral stenosis should be carefully sought, particularly in the female patient, because the association of these two obstructive lesions tends to diminish the physical findings of each. Mitral stenosis is easily missed and the severity of aortic stenosis underestimated. As with all valvular heart diseases, echocardiography is of great value in a situation like this.

Indications for surgery

In the adult patient valve replacement is indicated for symptoms or a systolic pressure gradient greater than 50–60 mmHg (lower when the left ventricle has failed), as without operation the outlook for these patients is poor. Critical coronary lesions can be bypassed at the same time. Asymptomatic children and young adults can be treated with valvotomy if the obstruction is severe, as the operative risk appears to be less than the risk of sudden death. This is only temporary but may postpone the need for valve replacement for many years.

Record 2

The *carotid pulses* are *normal*, the apical impulse is just palpable and not displaced. There are *no thrills*. There

---

*There may also be a presystolic impulse due to left atrial overactivity (this is also felt in moderately severe cases of hypertrophic obstructive cardiomyopathy). The result is a double apical impulse best felt in the left lateral recumbent position. Other signs which may be present include: a fourth heart sound; a single second sound or even paradoxical splitting of the second sound which are both due to prolonged left ventricular ejection.

is an *ejection systolic murmur* which is not (usually) harsh or loud and is audible in the aortic area but only faintly in the neck. The aortic component of the second sound is well heard. The blood pressure is normal (or may be hypertensive).

These findings suggest aortic sclerosis (gl.) (or minimal aortic stenosis) rather than significant aortic stenosis. (NB The differentiation of this from the other causes of a short systolic murmur include: mitral valve prolapse (gl.); trivial mitral incompetence and hypertrophic obstructive cardiomyopathy (gl.).)

9 / Aortic incompetence (lone)

Record

The pulse is regular* (give rate), of large volume and *collapsing* in character. The venous pressure is not raised but *vigorous arterial pulsations* can be seen in the neck (Corrigan's sign (gl.)†). The apex beat is *thrusting* in the anterior axillary line, in the sixth intercostal space. There is an *early diastolic murmur* audible down the left sternal edge and in the aortic area; it is *louder in expiration* with the patient *sitting forward*. (The blood pressure may be wide with a high systolic and low diastolic. In severe cases it may be 250–300/30–50.)

The diagnosis is aortic incompetence (now consider looking for *Argyll Robertson pupils*, *high-arched palate* or *marfanoid* appearance, or obvious features of an arthropathy especially *ankylosing spondylitis*. If these are not present the aortic incompetence is likely to be rheumatic in origin — rheumatic fever and infective endocarditis are the commonest identifiable causes).

The early diastolic murmur can be difficult to hear and is easily overlooked. It should be specifically sought with the patient sitting forward in expiration. Listen for the 'absence of silence' in the early part of diastole. The murmur is usually best heard over the mid-sternal region or at the lower left sternal edge. In some cases, particularly syphilitic aortitis, it is loudest in the aortic area. There is often an accompanying systolic murmur due to increased flow which does not necessarily indicate coexistent aortic stenosis (see p. 26).

If there is a mid-diastolic murmur at the apex it may be an Austin Flint murmur‡ or it may represent some associated mitral valve disease. These two may be clinically indistinguishable, though the presence of a loud first heart sound and an opening snap suggest the latter. Though the first heart sound in the Austin Flint may be loud, it is never palpable (i.e. no tapping impulse).

Causes of aortic incompetence

Rheumatic fever (gl.)

Infective endocarditis (usually occurs on a deformed valve)

Syphilitic aortitis (?Argyll Robertson pupils; there may be an aneurysm of the ascending aorta)

Ankylosing spondylitis (?male with fixed kyphosis and stooped 'question mark' posture — p. 268; aortic incompetence may also occur in the other seronegative arthropathies — psoriasis, ulcerative colitis (gl.) and Reiter's syndrome)

Rheumatoid arthritis (?hands, nodules)

Marfan's syndrome (gl.) (?tall with long extremities, arachnodactyly and high-arched palate, etc.)

Hurler's syndrome (gl.)

Severe hypertension (by causing aortic dilatation; complications of hypertension such as ascending aortic

---

*The pulse is usually regular unless there is associated mitral valve disease.

†Other physical signs which result from a large pulse volume and peripheral vasodilatation include de Musset's sign (the head nods with each pulsation) and Quincke's sign (capillary pulsation visible in the nail beds). Of greater clinical value is Duroziez's sign — the femoral artery is compressed and auscultated proximally with a stethoscope; a diastolic murmur implies retrograde flow and aortic incompetence of at least moderate severity.

‡The Austin Flint murmur occurs in severe aortic incompetence. It is probably attributable to: (i) the regurgitant jet interfering with the opening of the anterior mitral valve leaflet, and (ii) the left ventricular diastolic pressure rising more rapidly than the left atrial diastolic pressure.

aneurysm or dissecting aneurysm may also cause aortic incompetence)

Coarctation of the aorta (late complication)

Associated ventricular septal defect (loss of support for valve).

Indications for surgery

Although patients tolerate aortic incompetence longer than aortic stenosis (p. 22), the clinician's aim is to replace the valve *before* serious left ventricular dysfunction occurs. Every effort should be made to recognize any reduction in left ventricular function or reserve as early as possible. Serial chest X-rays, echocardiograms and radionuclear angiography will show a gradual increase in cardiac size. Radionuclear angiography can be particularly useful in showing evidence of early left ventricular dysfunction in asymptomatic patients. The left ventricular ejection fraction, though normal at rest, may show a subnormal rise during exercise. Aortic valve replacement may have to be undertaken as a matter of urgency in patients with infective endocarditis in whom the leaking valve causes rapidly progressive left ventricular dilatation.

10 / Mixed aortic valve disease

Record 1

The pulse is regular (give rate) and *slow rising* (may have a *bisferiens* character). The venous pressure is not raised. The apex beat is palpable 1 cm to the left of the midclavicular line as a *forceful, sustained heave*. There is a *systolic thrill* palpable at the apex, in the aortic area and also in the carotid. There is a *harsh ejection systolic murmur* in the aortic area radiating into the neck, the *aortic component* of the second sound is *soft*, and there is an *early diastolic murmur* down the *left sternal edge* audible when the patient is sitting forward in expiration.

The diagnosis is mixed aortic valve disease. Since the pulse is slow rising rather than collapsing, there is a systolic thrill, the second sound is soft and the apex has a forceful heaving quality, I think this is predominant aortic stenosis. (Systolic blood pressure will be low with a low pulse pressure.)

Record 2

The pulse is regular (give rate), of *large volume* and *collapsing* (may have a *bisferiens* character). The venous pressure is not raised. The apex beat is *thrusting* in the *anterior axillary line* in the sixth intercostal space. There is a harsh *ejection systolic murmur* in the aortic area radiating into the neck and an *early diastolic murmur* down the *left sternal edge* (loudest with the patient sitting forward in expiration).

The diagnosis is mixed aortic valve disease. Since the pulse is collapsing rather than plateau in character and the apex is displaced and thrusting, I think the predominant lesion is aortic incompetence. (Blood pressure will show a wide pulse pressure.)

Often mixed aortic murmurs will be due to either aortic stenosis with incidental aortic incompetence or severe aortic incompetence with a systolic flow murmur.* In such cases commenting on dominance is easy. Table 2.2 shows the factors in favour of a predominance of one lesion or the other. However, it may not be clear clinically which lesion is predominant—further investigation using cardiac catheter studies with left ventricular angiography and an aortogram to show the aortic regurgitation would be required to be certain. Echocardiography may help but the Doppler valve gradient is inaccurate in the presence of significant aortic incompetence.

*NB For the causes of aortic incompetence in this latter case see p. 24.

Table 2.2 Factors pointing to a predominant lesion in mixed aortic valve disease

	Aortic incompetence	Aortic stenosis
Pulse	Mainly collapsing	Mainly slow rising
Apex	Thrusting, displaced	Heaving, not displaced much
Systolic thrill	Absent	Present
Systolic murmur	Not loud, not harsh	Loud, harsh
Blood pressure		
Systolic	High	Low
Pulse pressure	Wide	Narrow

11 / Tricuspid incompetence

Record

The JVP is elevated (give height*) and shows *giant v waves*† which oscillate the earlobe (if the venous pressure is high enough) and which are diagnostic of tricuspid incompetence. (Now, if allowed, examine the heart, respiratory system and abdomen.‡)

The commonest cause of tricuspid incompetence is *not* organic, but dilatation of the right ventricle and of the tricuspid valve ring due to right ventricular failure in conditions such as:

Mitral valve disease

Cor pulmonale

Eisenmenger's syndrome (gl.)

Atrial septal defect (gl.)

Right ventricular infarction

Primary pulmonary hypertension (gl.)

Thyrotoxicosis.

Causes of primary tricuspid incompetence

Rheumatic heart disease (usually associated with tricuspid stenosis; almost invariably associated with other valvular disease—if there is pulmonary hypertension it may not be possible to differentiate organic from functional tricuspid incompetence on clinical grounds alone)

Infective endocarditis (especially intravenous drug addicts—recurrent septicaemia with pulmonary infiltrates should raise suspicion)

Congenital heart disease (e.g. Ebstein's anomaly (gl.))

Carcinoid syndrome (gl.) (flushing, diarrhoea, hepatomegaly, sometimes asthma; fibrous plaques on the endothelial surface of the heart are associated with tricuspid incompetence and pulmonary stenosis)

Myxomatous change (may be associated with mitral valve prolapse (gl.) or atrial septal defect)

Trauma.

---

* In centimetres vertically above the sternal angle, not the suprasternal notch or supraclavicular fossa (see Fig. 2.4). In tricuspid incompetence which is secondary to right ventricular dilatation, the venous pressure is usually of the order of 8–10 cm or more.

† These *v* waves are in fact *cv* waves because systole spans the time between *c* and *v* waves of the normal jugular pulse.

‡ In the *heart* you would expect to find the systolic murmur of tricuspid incompetence which may be louder on inspiration (Carvallo's sign) and augmented by the Müller manoeuvre (attempted inspiration against a closed glottis). There may be murmurs of associated or underlying disease of the heart valves, especially mitral. There may be a tricuspid diastolic murmur louder on inspiration and augmented by the Müller manoeuvre. This could be due to increased flow across the tricuspid valve or to concomitant tricuspid stenosis. In the *respiratory system* you would be looking for signs of the condition leading to underlying cor pulmonale. In the *abdomen* you may find forceful epigastric pulsations and hepatomegaly which is tender and pulsatile. In severe, longstanding tricuspid incompetence, ascites and signs of chronic liver disease (p. 62) can occur.

12 / Prosthetic valves

Record 1

There is a *midline sternotomy scar*. There is a *click at the first heart sound* (closing of the mitral prosthesis) and an *opening click* in diastole (this may occasionally be followed by a mid-diastolic flow murmur).

These clicks represent the opening and closing of a *mitral valve prosthesis*. (The pansystolic murmur ± signs of heart failure suggest it is leaking.)

Record 2

There is a *midline sternotomy scar*. The first heart sound is normal (unless there is accompanying mitral stenosis), and is followed by an *ejection click* (opening of the prosthesis), an *ejection systolic murmur* and a *click at* (as part of) *the second sound* (closing of the prosthesis).

These clicks suggest an *aortic valve prosthesis*. (The early diastolic murmur and collapsing pulse (?wide pulse pressure) suggest it is leaking.)

Complications of prosthetic valves

Thromboembolic disease (anticoagulants or anti-platelet agents reduce but do not abolish)

Infective endocarditis (always consider when leakage develops)

Leakage due to wear of the valve

Leakage due to inadequacy or infection (bacterial endocarditis) of valve siting

Near total or even total dehiscence of the valve from its siting (the valve will be seen to rock on X-ray screening when there is serious leakage)

Ball embolus (the ball of the Starr–Edwards valve)

Valve obstruction from thrombosis/fibrosis clogging up the valve mechanics

Haemolysis (aortic valve).

NB Porcine heterografts and cadavaric homografts do not cause clicks. They last on average 8–10 years and are therefore only used nowadays in the elderly.

13 / Ventricular septal defect

Note: the youthfulness of the patient is sometimes a clue to the diagnosis.

Record

The pulse is regular (give rate) and the venous pressure is not raised. The apex beat is (may be) palpable half-way between the midclavicular line and the anterior axillary line, and there is a *left parasternal heave* (there may be a systolic thrill). There is a *pansystolic murmur* at the lower left sternal edge which is also audible at the apex. (The pulmonary second sound may be loud due to pulmonary hypertension (gl.) and there may be an early diastolic murmur of secondary pulmonary incompetence.)

The diagnosis is ventricular septal defect.

Other features of ventricular septal defect

Maladie de Roger (gl.) (small haemodynamically insignificant hole, loud murmur, normal heart size, etc.; tends to close spontaneously)

Development of Eisenmenger's complex (gl.) (pulmonary hypertension with reversal of shunt) if a significant defect is left untreated

Susceptibility to subacute bacterial endocarditis (defects of all sizes—NB chemoprophylaxis)

Association with aortic incompetence in 5% of cases (10% in Japan)

Possibility of a mitral mid-diastolic flow murmur if shunt is large

May occur following acute myocardial infarction with septal rupture

Sometimes associated with Down's syndrome (gl.) and Turner's syndrome.

14 / Coarctation of the aorta

Record

The radial pulses (in this young adult with a well-developed upper torso) are regular, equal,* and of large volume (give rate). The *carotid pulsations* are *vigorous,*† and the JVP is not elevated (unless there is heart failure). The *femorals* are *delayed* and of *poor volume* (palpate the radial and femoral simultaneously). The *blood pressure* in the right arm is elevated at 190/110 mmHg (it will be *low in the legs*). There are *visible arterial pulsations*‡ and *bruits* can be heard over and around the *scapula, anterior axilla* and over the *left sternal border* (internal mammary artery). The cardiac impulse is heaving but not displaced (unless in failure). Systolic *thrills* are palpable over the collaterals and suprasternally. There is a *systolic murmur* which is loudest at the level of the *fourth intercostal space posteriorly* (the level of the coarctation), but is also audible in the *second intercostal spaces* close to the sternum (the murmur—if present—of the associated bicuspid aortic valve is often obscured by that from the coarctation).§

These findings suggest a diagnosis of coarctation of the aorta.

Male to female ratio is 2:1.

Other features and associations of coarctation of the aorta

Rib notching* and poststenotic dilatation on chest X-ray

Bicuspid aortic valve in 25% (site of infective endocarditis and may lead to coexisting aortic incompetence; diagnosis can be made by echocardiography)

Berry aneurysms of the circle of Willis (may cause death even in corrected cases)

Ventricular septal defect (?pansystolic murmur, etc. —p. 30)

Patent ductus arteriosus (gl.) (?machinery murmur, etc.)

Turner's syndrome (check for features of Turner's if your patient is female—webbed neck, increased carrying angle, short stature, etc. —p. 270)

Marfan's syndrome (gl.) (?tall, arachnodactyly, high arched palate, lens dislocation, etc.)

High mortality after the age of forty. Hypertension may not be cured even in corrected cases (low perfusion of kidneys may involve the renin–angiotensin system).

Other causes of rib notching

Neurofibromatosis (multiple neuromata on the intercostal nerves)

Enlargement of nerves (amyloidosis (gl.), congenital hypertrophic polyneuropathy)

Inferior vena cava obstruction

Blalock shunt (gl.) operation (left-sided unilateral rib notching)

Congenital.

---

*Rarely (2%) the coarctation is proximal to the origin of the left subclavian artery and the left arm pulses will be weaker than the right; rib notching will be unilateral and right sided.

†If you see vigorous carotid pulsations the likeliest cause is aortic incompetence (?collapsing pulse). The occasional patient, however, will have coarctation.

‡Collaterals are best observed with the patient sitting up and leaning forward with the arms hanging by the side.

§A continuous murmur in systole and diastole, arising from the dilated collaterals, may be heard over the back. An early diastolic murmur arising because of the dilated ascending aorta may be heard especially in older patients.

Chapter 3
Examine this patient's chest

Possible short cases include
Dullness at the lung base (p. 38)
Fibrosing alveolitis (p. 40)
Carcinoma of the bronchus (p. 46)
Bronchiectasis (p. 41)
Chronic bronchitis and emphysema (p. 43)
Pneumonia or chest infection (p. 42)
Pneumonectomy or lobectomy (p. 48)
Old tuberculosis
Radiation burn on the chest
Cor pulmonale (p. 45)
Superior vena cava obstruction (gl.)
Pancoast's syndrome (p. 46)
Pneumothorax (p. 50)
Systemic sclerosis (p. 176)
Ankylosing spondylitis (p. 268)
(Kypho)scoliosis.

Examination *routine*
While approaching the patient, asking for his permission to examine him and
settling him reclining at 45° to the bed with his chest bare, you should observe

   1 his **general appearance**. Note any evidence of *weight loss*. The features of
conditions such as superior vena cava obstruction, systemic sclerosis (p. 176)
and lupus pernio (gl.) may be readily apparent as should be severe kyphoscoliosis. However, *ankylosing spondylitis* is easily missed with the patient lying
down. Observe specifically whether the patient

   2 is **breathless** at rest or from the effort of removing his clothes,

   3 **purses his lips** (chronic small airways obstruction), or

   4 has central **cyanosis*** (cor pulmonale, fibrosing alveolitis, bronchiectasis).
Central cyanosis may be difficult to recognize; it is always preferable to look at
the oral mucous membranes (see below). Observe

---

* Occurs with a mean capillary concentration of $\geq 4\,g\,dl^{-1}$ of deoxygenated haemoglobin (or $0.5\,g\,dl^{-1}$ methaemoglobin). Alternatively, the presence of cyanosis may be supported by demonstrating a low arterial oxygen saturation (<85%) non-invasively with an ear oximeter applied to the antihelix of the ear. Central cyanosis is more readily detected in patients with polycythaemia than in those with anaemia—because of the low haemoglobin, patients with anaemia require a much lower oxygen saturation to have $4\,g\,dl^{-1}$ of unsaturated haemoglobin in capillary blood.

5 if the **accessory muscles** are being used during breathing (chronic small airways obstruction, pleural effusion, pneumothorax, etc.),

6 if there is generalized **indrawing** of the intercostal muscles (Fig. 3.1) or supraclavicular fossae (hyperinflation) or if there is indrawing of the lower ribs on inspiration (due to low, flat diaphragm in emphysema). Localized indrawing of the intercostal muscles suggests bronchial obstruction.

Listen to the breathing with unaided ears whilst you observe the chest wall and hands (but do not dither). This will allow a dual input whereby a collaboration of what you hear and what you see may help you form a diagnostic impression. You should listen to whether *expiration* is more *prolonged* than inspiration (normally the reverse), and difficult (chronic airways obstruction), whether it is *noisy* (breathlessness) and if there are any additional noises such as *wheezes* or *clicks*. Difficult and noisy inspiration is usually caused by obstruction in the major bronchi (mediastinal masses, retrosternal thyroid, bronchial carcinoma, etc.) while the more prolonged, noisy and often wheezy expiration is caused by chronic small airways obstruction (asthma, chronic bronchitis). While you are listening observe

7 the *movement* of the **chest wall**. It may be mainly *upwards* (emphysema) or *asymmetrical* (fibrosis, collapse, pneumonectomy, pleural effusion, pneumothorax). In the context of the examination it is particularly important to look for localized *apical flattening* suggestive of underlying fibrosis due to old tuberculosis or pneumonectomy (p. 48). You may also note a thoracotomy or thoracoplasty *scar* or the presence of *radiotherapy field markings* (Indian ink marks) or radiation *burns* on the chest (intrathoracic malignancy).

Check the hands for

8 **clubbing** (p. 200), *tobacco staining*, coal dust tattoos, or other conditions which affect the hands and may be associated with lung disease such as rheumatoid arthritis (nodules, p. 189) or systemic sclerosis (p. 176).

9 Feel the **pulse** and if it is **bounding**, or if the patient is cyanosed, check for a *flapping tremor* of the hands (CO_2 retention). If there is doubt about the

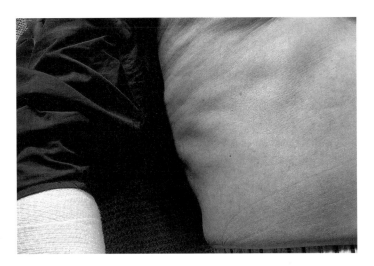

Fig. 3.1 Indrawing of the intercostal muscles in chronic obstructive airways disease.

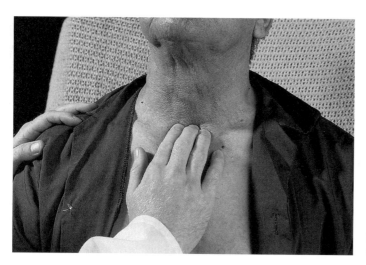

Fig. 3.2 Determining the position of the trachea.

presence of cyanosis you could at this point check the tongue and the buccal mucous membranes over the premolar teeth before moving to the neck to look for

10 raised venous pressure (cor pulmonale) or fixed distension of the neck veins (superior vena cava obstruction). Next examine

11 the **trachea**. Place the index and ring fingers on the manubrium sternae over the prominent points on either side (Fig. 3.2). Use the middle finger as the exploring finger to gently feel the tracheal rings to detect either *deviation* or a *tracheal tug* (i.e. the middle finger being pushed upwards against the trachea by the upward movement of the chest wall). Check the *notch–cricoid* distance (Fig. 3.3).*

12 Feel for **lymphadenopathy** (carcinoma, tuberculosis, lymphoma, sarcoidosis (gl.)) in the cervical region and axillae. As the right hand returns from the left axilla look for

13 the **apex beat** (difficult to localize if the chest is hyperinflated) which in conjunction with tracheal deviation may give you evidence of **mediastinal displacement** (collapse, fibrosis, pneumonectomy, effusion, scoliosis).

14 To look for **asymmetry** rest one hand lightly on either side of the front of the chest to see if there is any diminution of movement (effusion, fibrosis, pneumonectomy, collapse, pneumothorax). Next grip the chest symmetrically with the fingertips in the ribspaces on either side and approximate the thumbs to meet in the middle in a straight horizontal line in order

15 to assess **expansion** first in the inframammary (Fig. 3.4) and then in the supramammary regions. Note the distance between each thumb and the midline (may give further information about asymmetry of movement) and between both thumbs and try to express the expansion in centimetres (it is

---

* The length of trachea from the suprasternal notch to the cricoid cartilage is normally three or more finger breadths. Shortening of this distance is a sign of hyperinflation.

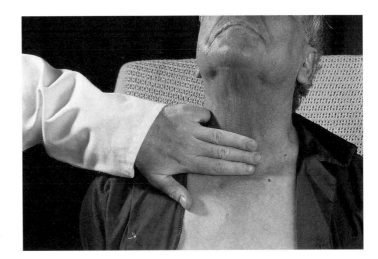

Fig. 3.3 Assessing the notch–cricoid distance.

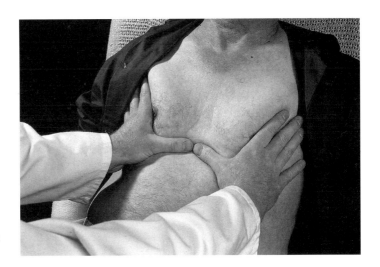

Fig. 3.4 Checking expansion on both sides.

better to produce a tape measure for a more accurate assessment of the expansion in centimetres) (Fig. 3.5). Comparing both sides at each level

16 **percuss** the chest from above downwards starting with the supraclavicular fossae and over the clavicles* and do not forget to percuss over the axillae. Few clinicians now regularly map out the area of cardiac dullness. In healthy people there is dullness behind the lower left quarter of the sternum which is lost together with normal liver dullness in hyperinflation. Complete palpation by checking for

17 **tactile vocal fremitus** with the ulnar aspect of the hand applied to the chest (Fig. 3.6).

18 Auscultation of the **breath sounds** should start *high* at the apices and you should remember to listen in the *axillae*. You are advised to cover both lung

* Percussion on the bare clavicle may cause discomfort to the patient.

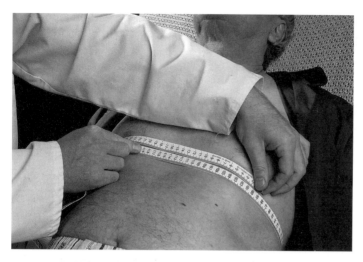

Fig. 3.5 Measuring expansion of the ribcage.

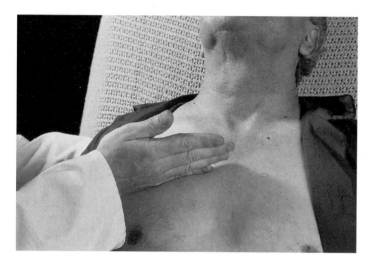

Fig. 3.6 Vocal fremitus—using the sensitive ulnar border.

fields first with the bell* before using the diaphragm (if for no other reason than that this allows you a chance to check the findings without appearing to backtrack!). In the nervousness of an examination harsh breathing heard with the diaphragm near a major bronchus (over the second intercostal space anteriorly or below the scapula near the midline posteriorly) may give an impression of bronchial breathing, particularly in thin people. Compare corresponding points on opposite sides of the chest. Ensure that the patient breathes with the mouth open, regularly and deeply, but not noisily. Auscultation is completed by checking

19 **vocal resonance** in all areas; **if** you have found an area of bronchial breathing (the sounds may resound close to your ears—aegophony) check

---

* Many physicians prefer to use the diaphragm in their routine examination of the chest though some believe that as the respiratory auscultatary sounds are usually of low pitch, the bell is preferable.

also for whispering pectoriloquy. The classic timings of crackles/crepitations of various origins are:

(a) *early inspiratory*: chronic bronchitis, asthma

(b) *early and mid-inspiratory and recurring in expiration*: bronchiectasis (altered by coughing)

(c) *mid/late inspiratory*: restrictive lung disease (e.g. fibrosing alveolitis*) and pulmonary oedema.

20 To examine the back of the chest sit the patient forward (it may help to cross the arms in front of the patient to pull the scapulae further apart) and repeat steps 14–19. You may wish to start the examination of the back by palpating for cervical nodes from behind (particularly the scalene nodes between the two heads of sternomastoid).

Though with sufficient practice this whole procedure can be performed rapidly without loss of efficiency, often in an examination you will only be asked to perform some of it—usually 'examine the back of the chest'. As always when forced to perform only part of the complete *routine*, be sure that the partial examination is no less thorough and professional. Be prepared to put on your 'wide-angled lenses' so as not to miss other related signs.

Though by now you will usually have sufficient information to present your findings, occasionally you will wish to check other features on the basis of the findings so far. Further purposeful examination gives an impression of confidence but it should not be overdone. For example, looking for evidence of Horner's syndrome, or wasting of the muscles of one hand† in a patient with apical dullness and a deviated trachea, will suggest professional keenness; whereas routinely looking at the eyes and hands after completion of the examination may only suggest to the examiner that you do not have the diagnosis and are hoping for inspiration! If you suspect airways obstruction the examiner may be impressed if you perform a bedside respiratory function test—the *forced expiratory time* (FET).‡

For *checklist* see p. 275.

---

* In fibrosing alveolitis late inspiratory crackles may become reduced if the patient is made to lean forward; thereby the compressed dependent alveoli (which crackle open in late inspiration) are relieved of the pressure of the lungs.

† A good *visual survey* may reveal such signs at the beginning.

‡ Ask the patient to take a deep breath in and then, on your command (timed with the second hand of your watch), to breathe out as hard and as fast as he can until his lungs are completely empty. A normal person will empty his lungs in less than 6 seconds (1 second for every decade of age, e.g. a normal 30-year-old will do it in 3 seconds). An FET of >6 seconds is evidence of airways obstruction. You need to practise this test with patients if it is to be slick. As with peak flow rate (PFR) and forced expiratory volume in 1 second (FEV_1) etc., it is important to make sure that certain patients, particularly females, *are* blowing as hard and as fast as they can ('don't worry about what you look like—give it everything you've got—like this'—give a demonstration) and empty their lungs completely ('keep going, keep going . . . keep going, well done!').

15 / Dullness at the lung base

Record
The pulse is regular and the venous pressure is not elevated. The trachea is central,* the expansion is normal, but the percussion note is *stony dull* at the R/L base(s), with *diminished* tactile *fremitus* and vocal *resonance*, and *diminished breath sounds*. There is (may be) an area of bronchial breathing above the area of dullness.

The diagnosis is R/L pleural effusion.

Causes of pleural effusion
> 35

Exudate (protein content >30 g l⁻¹)

1 *Bronchial carcinoma* (?nicotine staining, clubbing, radiation burns on chest, lymph nodes).
2 *Secondary malignancy* (?evidence of primary especially breast, lymph nodes, radiation burns).
3 *Pulmonary embolus and infarction* (?deep venous thrombosis; blood–stained fluid will be found at aspiration).
4 *Pneumonia* (bronchial breathing/crepitations, fever, etc.).
5 Tuberculosis.
6 Rheumatoid arthritis (?hands and nodules).
7 Systemic lupus erythematosus (SLE) (?typical rash).
8 Lymphoma (?nodes and spleen).
9 Mesothelioma (gl.) (asbestos worker, ?clubbing).

< 25

Transudate (protein content <30 g l⁻¹)

1 *Cardiac failure* (?jugular venous pressure (JVP) ↑, ankle and sacral oedema, large heart, tachycardia, S_3 or signs of a valvular lesion).
2 Nephrotic syndrome (gl.) (?generalized oedema, patient may be young).
3 Cirrhosis (?ascites, generalized oedema, signs of chronic liver disease — p. 62).

Other causes of pleural effusion
Meigs' syndrome (gl.) (ovarian fibroma)
Subphrenic abscess (?recent abdominal disease or surgery)
Peritoneal dialysis
Hypothyroidism (?facies, pulse, ankle jerks)

Pancreatitis (more common on the left; fluid has high amylase)
Dressler's syndrome (gl.) (recent myocardial infarction, ?pericardial friction rub)
Trauma
Asbestos exposure

---

* The trachea may be deviated if the effusion is very large. A large effusion without any mediastinal shift (clinically and on chest X-ray) raises the possibility of collapse as well as effusion.

Yellow nail syndrome (gl.) (yellowish-brown beaked nails usually associated with lymphatic hypoplasia)

Chylothorax (trauma or blockage of a major intrathoracic lymphatic — usually by a neoplastic process).

Other causes of dullness at a lung base

Raised hemidiaphragm (e.g. hepatomegaly, phrenic nerve palsy)

Basal collapse

Collapse/consolidation (if the airway is blocked by, for example, a carcinoma there may be no bronchial breathing)

Pleural thickening (e.g. old tuberculosis or old empyema or a mesothelioma).

16 / Fibrosing alveolitis

Record

There is *clubbing* of the fingers, (may be) *cyanosis*, and there are *fine inspiratory crackles* (or crepitations—whichever term you prefer as long as you know how they are caused) at both bases.

The likely diagnosis is (cryptogenic*) fibrosing alveolitis (CFA).

Conditions which may be associated with cryptogenic fibrosing alveolitis

Rheumatoid arthritis (?hands, nodules)

Systemic lupus erythematosus (?typical rash)

Systemic sclerosis (?typical mask-like facies, telangiectasia, sclerodactyly — p. 176)

Sjögren's syndrome (gl.) (?dry eyes and dry mouth)

Polymyositis (gl.) (?proximal muscle weakness and tenderness)

Dermatomyositis (gl.) (?heliotrope rash on eyes/hands and polymyositis)

Ulcerative colitis (gl.) (?colostomy)

Chronic active hepatitis (gl.) (?ictcrus, hepatosplenomegaly)

Raynaud's phenomenon (gl.)

Digital vasculitis.

Conditions in which alveolitis and pulmonary fibrosis occur

Sarcoidosis (gl.) (?erythema nodosum or history of; lupus pernio (gl.))

Extrinsic allergic alveolitis (?farmer, pigeon racer, etc.)

Asbestosis (gl.) (?lagger, etc.)

Silicosis (gl.) (?slate worker or granite quarrier, etc.)

Drug reactions (e.g. bleomycin, busulphan, nitrofurantoin, amiodarone)

Chemical inhalation (e.g. beryllium, mercury)

Poison ingestion (e.g. paraquat)

Radiation fibrosis

Mitral valve disease

Uraemia

Adult respiratory distress syndrome (complicating acute severe illness often with septicaemia).

---

* In the absence of an identifiable causal agent the fibrosing alveolitis is termed 'cryptogenic'. Occupational exposure to metal or wood dust is commoner in CFA patients than controls.

17 / Bronchiectasis

Record

This patient (who may be rather *underweight*, *breathless* and *cyanosed*) has *clubbing* of the fingers (not always present) and a frequent *productive cough* (the patient may cough in your presence;* there may be a *sputum pot* by the bed). There are (may be) *inspiratory clicks* heard with the unaided ear. There are *crepitations* over the . . . zone(s) (the area(s) where the bronchiectasis is) and (may be) widespread *rhonchi*.

The diagnosis could well be bronchiectasis. The frequent productive cough and inspiratory clicks are in favour of this. Other possibilities (clubbing and crepitations) are:

1 Carcinoma of the lung (?heavy nicotine staining, lymph nodes, etc.).
2 Fibrosing alveolitis* (marked sputum production and clicks are against this).
3 Lung abscess.

Possible causes of bronchiectasis

Respiratory infection in childhood (especially whooping cough, measles, tuberculosis)

Cystic fibrosis (gl.) (young, thin patient, may have malabsorption and steatorrhoea)

Bronchial obstruction due to foreign body, carcinoma, granuloma (tuberculosis, sarcoidosis (gl.)) or lymph nodes (e.g. tuberculosis)

Fibrosis (complicating tuberculosis, unresolved or suppurative pneumonia with lung abscess, mycotic infections or sarcoidosis)

Hypogammaglobulinaemia (congenital and acquired)

Allergic bronchopulmonary aspergillosis (proximal airway bronchiectasis)

Marfan's syndrome (gl.) (?tall, long extremities, high-arched palate)

Yellow nail syndrome (gl.) (?excessively curled yellow nails with bulbous fingertips; lymphoedema of extremities)

Congenital disorders such as sequestrated lung segments, bronchial atresia and Kartagener's syndrome.†

---

* It is worth asking the patient to 'give a cough' as it may help you differentiate bronchiectasis from fibrosing alveolitis.
† The features of Kartagener's syndrome are dextrocardia, situs inversus, infertility, dysplasia of frontal sinuses, sinusitis and otitis media. Patients have ciliary immotility.

18 / Chest infection/consolidation/ pneumonia

Record

There is reduced movement of the R/L side of the chest. There is *dullness* to percussion over . . . (describe where) with *bronchial breathing, coarse crepitations, whispering pectoriloquy* and a *pleural friction rub.*

These features suggest consolidation (say where).

Commonest causes of consolidation

Bacterial pneumonia (pyrexia, purulent sputum, haemoptysis, breathlessness)

Carcinoma (with infection behind the tumour; ?clubbing, wasting, etc. — p. 46)

Pulmonary infarction (fever less prominent, sputum mucoid, occasionally haemoptysis and blood-stained pleural effusion).

19 / Chronic bronchitis and emphysema

Note: usually patients will fall between the extremes of the classic *records* below.

Record 1

This thin man (with an anxious, drawn expression) presents the classic 'pink puffer' appearance. He has *nicotine staining* of the fingers. He is tachypnoeic at rest with *lip pursing* during expiration, which is *prolonged*. The suprasternal notch to cricoid distance is reduced (a sign of hyperinflation; normally >3 finger breadths). His chest is *hyperinflated, expansion* is mainly *vertical* and there is a *tracheal tug*. He uses his *accessory muscles* of respiration at rest and there is *indrawing* of the *lower ribs* on inspiration (due to a flattened diaphragm). The percussion note is hyper-resonant, obliterating cardiac and hepatic dullness, and the breath sounds are quiet (this is so in classic pure emphysema—frequently, though, wheezes are heard due to associated bronchial disease).

These are the physical findings of a patient with emphysema (inspiratory drive often intact).*

Record 2

This (male) patient (who smokes, lives in a foggy city, works amid dust and fumes, and has probably had frequent respiratory infections) presents the classic 'blue bloater' appearance. He has *nicotine staining* on the fingers. He is stocky and *centrally cyanosed* with suffused conjunctivae. His chest is *hyperinflated*, he uses his *accessory muscles* of respiration; there is *indrawing* of the *intercostal muscles* on inspiration and there is a *tracheal tug* (both signs of hyperinflation). His pulse is 80/min, the venous pressure is not elevated (may be raised with ankle oedema and hepatomegaly if cor pulmonale is present), the trachea is central, but the suprasternal notch to cricoid distance is reduced. *Expansion* is equal but *reduced* to 2 cm and the percussion note is resonant; on auscultation the expiratory phase is prolonged and he has widespread *expiratory rhonchi* and (maybe) coarse inspiratory crepitations. (His FET—p. 37—is 8 seconds.) There is no flapping tremor of the hands (unless he is in severe hypercapnoeic respiratory failure in which case ask to examine the fundi—? papilloedema).

These are the physical findings of advanced chronic bronchitis† (inspira-

---

*Emphysema is, however, a pathological diagnosis.
†Chronic bronchitis, though, is defined as sputum production (not due to specific disease such as bronchiectasis or tuberculosis) on most days for 3 months of the year on 2 consecutive years.

tory drive often reduced) producing **chronic small airways obstruction** (and, if ankle oedema, etc., right heart failure due to cor pulmonale).

Causes of emphysema

Smoking (usually associated with chronic bronchitis; mixed centrilobular and panacinar)

Alpha 1 antitrypsin deficiency (gl.) (?young patient; lower zone emphysema, panacinar in type; ?icterus, hepatomegaly, etc. of hepatitis or cirrhosis)

Coal dust (centrilobular emphysema—simple coal worker's pneumoconiosis—only minor abnormalities of gas exchange)

Macleod's (Swyer–James) syndrome (gl.)—rare (uni-lateral emphysema following childhood bronchitis and bronchiolitis with subsequent impairment of alveolar growth; breath sounds diminished on affected side).

Record **1** (continuation)

The decreased breath sounds over the . . . zone of the R/L lung of this patient with emphysema raises the possibility of an **emphysematous bulla.**

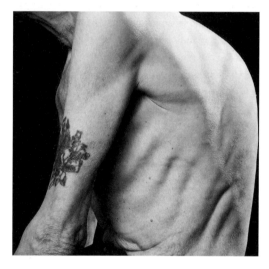

Fig. 3.7 Hyperinflated rib cage. Note indrawing of intercostal muscles.

20 / Cor pulmonale

Record

The patient's fingers are *nicotine-stained* and there is *central cyanosis*. The pulse is regular, the *venous pressure is raised* (give height) with prominent small *a* waves and giant *v* waves (if there is secondary tricuspid incompetence), and there is *ankle* and *sacral oedema*. *Expiration is prolonged and noisy*. The *accessory muscles* of respiration are in use at rest, and there is a *tracheal tug*. The trachea is central, expansion is equal, the percussion note is resonant, and tactile fremitus and vocal resonance are normal. There is a *left parasternal heave* and a palpable second heart sound* (?pansystolic murmur of tricuspid incompetence). There are (may be) widespread *expiratory rhonchi* and coarse inspiratory crepitations and the FET (see p. 37) is 8 seconds. (There is no *flapping tremor* of the hands—if there were you would want to examine the fundi for papilloedema.)

These findings suggest cor pulmonale due to chronic bronchitis and emphysema. (Right heart failure is often precipitated by acute infection.)

The auscultatory cardiac signs of pulmonary hypertension, some of which may be audible,* are:

Loud pulmonary second sound
Pulmonary early systolic ejection click
Right ventricular fourth heart sound.

Causes of pulmonary heart disease

Chronic obstructive bronchitis (with or without emphysema; by far the commonest cause—p. 43)

Recurrent pulmonary emboli (signs of pulmonary hypertension (gl.) without clinical evidence of other lung disease; ?deep venous thrombosis)

Primary pulmonary hypertension (gl.) (signs of pulmonary hypertension without clinical evidence of other lung disease; usually a female)

Non-pulmonary causes of alveolar hypoventilation (kyphoscoliosis, obesity, neuromuscular weakness)

Pansystolic murmur of functional tricuspid incompetence (giant *v* waves)

Early diastolic murmur of functional pulmonary incompetence (Graham Steell murmur (gl.)).

Lung diseases which only occasionally result in cor pulmonale include:

Progressive massive fibrosis (gl.) (?coal dust tattoos on the skin; chronic bronchitis is the commonest cause of cor pulmonale in miners)

Bronchiectasis (especially cystic fibrosis (gl.); ?clubbing, cyanosis, full sputum pot, productive cough, crepitations—p. 41)

Cryptogenic fibrosing alveolitis (?clubbing, cyanosis, basal crackles—p. 40)

Systemic sclerosis (hands, facies—p. 176)

Sarcoidosis (gl.) (?lupus pernio (gl.))

Asthma (severe and chronic; may be missed if the reversibility is not checked in chronic small airways obstruction).

---

* These findings, which may be prominent in cor pulmonale due to other causes, may be difficult to elicit in cor pulmonale where a barrel-shaped chest and hyperinflation are present, and the heart is enfolded by over-inflated lungs.

21 / Carcinoma of the bronchus

Record 1

There is *clubbing* of the fingers which are *nicotine-stained*. There is a hard *lymph node* in the R/L supraclavicular fossa. The pulse is 80/min and regular, and the venous pressure is not raised. The trachea is central, chest expansion normal, but the percussion note is *stony dull* at the R/L base and *tactile fremitus*, *vocal resonance* and *breath sounds* are all *diminished* over the area of dullness.

The likely diagnosis is carcinoma of the bronchus causing a *pleural effusion*.

Record 2

The patient is *cachectic*. There is a *radiation burn* on the R/L upper chest wall. There is *clubbing* of the fingers which are *nicotine-stained*. The pulse is 80/min, venous pressure is not elevated and there are no lymph nodes. The *trachea* is *deviated* to the R/L and *expansion* of the R/L upper chest is *diminished*. *Tactile vocal fremitus* and *resonance* are *increased* over the upper chest where the *percussion note is dull* and there is an area of *bronchial breathing*.

It is likely that this patient has had radiotherapy for carcinoma of the bronchus which is causing *collapse* and *consolidation of the R/L upper lung*.

Record 3

There is a *radiation burn* on the chest. There are *lymph nodes* palpable in the R/L axilla. The trachea is central. I did not detect any abnormality in expansion, vocal fremitus, vocal resonance or breath sounds, but there is *wasting* of the *small muscles* of the R/L *hand*, and *sensory loss* (plus pain) over the *T1** dermatome. There is a R/L *Horner's syndrome* (p. 180).

The diagnosis is *Pancoast's syndrome* (due to an apical carcinoma of the lung involving the lower brachial plexus and the cervical sympathetic nerves).

Other complications of carcinoma of the bronchus

1 Other local effects such as:

Superior vena cava obstruction (gl.) (?oedema of the face and upper extremities, suffusion of eyes, fixed engorgement of neck veins and dilatation of superficial veins, etc.)

Stridor (often associated with superior vena cava obstruction; dysphagia may occur)

2 Metastases and their effects (pain, ?hepatomegaly, neurological signs, etc.)

3 Non-metastatic effects such as:

Hypertrophic pulmonary osteoarthropathy (?clubbing plus pain and swelling of wrists and/or ankles—subperiosteal new bone formation on X-ray)

Neuropathy (peripheral neuropathy—sensory, motor or mixed; cerebellar degeneration and encephalopathy; proximal myopathy, polymyositis (gl.),

---

* The weakness, sensory loss and especially pain may be more widespread (C8, T1, T2).

dermatomyositis (gl.), reversed myasthenia—Eaton–Lambert syndrome (gl.)†)

Endocrine (inappropriate antidiuretic hormone, ectopic adrenocorticotrophic hormone (ACTH), ectopic parathormone or parathormone-related peptide,‡ carcinoid (gl.))

Gynaecomastia (if rapidly progressive and painful may be a human chorionic gonadotrophin (hCG) secreting tumour)

Thrombophlebitis migrans (gl.) (?deep venous thrombosis)

Non-bacterial thrombotic endocarditis

Anaemia (usually normoblastic; occasionally leucoerythroblastic from bone marrow involvement)

Pruritus

Herpes zoster (p. 235)

Acanthosis nigricans (gl.) (grey-brown/dark brown areas in the axillae and limb flexures, in which skin becomes thickened, rugose and velvety with warts)

Erythema gyratum repens (irregular wavy bands with a serpiginous outline and marginal desquamation on the trunk, neck and extremities).

Record 4 (lobectomy)

There is a R/L *thoracotomy scar*. The *trachea is deviated* to the R/L. On the R/L side *chest expansion is diminished*, the percussion note is more resonant and the breath sounds are harsher. The patient has had a R/L lobectomy to remove a tumour, resistant lung abscess or localized area of bronchiectasis.

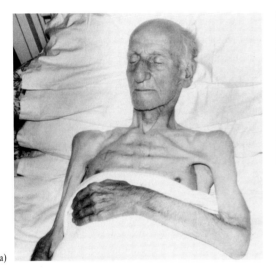

(a)

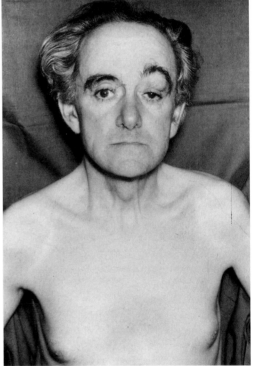

(b)

Fig. 3.8 (a) Cachexia due to carcinoma of the bronchus (note radiotherapy ink marks). (b) Pancoast's tumour (note gynaecomastia and left Horner's syndrome).

† This can be skilfully, and somewhat theatrically, demonstrated by activating a previously absent or feeble biceps reflex after you have made the patient flex his forearm against resistance. In the Eaton–Lambert syndrome the activity would increase the reflex, in contrast with myasthenia gravis where the reflex would be unaffected.

‡ Hypercalcaemia may also be due to bone secondaries.

22 / Pneumonectomy/lobectomy

Note: if you are asked to discuss the chest X-ray of a pneumonectomy short case, it would usually show a 'white out' on one side, deviated trachea and compensatory hyperinflation on the other.

Record 1

There is a **deformity of the chest with** *flattening* on the R/L and a *thoracotomy scar* on that side. The **trachea is** *deviated* to the R/L and the apex beat is *displaced* in the same direction. On the R/L *expansion* is reduced, the **percussion note is** *dull* and the *breath sounds are diminished*. There is an **area of bronchial breathing in the** R/L upper zone (over the grossly deviated trachea).

These findings suggest a R/L pneumonectomy.

In the patient with lobectomy, as opposed to total pneumonectomy, the signs will be more confined. For example see *record 2*.

Record 2

There is a *deformity* of the chest with the left lower ribs *pulled in* and a left-sided *thoracotomy scar*. The *trachea* is central (may be displaced) but the *apex beat* is displaced to the left. The percussion note is *dull* over the left lower zone and *breath sounds are diminished* in this area.

These signs suggest a left lower lobectomy.

Surgical resection and the lung

Surgery has little role in the management of *small cell carcinoma*. In others, after a full assessment which includes clinical examination, lung function tests, bone and liver biochemistry, isotope bone scan, ultrasound or computerized tomography (CT) scan of the liver, mediastinal CT scan and, if necessary, mediastinoscopy, 25% of *non-small cell* lung cancers will be suitable for attempted surgical resection. The operative mortality for lobectomy is about 2–4% and this rises to about 6% for total pneumonectomy, which may be required if the tumour involves both divisions of a main bronchus or more than one lobe.

Surgical resection is often required for *solitary pulmonary nodules* of uncertain cause. The possibility of undiagnosed small cell cancer in this instance is not necessarily a reason for avoiding thoracotomy; resection of small cell lung cancer presenting as a solitary pulmonary nodule may have a 5-year survival compa-

rable to that of other forms of nodular bronchogenic carcinoma treated surgically (approximately 25%).

Surgical resection is indicated in the **treatment of** *bronchiectasis* (p. 41) when other forms of treatment have failed to control symptoms, particularly if it is localized and if recurrent haemoptysis is present.

Old tuberculosis

In the days before antituberculous chemotherapy, tuberculosis was sometimes treated surgically:

Record 3

The **trachea is** *deviated* to the R/L. The R/L upper chest shows *deformity* with *decreased expansion, dull percussion note, bronchial breathing* and *crepitations*. The **apex beat** is (may be) *displaced* to the R/L. There is a *thoracotomy scar* posteriorly with evidence of **rib resections.**

The patient has had a R/L thoracoplasty for treatment of tuberculosis before the days of chemotherapy.

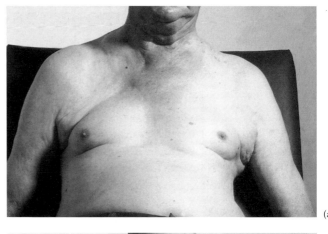

(a)

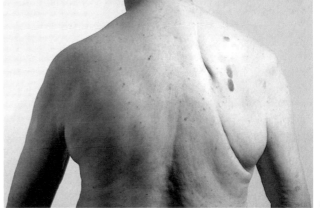

(b)

Fig. 3.9 (a) Deformity of the right chest with flattening. (b) Right-sided thoracotomy scar on the back.

23 / Pneumothorax

Record

The R/L *side* of the chest (of this tall, thin, young adult male—old patients are usually bronchitic) *expands poorly* compared with the other side. Though the *percussion note* on the R/L side is *hyper-resonant*, the tactile fremitus, vocal resonance and *breath sounds* are all *diminished* (large pneumothorax of one side may push the *trachea* and apex beat to the opposite side).

These findings suggest a pneumothorax of the R/L side.

Male to female ratio is 6 : 1.

A 'crunching' sound in keeping with the heart beat may be heard when the pneumothorax is small.

Treatment is not required in a healthy individual with a small pneumothorax (i.e. if only a quarter of one side is affected). Drainage is indicated for:

Larger pneumothorax associated with dyspnoea, increasing in size or not resolving after 1 week

Tension pneumothorax

Pneumothorax complicating underlying severe chronic bronchitis with emphysema

Pneumothorax exacerbating acute severe asthma (hence chest X-ray mandatory in acute severe asthma).

When drainage is indicated, simple aspiration (with a plastic cannula, syringe and three-way tap so that aspirated air can be voided) should usually be attempted before resorting to inter-costal drainage via a tube attached to an underwater seal. Tension pneumothorax should be released urgently by stabbing an intravenous cannula through the chest wall at the second intercostal space, midclavicular line, pending the insertion of an intercostal drain.

Recurrent spontaneous pneumothorax is treated by obliteration of the pleural space (pleurectomy; application of irritating substances into the pleural cavity; scarification of the pleura followed by intrapleural suction).   *Pleurodesis*

Causes of pneumothorax

Traumatic

Penetrating chest wounds

Iatrogenic (chest aspiration, intercostal nerve block, subclavian cannulation, transbronchial biopsy, needle aspiration lung biopsy, positive pressure ventilation)

Chest compression injury (including external cardiac massage).

Spontaneous

Primary (a common cause in young men*)

Secondary

Chronic obstructive pulmonary disease

Asthma

Congenital cysts and bullae

Pleural malignancy

Rheumatoid lung disease (p. 189)

Bacterial pneumonia (p. 42)

Tuberculosis

Cystic fibrosis (gl.)

Tuberous sclerosis (gl.)

Endometriosis of the pleura

Marfan's syndrome (gl.)

Sarcoidosis (gl.)

Histiocytosis X (gl.)

Whooping cough

Oesophageal rupture

Pneumocystis carinii pneumonia.

---

* The risk of a second pneumothorax in a young adult following the first episode is of the order of 25%. After a second episode, the risk increases to the order of 50%.

Chapter 4
Examine this patient's abdomen

Possible short cases include
Hepatosplenomegaly (not chronic liver disease) (p. 61)
Splenomegaly (p. 59)
Polycystic kidneys (p. 64)
Chronic liver disease (p. 62)
Hepatomegaly (without chronic liver disease or splenomegaly) (p. 58)
Ascites (p. 68)
Single palpable kidney
Miscellaneous abdominal masses (p. 66)
Hepatosplenomegaly and generalized lymphadenopathy
Hepatomegaly and generalized lymphadenopathy
Primary biliary cirrhosis (p. 70)
Crohn's disease (p. 72).

Other diagnoses could be: aortic aneurysm, haemochromatosis (gl.), poly-cystic kidneys and a transplanted kidney, splenomegaly and generalized lymphadenopathy, abdominal lymphadenopathy and postsplenectomy.

Examination *routine*
Analysis of the above list reveals that in nearly 80% of cases the findings in the abdomen relate to a palpable spleen, liver or kidneys. Bearing this in mind you should approach the right-hand side of the patient and position him so that he is lying supine on one pillow (if comfortable), with the whole abdomen and chest in full view. Ideally the genitalia should also be exposed but to avoid embarrassment to patients, who, in examina-tions, are volunteers and whose genitals are usually normal, we suggest that you ask the patient to lower his garments and ensure that these are pulled down to a level about halfway between the iliac crest and the sym-physis pubis. While these preparations are being made you should be performing

1 a *visual survey* of the patient. Amongst the many relevant physical signs that you may observe in these few seconds are pallor, pigmentation, jaundice, spider naevi, xanthelasma, parotid swelling, gynaecomastia, scratch marks, tattoos, abdominal distension, distended abdominal veins, an abdominal swelling, herniae and decreased body hair. If you use the following *routine* most of these will also be noted during your subsequent examination but at this stage you should particularly note any

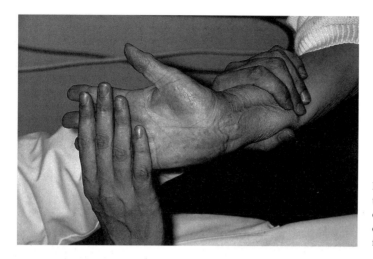

Fig. 4.1 Eliciting a flapping tremor — the patient is unable to maintain extension once you let go. Note palmar erythema in this patient with liver failure.

2 **pigmentation**. As the patient is being correctly positioned,
3 *quickly* **examine the hands*** for
  (a) Dupuytren's contracture (gl.),
  (b) clubbing,
  (c) leuconychia,
  (d) palmar erythema, and
  (e) a flapping tremor (if relevant) (Fig. 4.1).†

After asking you to examine the abdomen many examiners would like, and *expect*, you to concentrate on the abdomen itself without delay, and yet they will not forgive you for missing an abnormal physical sign elsewhere. This emphasizes the importance of a good *visual survey*; a trained eye will miss nothing important on the face or in the hands while the patient is being properly positioned with the hands by his side. Thus, steps 1–3 need not occupy you for more than a few seconds; you may wish to omit steps 5 and 6 if there is no visible abnormality, and steps 7–11 can be completed as part of the *visual survey*.

4 Pull down the **lower eyelid** to look for *anaemia*. At the same time check the sclerae for *icterus* and look for *xanthelasma*. The guttering between the eyeball and the lower lid is the best place to look for pallor or for any discoloration (e.g. cyanosis, jaundice, etc.).

5 Look at the lips for cyanosis (cirrhosis of the liver) and shine your pen torch into the **mouth** looking for swollen lips (Crohn's) (Fig. 4.2), telangiectasis (Osler–Weber–Rendu), patches of pigmentation (Peutz–Jeghers (gl.)) and mouth ulcers (Crohn's).

---

* For a full list of the signs that may be visible in the hands in chronic liver disease, see p. 62.
† A flapping tremor, or an involuntary flexion of all metacarpophalangeal joints when the patient is asked to keep the hands extended (Fig. 4.1), is usually present in advanced liver and respiratory failure. In either case the patient's mental state is obtunded and the patient is less likely to be used as a short case, but it would be unwise to rely on that assumption.

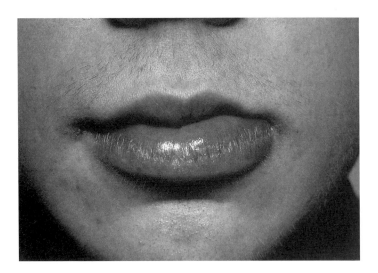

Fig. 4.2 Crohn's lips (orofacial granulomatosis).

6 Palpate the neck and supraclavicular fossae for *cervical lymph nodes.** If you do find lymph nodes you should then proceed to examine the axillae and groins for evidence of generalized lymphadenopathy (lymphoma, chronic lymphatic leukaemia (gl.)). As you move from the neck to the chest, check for

7 gynaecomastia (palpate for glandular breast tissue in obese subjects),

8 spider naevi (may have been noted already on hands, arms and face and may also be present on the back), and

9 scratch marks (may have been noted on the arms, and may also be found on the back and elsewhere). Next,

10 look at the chest (in the male) and in the axillae for **paucity of hair** (if diminished note facial hair in the male; pubic hair if not visible, may be noted later).

11 Observe the abdomen in *three segments* (epigastric, umbilical and suprapubic) for any visible signs such as *pulsations*, generalized *distension* (ascites) (Fig. 4.3) or a *swelling* in one particular area. Note any scars or fistulae (previous surgery; Crohn's). Look for distended *abdominal* veins (the flow is away from the umbilicus in portal hypertension but upwards from the groin in inferior vena cava obstruction).

With practise the examination to this point can be completed very rapidly and will provide valuable information which may be overlooked if proceeding carelessly straight to palpation of the abdomen. If the examiner insists that you start with abdominal palpation† it suggests that there is little to be found elsewhere, but you should nevertheless be prepared to use your 'wide-angled lenses' in order not to miss any of the above features.

---

* The supraclavicular lymph nodes, particularly on the left side, may be enlarged with carcinoma of the stomach (*Troisier's sign* (gl.); NB *Virchow's node* (gl.) behind the left sternoclavicular joint) or carcinoma of any other abdominal organ or with carcinoma of the bronchus.

† Some examiners admit to being irritated at seeing students examine normal hands for a long time after being asked to examine the abdomen. They argue that the information obtainable from the face, mouth and hands can be gathered without delay during the inspection part of the examination.

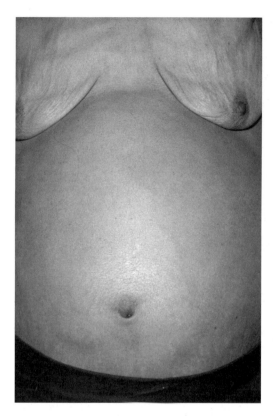

Fig. 4.3 Ascites. Note the everted umbilicus and prominent veins.

12 Palpation of the abdomen should be performed in an orthodox manner; any temptation to go straight for a visible swelling should be resisted. Put your palm gently over the abdomen and ask the patient if he has any tenderness and to let you know if you hurt him. First systematically examine the whole of the abdomen with *light palpation*. Palpation should be done with the *pulps* of the fingers rather than the tips, the best movement being a gentle flexion at the metacarpophalangeal joints with the hand flat on the abdominal wall (Fig. 4.4). Next, examine specifically for the *internal organs*. For both liver and spleen start in the right iliac fossa (you cannot be frowned upon for following this orthodox procedure*), working upwards to the right hypochondrium in the case of the *liver* and diagonally across the abdomen to the left hypochondrium in the case of the *spleen*. The organs are felt against the radial border of the index finger and the pulps of the index and middle fingers as they descend on inspiration, at which time you can gently press and move your hand upwards to meet them. The *kidneys* are then sought by bimanual palpation of each lateral region (Fig. 4.5). Palpation of the internal organs may be difficult if there is ascites. In this case the technique is to press quickly, flexing at the wrist

*Even though it is the time-honoured orthodox procedure, many clinicians, these days, are opposed to this practice. They argue that a grossly enlarged spleen will be picked up on the initial light palpation which makes the approach from the right iliac fossa unnecessary. If they do not feel a mass in the left hypochondrium on initial palpation, they start deep palpation a few centimetres below the left costal edge.

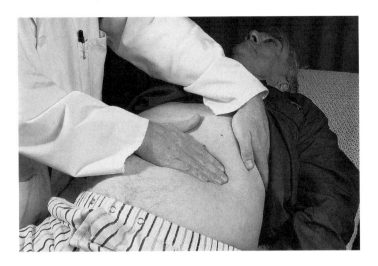

Fig. 4.4 Palpating the spleen.

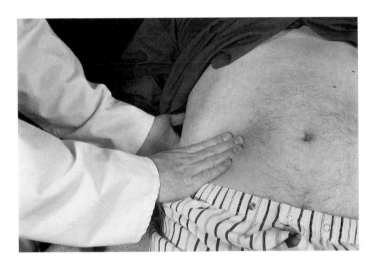

Fig. 4.5 Bimanual palpation of the kidney. Gently press the left hand under the loin and the kidney can be felt between the two hands as the patient breathes in.

joint, to displace the fluid and palpate the enlarged organ ('dipping' or 'ballot-ting'). In a patient well chosen for an examination, a mass in the left hypochon-drium may present a problem of identification; the examiner (testing your confidence) may ask you if you are sure that it is a spleen and not a kidney or vice versa. Do not forget to establish whether you can *get above* the mass and *separate* it from the costal edge, whether you can *bimanually* palpate it and whether the percussion note over it is *resonant* (all features of an enlarged kidney, see also p. 59). Palpate *deeply* with the pulps to look for the *ascending* and *descending colons* in the flanks, and use *gentle* palpation to feel for an *aortic aneurysm* in the midline. Complete palpation by feeling for *inguinal lymph nodes*, noting obvious herniae and, at the same time, adding information about the distribution and thickness of pubic hair to that already gained about the rest of the body hair.

13 Percussion must be used from the nipple downwards on both sides to locate the upper edge of the liver on the right and the spleen on the left (NB the left lower lateral chest wall may become dull to percussion before an enlarged spleen is palpable). The lower palpable edges of the spleen and liver should be defined by percussion in an orthodox manner, proceeding from the resonant to dull areas. If you suspect free fluid in the peritoneum you must establish its presence by demonstrating

14 shifting dullness. Initially check for *stony dullness* in the flanks. There is no need to continue with the procedure of demonstrating shifting dullness if this is not present. By asking the patient with ascites to turn on his side you can shift the dullness from the upper to the lower flank (Fig. 4.6). Before you conclude the palpation and percussion of the abdomen, ask yourself whether you have found anything abnormal. If there are no abnormal physical signs make sure that you have not missed a polycystic kidney or a palpable splenic edge (or occasionally a mass in the epigastrium or iliac fossae); during your auscultation listen carefully for a bruit over the aorta and renal vessels. Generally speaking

15 auscultation has very little to contribute in the examination setting, but as part of the full *routine* you should listen to the bowel sounds, check for renal

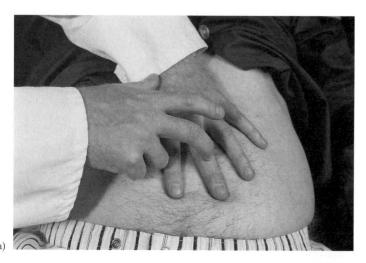

(a)

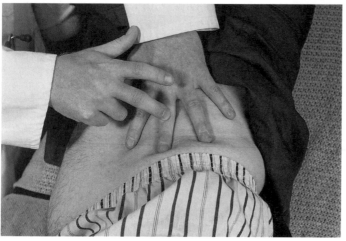

(b)

Fig. 4.6 Shifting dullness. (a) Percuss towards the flank; if *stony dull* turn the patient over on the opposite side.
(b) The stony dullness will no longer be present. Now percuss towards the dependent midline where the dullness caused by free fluid in the peritoneum should have shifted.

artery bruits and for any other sounds such as a rub over the spleen or kidney or a venous hum (both excessively rare).

Examination of the

16 external genitalia is not usually required in an examination for the reasons given above, and we have never heard of a case where

17 a rectal examination was required. You should, however, comment that you would like to complete your examination of the abdomen by examining the external genitalia (especially in the male with chronic liver disease — small testes; or cervical lymphadenopathy — drainage of testes to para-aortic and cervical lymph nodes) and rectum. You may of course never get this far since the examiner may interrupt you at an appropriate stage to ask for your findings.

For *checklist* see p. 275.

24 / Hepatomegaly (without splenomegaly)

Record

The liver is palpable at . . . cm below the right costal margin (*?icterus, ascites,* signs of *cirrhosis* (do not miss gynaecomastia), *pigmentation, lymph nodes*).

Common causes

1 Cirrhosis—usually alcoholic (?spider naevi, gynaecomastia, etc. —p. 62).
2 Secondary carcinoma (?hard and knobbly, cachexia, evidence of primary).
3 Congestive cardiac failure (?jugular venous pressure (JVP) ↑, ankle oedema, *S3* or cardiac murmur; tender pulsatile liver with giant *v* waves in the JVP in tricuspid incompetence).

Other causes of hepatomegaly

Infections such as hepatitis A, glandular fever, Weil's disease (gl.) and hepatitis B (remember hepatitis serology heads the list of investigations in icterus of uncertain cause)

Primary tumours both malignant (hepatoma may complicate cirrhosis) and benign (liver cell adenoma is associated with oral contraceptive use)

Lymphoproliferative disorders (?lymph nodes)

Primary biliary cirrhosis (?middle-aged female, scratch marks, xanthelasma, etc. —p. 70)

Haemochromatosis (gl.) (?male, slate-grey pigmentation, etc.)

Sarcoidosis (gl.) (?erythema nodosum or history of; lupus pernio (gl.); chest signs)

Amyloidosis (gl.) (?rheumatoid arthritis or other underlying chronic disease—see footnote, p. 61)

Hydatid cyst (gl.) (?Welsh connection—NB patient's name)

Amoebic abscess (?tropical connection—name, appearance)

Budd-Chiari syndrome (gl.) (?icterus, ascites, tender hepatomegaly)

Riedel's lobe (gl.)

Emphysema (apparent hepatomegaly).

Hard and knobbly hepatomegaly— possible causes

Malignancy—primary or secondary

Polycystic liver disease (?kidneys—p. 64)

Macronodular cirrhosis (following hepatitis B with widespread necrosis)

Hydatid cysts (may be eosinophilia; rupture may be associated with anaphylaxis)

Syphilitic gummas (late benign syphilis; there is usually hepatosplenomegaly and anaemia; rapid response to penicillin).

25 / Splenomegaly (without hepatomegaly)

Record

The spleen is palpable at . . . cm.

Or

There is a *mass* in the *left hypochondrium*. On palpation I *cannot get above* the mass, it has a *notch*, and on inspiration moves diagonally across the abdomen. The *percussion note is dull* over the left lower lateral chest wall and over the mass.

   I think this is the spleen enlarged at . . . cm. Likely causes* to be considered are:

Very large spleen†

1 Chronic myeloid leukaemia (gl.) (Philadelphia chromosome positive in 90%).

2 Myelofibrosis (gl.).

And in other parts of the world:

3 Chronic malaria (gl.).

4 Kala-azar (gl.).

Spleen enlarged 4–8 cm (2–4 finger breadths)

1 Myeloproliferative disorders‡ (e.g. chronic myeloid leukaemia and myelofibrosis).

2 Lymphoproliferative disorders§ (e.g. lymphoma (gl.) and chronic lymphatic leukaemia (gl.)).

---

* To help you remember some common causes to mention in an examination we have given the three or four most common causes of a spleen of a particular size. An alternative way of dividing up splenomegaly which can be found in many textbooks is:
1 Infectious and inflammatory splenomegaly (e.g. subacute bacterial endocarditis, infectious mononucleosis, sarcoidosis)
2 Infiltrative splenomegaly
   (a) benign (e.g. Gaucher's, amyloidosis)
   (b) neoplastic (e.g. leukaemias, lymphoma)
3 Congestive splenomegaly (e.g. cirrhosis, hepatic vein thrombosis)
4 Splenomegaly due to reticuloendothelial hyperplasia (e.g. haemolytic anaemias, immune thrombocytopenias).
† *Gaucher's* disease and *rapidly progressive lymphoma* (especially high-grade lymphoma) may also cause a huge spleen. *Chronic congestive splenomegaly* (Banti's syndrome = splenomegaly, pancytopenia, portal hypertension and

gastrointestinal bleeding) may also cause massive splenomegaly. A huge spleen developing in a patient with *polycythaemia rubra vera* is usually due to the development of myelofibrosis (?pallor, cf. plethora of polycythaemia).
‡ When listing the causes of splenomegaly or hepatosplenomegaly in the limited time of an examination, to use the term 'myeloproliferative disorders' in its broadest interpretation is a useful way of covering several conditions in one phrase. If asked to explain it (unlikely), one strict definition covers a group of related disorders of haemopoietic stem cell proliferation: chronic myeloid leukaemia (CML), myelofibrosis, polycythaemia rubra vera and essential thrombocythaemia. The term can be used more broadly to cover acute myeloid leukaemia as well. A small spleen is more likely to be due to acute leukaemia than CML or myelofibrosis because splenic enlargement in the latter conditions is *often already marked at the time of presentation.*

3 Cirrhosis of the liver with portal hypertension (spider naevi, icterus, etc. — p. 62).

Spleen just tipped or enlarged 2–4 cm (1–2 finger breadths)

1 Myeloproliferative disorders.‡
2 Lymphoproliferative disorders§ (?palpable lymph nodes).
3 Cirrhosis of the liver with portal hypertension.
4 Infections such as:
    (a) glandular fever (?throat, lymph nodes)
    (b) infectious hepatitis (?icterus)
    (c) subacute bacterial endocarditis (?heart murmur, splinter haemorrhages, etc.).

Other causes of splenomegaly

Polycythaemia rubra vera (gl.) (?plethoric, middle-aged man)

Brucellosis (gl.) ('examine this farmer's abdomen')

Sarcoidosis (gl.) (?erythema nodosum or history of; lupus pernio (gl.); chest signs)

Haemolytic anaemia (gl.) (?icterus)

Pernicious anaemia and other megaloblastic anaemias (?pallor; NB subacute combined degeneration of the cord (SACD) — p. 114; NB associated organ-specific autoimmune diseases, especially autoimmune thyroid disease, diabetes, Addison's, vitiligo, hypoparathyroidism (gl.) — see p. 214)

Idiopathic thrombocytopenic purpura (?young female, purpura)

Felty's syndrome (gl.) (?hands, nodules)

Amyloidosis (gl.) (?underlying chronic disease, other organ involvement — see p. 61)

Systemic lupus erythematosus (SLE) (?typical rash)

Lipid storage disease (spleen may be enormous — e.g. Gaucher's (gl.))

Myelomatosis (gl.)

Chronic iron deficiency anaemia

Thyrotoxicosis

Other infections (subacute septicaemia, typhoid, disseminated tuberculosis, trypanosomiasis, echinococcosis)

Other causes of congestive splenomegaly* (hepatic vein thrombosis, portal vein obstruction, schistosomiasis (gl.), congestive heart failure).

§ The lymphoproliferative disorders are chronic lymphatic leukaemia, lymphoma, myelomatosis, Waldenström's macroglobulinaemia, acute lymphatic leukaemia and hairy cell leukaemia. Of these, the first two and Waldenström's macroglobulinaemia are usually associated with lymphadenopathy and hepatomegaly. Multiple myeloma seldom causes palpable spenomegaly.

26 / Hepatosplenomegaly

Record

There is hepatosplenomegaly, the *spleen* is enlarged . . . cm below the left costal margin. The *liver* is palpable at . . . cm below the right costal margin; it is non-tender, firm and smooth (now look for clinical *anaemia, lymphadeno-pathy* and signs of *chronic liver disease*).

Likely causes to be considered are:

No other signs or clinical anaemia only

1 Myeloproliferative disorders (p. 60).
2 Lymphoproliferative disorders (p. 60).
3 Cirrhosis of the liver with portal hypertension (less likely if there are no other signs of chronic liver disease).

Hepatosplenomegaly plus palpable lymph nodes*

1 Chronic lymphatic leukaemia (gl.).
2 Lymphoma (gl.).
Other conditions to be considered would include infectious mononucleosis (?throat), infective hepatitis (?icterus) and sarcoidosis (gl.).

Signs of chronic liver disease

Cirrhosis of the liver with portal hypertension (p. 62).

Other causes of hepatosplenomegaly

Hepatits B or C† (?icterus, tattoo marks, needle marks)
Brucellosis (gl.) ('examine this farmer's abdomen')
Weil's disease (gl.) (?icterus, sewerage worker or fell into a canal)
Toxoplasmosis (glandular fever-like illness)
Cytomegalovirus infection (glandular fever-like illness)
Pernicious anaemia and other megaloblastic anaemias (NB SACD—p. 114; NB associated organ-specific autoimmune disease—p. 214)
Storage disorders (e.g. Gaucher's (gl.)—spleen is often huge; glycogen storage disease)

Amyloidosis (gl.) (?underlying chronic disease)‡
Other causes of portal hypertension (e.g. Budd–Chiari syndrome (gl.) = hepatic vein thrombosis—see pp. 62 and 68)
Infantile polycystic disease (in some variants of this, children have relatively mild renal involvement but hepatosplenomegaly and portal hypertension).

Common causes on a worldwide basis

Malaria (gl.)
Kala-azar (gl.)
Schistosomiasis (gl.)
Tuberculosis.

*These conditions can also occur without palpable lymph nodes.
†NB Hepatitis serology heads the list of investigations of icterus of uncertain cause.
‡Though hepatosplenomegaly can occur in primary and myeloma-associated amyloidosis, it is commoner in the secondary form. Other organs particularly involved in secondary amyloidosis are kidneys (nephrotic syndrome

(gl.)), adrenals (clinical adrenocortical failure may occur) and alimentary tract (rectal biopsy). Conditions associated with secondary amyloidosis include rheumatoid arthritis (including juvenile type), tuberculosis, leprosy (gl.), chronic sepsis, Crohn's disease, ulcerative colitis (gl.), ankylosing spondylitis, paraplegia (bedsores and urinary infection), malignant lymphoma and carcinoma. See also footnote on p. 101.

27 / Chronic liver disease

Record

The patient is *icteric*, *pigmented* and *cyanosed* (due to pulmonary venous shunts). He has *clubbing, leuconychia, palmar erythema, Dupuytren's contracture* (gl.)* and there are several *spider naevi*. He has a flapping tremor of the hands (suggesting some portosystemic encephalopathy). There are scratch marks on the forearms and back, and there is purpura. There is *gynaecomastia, scanty body hair* and his *testes are small*. There is 5 cm *hepatomegaly* and 3 cm *splenomegaly*. He has *ascites* and *ankle oedema*, and there are *distended abdominal veins* in which the flow is away from the umbilicus.

The diagnosis is likely to be cirrhosis of the liver with portal hypertension.

Possible causes

1 Alcohol.

2 Viral hepatitis
  (a) hepatitis B (?health or clinical laboratory worker)
  (b) hepatitis C (the major cause of post-transfusion hepatitis)
  (c) hepatitis D (unusual; requires antecedent or simultaneous hepatitis B virus infection).

3 Lupoid hepatitis (pubertal or menopausal female, steroid responsive; associated with diabetes, inflammatory bowel disease, thyroiditis and pulmonary infiltrates; ?smooth muscle antibodies).

4 Primary biliary cirrhosis (middle-aged female, scratch marks, xanthelasma; ?antimitochondrial antibody — p. 70).

5 Haemochromatosis (gl.) (male, slate-grey pigmentation).

6 Cryptogenic.

Other causes

Cardiac failure (?JVP ↑, *v* waves, *S3* or a valvular lesion, tender pulsatile liver if tricuspid incompetence)

Constrictive pericarditis† (JVP raised, abrupt *x* and *y* descent, loud early *S3* ('pericardial knock' — a valuable sign but only present in <40% of cases) though heart sounds are often normal, slight 'paradoxical pulse', *no signs in lung fields*, chest X-ray may show calcified pericardium; rare but important cause of ascites as response to treatment may be dramatic)

Budd–Chiari syndrome (gl.) (in the acute phase ascites develops rapidly with pain, there are no cutaneous signs of chronic liver disease and the liver is

---

*Twenty signs which may be present in the hands of the patient with chronic liver disease are clubbing, Dupuytren's contracture, palmar erythema, spider naevi, flapping tremor, leuconychia, scratch marks, icterus, pallor, pigmentation, cyanosis, xanthomata, purpura, koilonychia (gl.), paronychia, abscesses, oedema, muscle wasting, tattoos (?HBsAg-positive), needle marks (intravenous drug abuse — more likely in antecubital fossa).

† The spleen may be palpable. In the absence of evidence of *bacterial endocarditis* or *tricuspid valve disease*, the presence of splenomegaly in a patient with congestive heart failure should arouse suspicion of *constrictive pericarditis* or *pericardial effusion with tamponade*.

smoothly enlarged and tender; if the inferior vena cava is involved there is no hepatojugular reflux)

Biliary cholestasis (bile obstruction with or without infection)

Toxins and drugs (methotrexate, methyldopa, isoniazid, carbon tetrachloride, amiodarone, aspirin, phenytoin, propylthiouracil, sulphonamides)

Wilson's disease (gl.) (?Kayser–Fleischer rings (gl.), tremor, rigidity, dysarthria)

Alpha 1 antitrypsin deficiency (gl.) (?lower zone emphysema)

Other metabolic causes (galactosaemia (gl.), tyrosinaemia, type IV glycogenosis).

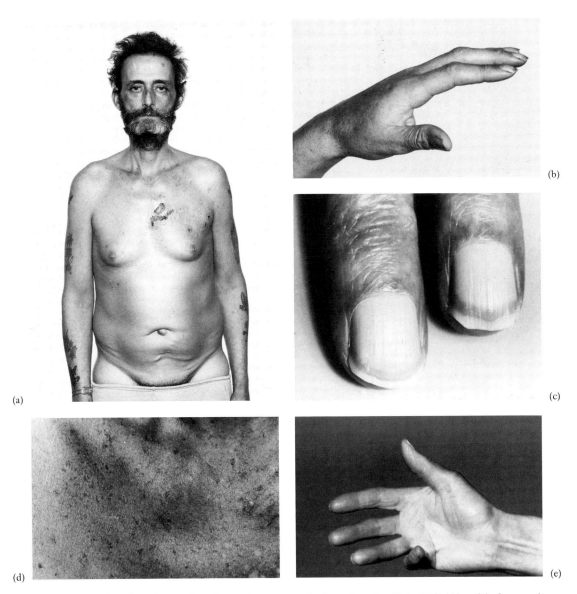

(a)

(b)

(c)

(d)

(e)

Fig. 4.7 (a) Note from above downwards: spider naevi, herpes zoster (debilitated patient), gynaecomastia, tattoo marks, everted umbilicus, swelling of the flanks, abdominal wall veins and paucity of hair. (b) Clubbing of the fingers and leuconychia (same patient as (a)). (c) Leuconychia. (d) Spider naevi (close up). (e) Dupuytren's contracture.

28 / Polycystic kidneys

Record

There are *bilateral masses* in the *flanks* which are *bimanually ballotable*. I can *get above* them and the percussion note is *resonant* over them.* I suspect, therefore, that they are renal masses and a likely diagnosis is polycystic kidneys (?*uraemic facies*; the *blood pressure* may be raised). The *arteriovenous fistula/shunt* on his arm indicates that the patient is being treated with haemodialysis (about 5% develop renal failure).

Other causes of bilateral renal enlargement

1 Bilateral hydronephrosis.
2 Amyloidosis (gl.) (?underlying chronic disease, hepatosplenomegaly, etc. — see p. 61).
3 Tuberous sclerosis (gl.) (?adenoma sebaceum).
4 Von Hippel–Lindau disease.†

Polycystic disease of the liver in adults may cause a nodular liver enlargement (liver function may be normal despite massive hepatomegaly). About 50% have renal involvement. Cystic liver is a major feature of infantile polycystic disease (autosomal recessive) but a minor feature of adult polycystic kidney disease (autosomal dominant).

Other features of adult polycystic kidney disease

Cysts may also occur in other organs—most important are sacular aneurysms (berry aneurysms) of the cerebral arteries (10%) which, in combination with the hypertension, leads to serious risk of intracranial haemorrhage (cause of death in 10% of cases according to some authorities). There may be focal neurological defects

Mitral valve prolapse (gl.) may occur in 25% as a further manifestation of the systemic collagen defect. Patients often have palpitations and atypical chest pain

It may present with flank pains, bleeding, urinary tract infection, nephrolithiasis or obstructive uropathy

Renal cell carcinoma may be more common than in the general population but this is uncertain.

---

* Look for abdominal scars from previous peritoneal dialysis or cyst aspiration. The latter is performed to relieve obstruction of the outflow tract by the cyst, intractable pain or haematuria.

† An autosomal dominant condition in which patients develop retinal haemangiomata, cerebellar haemangioblastomata and phaeochromocytomata (gl.). Hepatic, renal, pancreatic and epididymal cysts may occur.

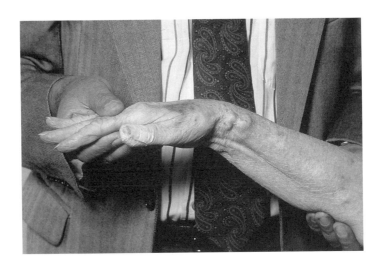

Fig. 4.8 Arteriovenous shunt.

29 / Abdominal mass

Record 1
In this young (?somewhat pale-looking) adult patient there is a freely mobile 5 × 4 cm (measure) firm non-tender mass in the *right iliac fossa*. None of the abdominal organs is enlarged, and there are no fistulae.

The diagnosis could be Crohn's disease (p. 72).

Other causes of a mass in the right iliac fossa
1 Ileocaecal tuberculosis (?ethnic origin, chest signs).
2 Carcinoma of the caecum (?older person, non-tender and hard mass, lymph nodes).
3 Amoebic abscess (?travelled abroad).
4 Lymphoma (?hepatosplenomegaly, lymph nodes elsewhere).
5 Appendicular abscess.
6 Neoplasm of the ovary.
7 Ileal carcinoid (rare).

Record 2
A freely mobile tender 6 × 5 cm mass is palpable in the *left iliac fossa* in this elderly patient. None of the other organs is palpable.

It is probably a diverticular abscess (usually tender).

Other causes of a mass in the left iliac fossa
1 Carcinoma of the colon (?non-tender, hepatomegaly).
2 Neoplasm of the left ovary.
3 A faecal mass (no other signs).
4 Amoebic abscess.

Record 3
In this thin and pale patient there is a round, hard 8 × 6 cm non-tender mass with ill-defined edges in the *epigastrium*. It does not move with respiration. Neither the liver nor the spleen is enlarged (check neck for lymph nodes).

The probable diagnosis is a neoplasm such as:
1 Carcinoma of the stomach (?Troisier's sign (gl.)).
2 Carcinoma of the pancreas (?icterus. NB Courvoisier's sign (gl.)).
3 Lymphoma (?generalized lymphadenopathy, spleen).

Record 4

In this elderly patient there is a *pulsatile* (pulsating anteriorly as well as transversely), 6 × 4 cm firm mass* palpable 2 cm above the umbilicus and reaching the epigastrium. Both femoral pulses are palpable just before the radials (no evidence of dissection) and there are no bruits heard either over the mass or over the femorals. (Look for evidence of peripheral vascular insufficiency in the feet.)

This patient has an aneurysm of his abdominal aorta (the commonest cause is arteriosclerosis).†

If you find a mass in either upper quadrant you should define its:

Size

Shape

Consistency

Whether you can get above it

Whether it is bimanually ballotable

Whether it moves with respiration

Whether it is tender.

In either upper quadrant it has to be differentiated from a renal mass (p. 64); if in the left hypochondrium it has to be differentiated from a spleen (p. 59) and in the right hypochondrium from a liver (p. 58). Other causes of an upper quadrant mass include:

Carcinoma of the colon

Retroperitoneal sarcoma

Lymphoma (gl.) (?generalized lymphadenopathy, spleen)

Diverticular abscess (?tender).

---

*Pulsations without a mass may be transmitted from a normal aorta. A mass from a neighbouring structure may overlie the aorta and transmit (only anterior) pulsations.

†Mycotic aneurysms are a major complication (2.5% of patients with valvular infections) of infective endocarditis and are most commonly associated with relatively non-invasive organisms such as *Streptococcus viridans*. They may occur at any age, either during the active phase or months (sometimes years) after the endocarditis has been successfully treated. More common sites of mycotic aneurysms are the brain (2–6% of all aneurysms in the brain), sinuses of Valsalva, and ligated ductus arteriosus. Clinical manifestations of abdominal aortic aneurysms (e.g. backache) appear after the lesions have started to leak slowly. Surgical treatment is almost always indicated.

30 / Ascites

Record

There is *generalized swelling* of the abdomen and the umbilicus is *everted*. The flanks are *stony dull* to percussion but the centre is resonant (floating, gas-filled bowel). The dullness is *shifting* and a *fluid thrill* can be demonstrated (in tense, large ascites).

This is ascites.

Usual causes

1 Cirrhosis with portal hypertension (?hepatomegaly, icterus, spider naevi, leuconychia, etc. — p. 62).

2 Intra-abdominal malignancy (especially ovarian and gastrointestinal — ?hard knobbly liver, mass, cachexia, nodes, e.g. Troisier's sign (gl.)).

3 Congestive cardiac failure (?JVP↑, ankle and sacral oedema, hepatomegaly (pulsatile if tricuspid incompetence), large heart, tachycardia, *S3* or signs of the cardiac lesion).

Other causes

Nephrotic syndrome (gl.) (?young, underlying diabetes (fundi), evidence of chronic disease underlying amyloid, evidence of collagen disease, etc.)

Other causes of hypoalbuminaemia (e.g. malabsorption)

Tuberculous peritonitis* (?ethnic origin, chest signs)

Constrictive pericarditis (JVP raised, abrupt *x* and *y* descent, loud early *S3* ('pericardial knock') though heart sounds often normal, slight 'paradoxical' pulse, *no signs in lung fields*; chest X-ray may show calcified pericardium; rare but important as response to treatment may be dramatic)

Budd–Chiari syndrome (gl.) (ascites develops rapidly with pain, icterus but no signs of chronic liver disease, smoothly enlarged tender liver; causes include tumour infiltration, oral contraceptives, polycythaemia rubra vera (gl.), ulcerative colitis (gl.) and severe dehydration)

Myxoedema (?facies, ankle jerks, etc. — very rare)

Meigs' syndrome (gl.) (ovarian fibroma — important as easily correctable by surgery)

Pancreatic disease

Chylous ascites (due to lymphatic obstruction — milky fluid).

---

*NB Tuberculous peritonitis may attack debilitated alcoholics. Therefore it should always be considered when ascites is present in a cirrhotic. Fever or abdominal pain are suggestive but may not be present. Examination of the ascitic fluid may help — an exudative protein content ($>25 \, \mathrm{g \, l^{-1}}$) with lymphocytes is also suggestive. Staining of the fluid for acid-fast bacilli (AFB) is rarely positive and culture is only positive in somewhat less than 50%. Diagnostic procedures include peritonoscopy (bowel adhesions may cause difficulty) and open peritoneal biopsy.

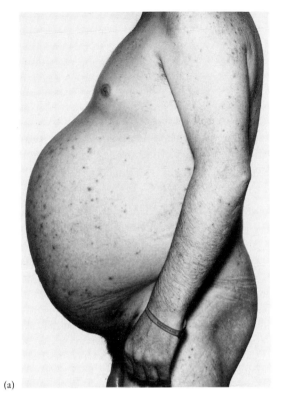

(a)

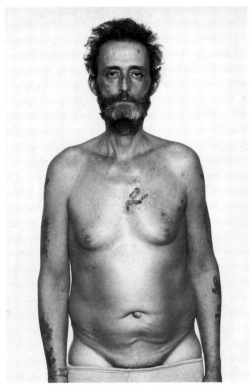

(b)

Fig. 4.9 (a) Gross ascites. (b) Residual ascites in another patient on treatment with diuretics (see also p. 63).

31 / Primary biliary cirrhosis

Record

This middle-aged lady is *icteric* (may not be) with *pigmentation* of the skin. There are *excoriations* (due to scratching) and she has *xanthelasma* (other xanthomata frequently occur over joints, skin folds and at sites of trauma). The liver is enlarged . . . cm (may be very large; there may be splenomegaly).

The clinical diagnosis is primary biliary cirrhosis (there may be *clubbing*). The scratch marks are due to *pruritus* (the predominant presenting symptom).

HLA phenotypes B8 and C4B2 = threefold increase in risk
Serum antimitochondrial antibody positive in 95–99%
Smooth muscle antibody positive in 50%
Antinuclear factor positive in 20%.

Impaired biliary excretion of copper occurs with excessive copper deposition in the liver. This may not be an important factor in the pathogenesis of the progressive liver disease, but it can be helpful in the diagnosis—sometimes differentiation from chronic active hepatitis (gl.) (25% have antimitochondrial antibody) can be difficult (clinically and histologically) and the issue can be resolved by staining the biopsy specimen for copper. Kayser–Fleischer rings (gl.) occasionally occur. Penicillamine (immunological, antifibrotic, as well as chelating effects) has been used in advanced disease but there is no evidence that it improves survival. Immunosuppressive agents (including corticosteroids, azathioprine, methotrexate and cyclosporin A) and antifibrotics (e.g. colchicine) may have a small effect. Ursodeoxycholic acid improves serum biochemistry, decreases the rate of referral for liver transplantation and reduces pruritis, but no effect on histology or survival has yet been convincingly demonstrated. Supplements of fat-soluble vitamins, calcium and phosphate are given in view of malabsorption. The pruritus often responds to cholestyramine (taken before and after meals), though phenobarbitone, rifampicin, opiate antagonists (e.g. naloxone) or propofol may also help. Resistant pruritus responds to norethandrolone but this deepens jaundice. Physical intervention (bile diversion, haemoperfusion, charcoal column perfusion or plasmapheresis) may also help severe pruritis. Liver transplantation has been used successfully but there is increasing evidence that the disease may recur in the transplanted liver.

The patient is at risk of

Bleeding oesophageal varices
Steatorrhoea and malabsorption, leading to
Osteomalacia.

Associated conditions*

Sjögren's syndrome (gl.)
Systemic sclerosis
CRST syndrome (see p. 176)
Rheumatoid arthritis
Hashimoto's thyroiditis (gl.)
Renal tubular acidosis (gl.)
Coeliac disease (gl.)
Dermatomyositis (gl.).

*The incidental finding of a raised alkaline phosphatase in patients with the conditions on this list should raise the suspicion of an associated primary biliary cirrhosis.

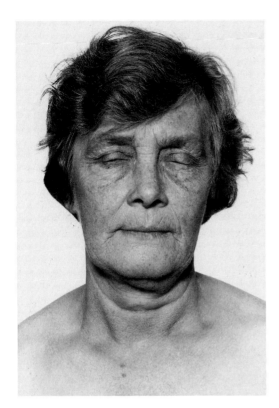

Fig. 4.10 Note xanthelasma, pigmentation and spider naevi.

32 / Crohn's disease

Record 1

The *multiple laparotomy scars* suggest a chronic, relapsing, abdominal condition which has led to crises requiring surgical intervention on several occasions. In view of the associated *fistula* formation, Crohn's disease is likely.

Record 2

The chronically *swollen lips* (granulomatous infiltration) and history of chronic diarrhoea are suggestive of Crohn's disease (examine inside the *mouth for ulcers* which vary in size).

Record 3

There is a (characteristic) *dusky blue discoloration* of the perianal skin. There are *oedematous skin tags* (which look soft but are very firm), there is *fissuring*, *ulceration* and *fistula* formation.

The diagnosis is perianal Crohn's disease (may antedate disease elsewhere in the bowel).

Record 4
Right iliac fossa mass —see p. 66.

Other physical signs in Crohn's disease
Fever
Anaemia (malabsorption, chronic disease and gastrointestinal blood loss)
Clubbing
Arthritis (including sacroiliitis)
Erythema nodosum (p. 233)

Pyoderma gangrenosum (gl.)
Iritis
Ankle oedema (hypoproteinaemia).

Other causes of anal fistulae (rare)
Simple fistula from an abscess of an anal gland
Tuberculosis
Ulcerative colitis (gl.)
Carcinoma of the rectum.

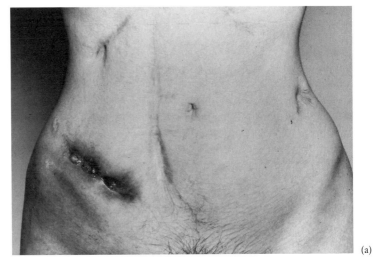

(a)

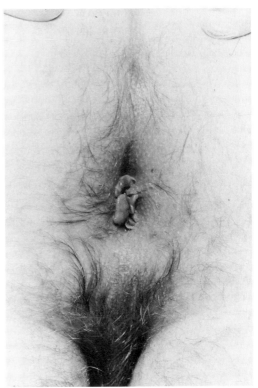

(b)

(c)

Fig. 4.11 (a) Multiple scars and fistulae. (b) Crohn's lips. (c) Perianal lesions.

Chapter 5
Examine this patient's visual fields

Possible short cases include

Homonymous hemianopia
Bitemporal hemianopia
Optic atrophy (p. 145).
Unilateral hemianopia
Partial field defect in one eye due to retinal artery branch occlusion
Quadrantic field defect (homonymous, bitemporal or unilateral)
Acromegaly (p. 257).

Examination *routine*

Ask the patient to sit upright on the side of the bed while you position yourself in visual confrontation about 1 metre away (Fig. 5.1). This apposition will help you to test the visual fields of his left and right eyes against those of your right and left, respectively. As he is doing this perform

1 a *visual survey* (acromegaly, hemiparesis, cerebellar signs in multiple sclerosis) of the patient. Test both temporal fields together so that you do not miss any *visual inattention*. Ask the patient to look at your eyes while you place your index fingers just inside the outer limits of your temporal fields. Then move your fingers in turn and then both at the same time, and ask him:

'Point to the finger which moves'.

If there is visual inattention, the patient will only point to one finger when you move both at the same time. Next test each eye individually and ask him to cover his right eye with his right index finger, and close your left eye:

'Keep looking at my eye'.

2 Examine his **peripheral visual fields**. Test his left temporal vision against your right temporal by moving your wagging finger from the periphery towards the centre:

'Tell me when you see my finger move'.*

The temporal field should be tested in the horizontal plane and by moving your finger through the upper and lower temporal quadrants. Change hands and repeat on the nasal side. By comparing his visual field with your own, any

---

*This will pick up most gross visual field defects rapidly. Moving objects are more easily detected and therefore your moving finger will be immediately noticed by the patient as it moves out of the blind area into his field of vision. Remember that his area of blindness to a stationary object may be greater than that to a moving object. In the dysphasic patient you should ask him to point at the moving finger when he sees it rather than telling you he sees it.

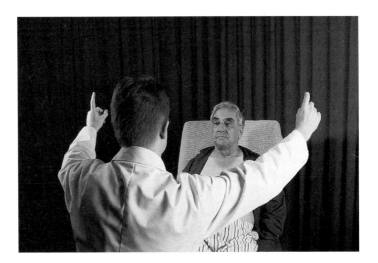

Fig. 5.1 Confrontation—testing the patient's visual fields against your own.

areas of field defect are thus mapped out. The visual fields of his right eye are similarly tested.

3 A **central scotoma** is tested for with a red-headed hat pin (see Fig. 6.2, p. 80). If you have already found a field defect which does not require further examination, or if the examiner does not wish you to continue, he will soon stop you. Otherwise comparing your right eye with his left, as before, move the red headed pin from the temporal periphery through the central field to the nasal periphery, asking the patient:

'Can you see the head of the pin? What colour is it? Tell me if it disappears or changes colour'.

If there is no scotoma find his blind spot and compare it with your own.

Having found the field defect, look for

4 **additional features** (e.g. acromegaly, hemiparesis, nystagmus and cerebellar signs) if appropriate. Recall the possible causes for each type of field defect as this question, at the end of the case, is almost inevitable (see p. 76).

For *checklist* see p. 276.

33 / Visual field defect

Record 1

There is a *homonymous hemianopia*. This suggests a lesion of the *optic tract* behind the optic chiasma (with sparing of the macula and hence normal visual acuity).

Likely causes

1 Cerebrovascular accident (?ipsilateral hemiplegia, atrial fibrillation, heart murmurs or bruits, hypertension).
2 Tumour (?ipsilateral pyramidal signs, papilloedema).

Record 2

There is a *bitemporal* visual field defect worse on the R/L side. This suggests a lesion at the *optic chiasma*. (NB There may be optic atrophy, sometimes with a central scotoma, on the R/L side due to simultaneous compression of the optic nerve by the lesion.)

Possible causes

1 Pituitary tumour (?acromegaly, hypopituitarism, gynaecomastia, galact-orrhoea (gl.), menstrual disturbance, etc.).
2 Craniopharyngioma (gl.) (?calcification on skull X-ray).
3 Suprasellar meningioma (gl.).
4 Aneurysm.
Rarer causes are glioma, granuloma and metastasis.

Record 3

The visual fields are considerably constricted, the central field of vision being spared. This is *tunnel vision.** I would like to examine the fundi, looking for evidence of retinitis pigmentosa, glaucoma (gl.) (pathological cupping) or widespread choroidoretinitis. (Hysteria may occasionally be a cause; papilloedema causes enlargement of the blind spot and peripheral constriction.)

Record 4

There is a *central scotoma*. (NB The discs may be pale (atrophy), swollen and pink (papillitis) or normal (retrobulbar neuritis).)

Causes to be considered

Demyelinating diseases (?nystagmus, cerebellar signs, etc.; however, multiple sclerosis frequently causes retrobulbar neuritis without other signs)

*The Committee on the Safety of Medicine has received reports of visual field defects associated with the anti-epileptic drug *vigabatrin* including three cases of severe, symptomatic, persistent visual field constriction (tunnel vision).

Compression†

Ischaemia

Leber's optic atrophy (gl.) (males : females = 6 : 1)

Toxins (e.g. methyl alcohol)

Macular disease

Nutritional (famine, etc., tobacco–alcohol amblyopia, vitamin B$_{12}$ deficiency, diabetes mellitus).

Record 5

There is *homonymous upper quadrantic visual field loss.* This suggests a lesion in the temporal cortex.

NB Field defects may sometimes originate from retinal damage, e.g. occlusion of a branch of the retinal artery or a large area of choroidoretinitis.

---

† There may be clues as to the site of the compression. (i) A lesion in the frontal lobe which compresses the optic nerve may cause dementia. (ii) It may also cause contralateral papilloedema (*Foster–Kennedy syndrome* (gl.) due to a frontal tumour or aneurysm, e.g. olfactory groove meningioma). (iii) A lesion in front of the chiasma involving crossing fibres that loop forward into the opposite optic nerve may cause a contralateral upper temporal quadrantic field defect. (iv) A lesion at the chiasma may cause a bitemporal field defect. (v) A lesion at the lateral chiasma (pituitary tumour, aneurysm, meningioma) involving the terminal optic tract as well as the optic nerve may cause a homonymous hemianopia.

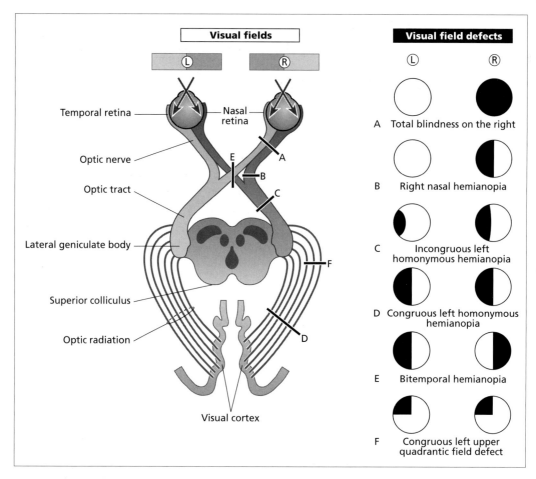

Fig. 5.2 The visual pathways and visual field defects resulting from different lesions. If there is exact overlap of the field defects from both eyes the defect is said to be congruous. If not, it is incongruous. The defects in B and E above are incongruous. Though the complete homonymous hemianopia in D is congruous, lesions of the optic tract (C), which are comparatively rare, produce characteristic incongruous visual changes. The fibres serving identical points in the homonymous half fields do not fully commingle in the anterior optic tract so lesions encroaching on this structure produce incongruous and usually incomplete homonymous hemianopias. Lesions of the geniculate ganglia, visual radiations or visual cortex produce congruous visual field defects. F represents a lesion of the temporal loop of the optic radiation.

Chapter 6
Examine this patient's cranial nerves

Note: in a short case examination, a student may be given this instruction (rarely) either because there is something obvious (facial asymmetry, ptosis, palatal palsy, etc.) or because the examiner wishes to test whether the student has a structured approach to the task. If you see something obvious then you may consider homing in on that, otherwise you should follow the *routine* given below.

Possible short cases include
Bulbar palsy (p. 85)
Cerebellopontine angle syndrome (gl.)
Myasthenia gravis (p. 162)
Ocular palsy (p. 155)
VIIth nerve palsy (p. 173)

Examination *routine*
It is one of the most feared instructions but at the same time it can provide an opportunity to score highly. More than in any other system, the well-rehearsed student can appear competent and professional compared to the unrehearsed. Detailed examination of the individual nerves is not usually required but rather a quick and efficient screen like that used by neurologists at the bedside or in out-patients (it is well worth attending neurology out-patients to watch quick and efficient examination techniques, if for nothing else). Not only can you look good but also the abnormalities are usually easy to detect. Although it is to be hoped that your practised *routine* will not miss out any nerves, it is preferable to perform a smooth, professional examination, which accidentally misses out a nerve, than to test your examiner's patience through a hesitant and meditative examination which takes a long time to start and may never finish! Since the examination is most easily carried out face to face with the patient it is best, if possible, to get him to sit on the edge of the bed facing you. First

1 take a good general and *quick* **look** at the patient; in particular his face, for any obvious abnormality. Next ask him about

2 his **sense of smell and taste:**
   'Do you have any difficulty with your sense of smell?' (I)

Although you should have the ability to examine taste and smell formally if equipment is provided, usually questioning (or possibly the judicious use of a bedside orange) is all that is required. All the examination referable to the eyes is best performed next. Unless there is a Snellen's chart available ask the patient to look at the clock on the wall or some newspaper print to give you a good idea of his

3 **visual acuity**:

'Do you have any difficulty with your vision?'

'Can you see the clock on the wall?' (if he has glasses for long sight he should put them on).

'Can you tell me what time it says?' (II)

A portable Snellen's chart will enable you to perform a more formal test (Fig. 6.1) (see Appendix 4). Now test

4 **visual fields** (see p. 74), including for *central scotoma*, with a red-headed hat pin (Fig. 6.2). Follow this by examining

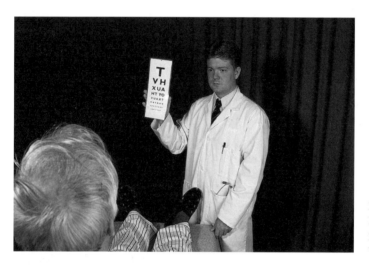

Fig. 6.1 A portable Snellen's chart held approximately 2 m from the patient's eyes (just beyond the end of the bed) (see Appendix 4).

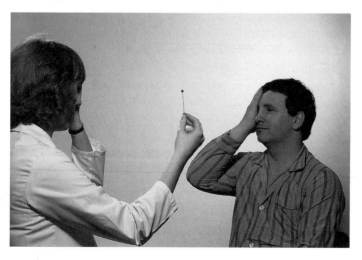

Fig. 6.2 Testing central vision for the presence of a scotoma.

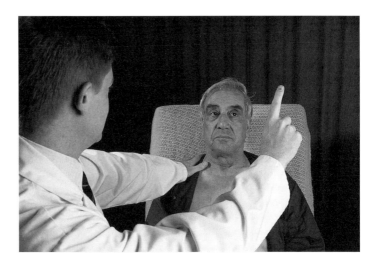

Fig. 6.3 Follow the eye movements and ask if there is diplopia in any direction.

5 **eye movements** (move your finger in the shape of a cross, from side to side then up and down) (Fig. 6.3):

'Look at my finger; follow it with your eyes' (III, IV, VI)

asking the patient at the extremes of gaze whether he sees one or two fingers. If he has diplopia establish the extent and ask him to describe the 'false' image. As you test eye movements note at the same time any

6 **nystagmus** (VIII, cerebellum or cerebellar connections) or

7 **ptosis** (III, sympathetic).

Remember that either extreme abduction of the eyes or gazing at a finger that is too near can cause nystagmus in normal eyes (optikokinetic). Now examine

8 the **pupils** for the direct and consensual *light reflex* (II → optic tract → lateral geniculate ganglion → Edinger–Westphal nucleus of III → fibres to ciliary muscle) (Fig. 6.4) and for the *accommodation–convergence* reflex (cortex → III) with your finger just in front of his nose:

'Look into the distance'.

Now look at my finger' (see also footnote, p. 151).

Finally examine the optic discs (II) by

9 **fundoscopy** (this can be left until last if you prefer). Having finished examining the eyes examine

10 **facial movements**:

'Raise your eyebrows'. ⎫
'Screw your eyes up tight'. ⎪
'Puff your cheeks out'. ⎬ VII
'Whistle'. ⎪
'Show me your teeth'. ⎭

'Clench your teeth'—feel masseters and temporalis. ⎫ motor V
'Open your mouth; stop me closing it' ⎭

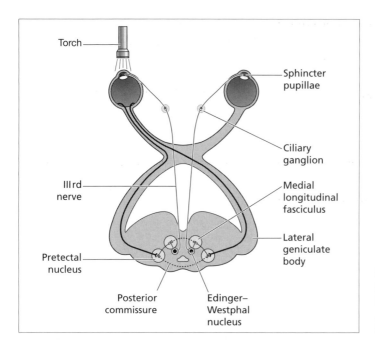

Fig. 6.4 Pupillary reflex pathway (reproduced with permission from F. Plum & J.B. Posner, *Diagnosis of Stupor and Coma*, 3rd edn, 1982, FA Davis).

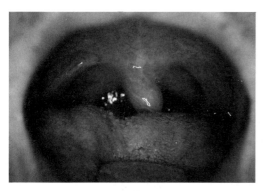

Fig. 6.5 Palatal movement. Note deviation of the uvula to the left (right Xth cranial nerve palsy).

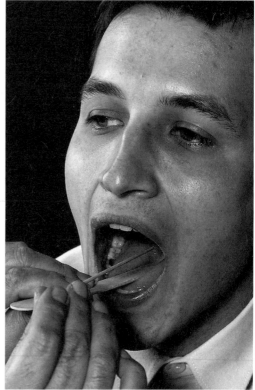

Fig. 6.6 Testing the gag reflex—afferent IXth nerve, efferent Xth nerve.

11 then **palatal movement** (Fig. 6.5):

'Keep your mouth open; say aah' (IX, X)

12 and **gag reflex***—touch the back of the pharynx on both sides with an orange stick (IX, X) (Fig. 6.6). Look at

13 the **tongue** as it lies in the floor of the mouth for *wasting* or *fasciculation* (XII):

'Open your mouth again'

then get the patient to:

'Put your tongue out'—note any deviation†—'waggle it from side to side'. (XII)

14 Test the **accessory nerve**:‡

'Shrug your shoulders; keep them shrugged'—push down on the shoulders. (XI)

'Turn your head to the left side—now to the right'—feel for the sternomastoid muscle on the side opposite to the turned head.

Finally test

15 **hearing:**

'Any problem with the hearing in either ear?'

'Can you hear that?'—rub your finger and thumb together in front of each

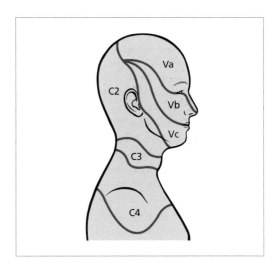

Fig. 6.7 Dermatomes in the head and neck.

* This can be unpleasant but it is important if there is a deficit, so ask the examiner's permission, explain to the patient and ask for his permission as well.

† In unilateral facial paralysis the protruded tongue, though otherwise normal, may deviate so that unilateral hypoglossal paralysis is suspected (see p. 173). In unilateral lower motor neurone XIIth nerve palsy there is wasting (?fasciculation) on the side of the lesion and the tongue curves to that side.

‡ Painless neck weakness has only four causes: myasthenia gravis (p. 162), dystrophia myotonica (p. 209), polymyositis (gl.) and motor neurone disease (p. 110).

ear in turn (VIII—proceed to the **Rinné and Weber tests*** if there is any abnormality, and look in the ear if you suspect disease of the external ear, perforated drum, wax, etc.), and

16 test **facial sensation** including *corneal reflex* (sensory V—Fig. 6.7).

For *checklist* see p. 276.

---

* *Weber test*: sound from a vibrating tuning fork held on the centre of the forehead is conducted towards the ear if it has a conductive defect (e.g. wax or otitis media) and away from the ear if it has a nerve deafness. *Rinné test*: a positive test (normal) is when the sound of the tuning fork is louder by air conduction (prongs by external auditory meatus) than by bone conduction (base of fork on mastoid process). Negative is abnormal.

34 / Bulbar palsy

Record

The *tongue is flaccid* and *fasciculating* (it is wasted, wrinkled, thrown into folds and increasingly motionless). The *speech is indistinct* (flaccid dysarthria), lacks modulations and has a *nasal twang*, and *palatal movement is absent*. There is (may be) saliva at the corners of the mouth (and while the patient talks he may be seen to pause periodically to gulp the secretions that have accumulated meanwhile in the pharynx; there may be dysphagia and nasal regurgitation).

This is bulbar palsy.

Possible causes

1 Motor neurone disease (?muscle fasciculation, absence of sensory signs, etc. —p. 110).
2 Syringobulbia (?nystagmus, Horner's, dissociated sensory loss, etc.).
3 Guillain–Barré syndrome (gl.) (?generalized including facial flaccid paralysis, absent reflexes, peripheral neuropathy or widespread sensory defect; monitor peak flow rate).
4 Poliomyelitis.
5 Subacute meningitis (carcinoma, lymphoma (gl.), etc.).
6 Neurosyphilis.

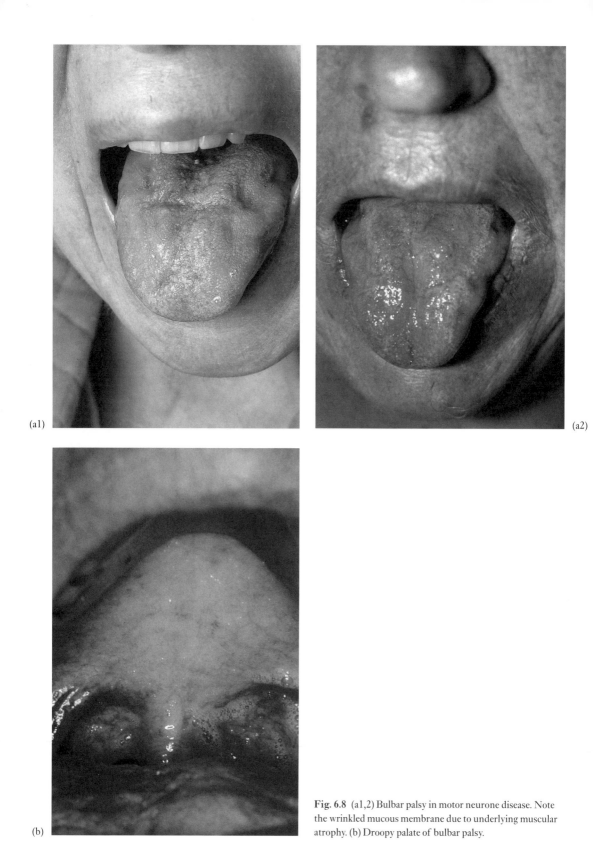

(a1)

(a2)

(b)

Fig. 6.8 (a1,2) Bulbar palsy in motor neurone disease. Note the wrinkled mucous membrane due to underlying muscular atrophy. (b) Droopy palate of bulbar palsy.

35 / Pseudobulbar palsy

Record

There is monotonous, slurred, high–pitched, 'Donald Duck' *dysarthria* and the patient *dribbles persistently* from the mouth (he has dysphagia and may have nasal regurgitation). He *cannot protrude his tongue* which lies on the floor of the mouth and is *small and tight. Palatal movement is absent,* the *jaw jerk is exaggerated* and he is *emotionally labile.*

The diagnosis is pseudobulbar palsy (?bilateral generalized spasticity and extensor plantar responses).

Commonest cause

Bilateral cerebrovascular accidents of the internal capsule.

Other causes

Multiple sclerosis
Motor neurone disease
High brainstem tumours
Head injury.

Chapter 7
Examine this patient's arms

Possible short cases include:
Wasting of the small muscles of the hand (p. 192)
Motor neurone disease (p. 110)
Hemiplegia (p. 103)
Cerebellar syndrome (p. 92)
Cervical myelopathy (p. 106)
Neurofibromatosis (p. 219)
Muscular dystrophy (gl.)
Psoriasis (p. 195)
Purpura due to steroids (p. 228)
Parkinson's disease (p. 260)
Syringomyelia (gl.)
Lichen planus (gl.)
Pseudoxanthoma elasticum (gl.)
Old polio (p. 112)
Rheumatoid arthritis (p. 189)
Axillary vein thrombosis
Ulnar nerve palsy (p. 198)
Pancoast's syndrome (p. 46)
Herpes zoster (p. 235)
Polymyositis (gl.)
Mycosis fungoides (gl.)

Examination *routine*

Consideration of the above list reveals that the vast majority (over 80%) of conditions behind this instruction are neurological with a handful of spot diagnoses which will usually be obvious. If the diagnosis is not an obvious 'spot' (and you should make sure that you would recognize each on the list—see individual short cases) your *routine* should commence in the usual way by scanning the whole patient but in particular looking at

1 the **face** for obvious abnormalities such as *asymmetry* (hemiplegia), *nystagmus* (cerebellar syndrome), *wasting* (muscular dystrophy), sad, immobile, unblinking facies (*Parkinson's disease*) or *Horner's syndrome* (syringomyelia, Pancoast's syndrome). You may return to seek a less obvious Horner's or nystagmus later, if necessary. In search of obvious abnormalities run your eyes down to

2 the **neck** (pseudoxanthoma elasticum, lymph nodes), and then scan down the arms looking in particular at

3 the **elbows** which should be particularly inspected for *psoriasis, rheumatoid nodules* and *scars* or *deformity* underlying an ulnar nerve palsy. Before picking up the hands look for

4 a **tremor** (Parkinson's disease), then briefly inspect

5 the **hands** in the same way as you have practised under 'Examine this patient's hands', looking at:

    (a) the joints (swelling, deformity),

    (b) nail changes (pitting, onycholysis (gl.), clubbing, nail-fold infarcts), and

    (c) skin changes (colour, consistency, lesions).

If you have not already been led towards a diagnosis requiring specific action, start a full neurological examination by studying first

6 the **muscle bulk** in the upper arms, lower arms and hands, bearing in mind that in about one-quarter of cases there will be wasting of the small muscles of the hands (see p. 192), and in one-fifth of cases there will be motor neurone disease which means wasting and

7 **fasciculation**.

8 Test the **tone** in the arms by passively bending the arm (with the patient relaxed) to and fro in an irregular and unexpected fashion, and in the hands by flexing and extending all the joints, including the wrist in the classic 'rolling wave' fashion used to detect cog-wheel rigidity (Parkinson's disease).

9 Ask the patient:

    'Hold your **arms out in front** of you' (look for *winging* of the scapulae, involuntary movements or the *myelopathy hand sign**).

    'Now close your eyes' (look for *sensory wandering*—parietal drift or pseudoathetosis—Fig. 8.4c, p. 107).

Next test

10 **power**:

    (a) 'Put your arms out to the side' (demonstrate this to the patient yourself—arms at 90° to your body with elbows flexed); 'Stop me pushing them down' (deltoid—C5)

    (b) 'Bend your elbow; stop me straightening it' (biceps—C5,6)

    (c) 'Push your arm out straight'—resist elbow extension (triceps—C7)

    (d) 'Squeeze my fingers'—offer two fingers (C8,T1)†

    (e) 'Hold your fingers out straight' (demonstrate); 'Stop me bending them' (if the patient can do this there is nothing wrong with motor C7 or the radial nerve)

    (f) 'Spread your fingers apart' (demonstrate); 'Stop me pushing them together' (dorsal interossei—ulnar nerve)

---

* With the hands outstretched and supinated, passive abduction of the little finger indicates a pyramidal lesion or ulnar nerve palsy (sensory testing should distinguish). The sign is common in, but not specific for, cervical pyramidal lesions—as the lesion becomes more severe, adjacent fingers also passively abduct.

† See footnote, p. 186.

(g) 'Hold this piece of paper between your fingers; stop me pulling it out' (palmar interossei—ulnar nerve)

(h) 'Point your thumb at the ceiling; stop me pushing it down' (abductor pollicus brevis—median nerve)

(i) 'Put your thumb and little finger together; stop me pulling them apart' (opponens pollicis—median nerve).

11 Test **coordination**

(a) 'Can you do this?'—demonstrate by flexing your elbows at right angles and then pronating and supinating your forearms as rapidly as possible

(b) 'Tap quickly on the back of your hand' (demonstrate)

(c) 'Touch my finger; touch your nose; backwards and forwards quickly and neatly' (demonstrate if necessary—vary the target).

12 Check the biceps (C5,6), triceps (C7), supinator (C5,6) and finger (C8) **reflexes.**

13 Finally perform a **sensory screen** with *light touch* and *pinprick* bearing in mind the dermatomes shown in Fig. 7.1 and the areas of sensation covered by the ulnar, median and radial nerves in the hand (see Fig. 14.1, p. 186). Finally, check *vibration* and *joint position* sense.

We leave you to consider where else you could look with each of the conditions given on the list in order to find additional information (see individual short cases). For example, you could look for nystagmus should you find cerebellar signs, or for a Horner's syndrome should you suspect syringomyelia or Pancoast's syndrome.

For *checklist* see p. 276.

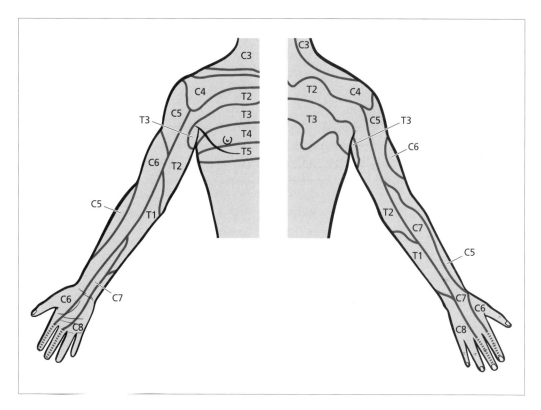

Fig. 7.1 Dermatomes in the upper limb. There is considerable variation and overlap between the cutaneous areas supplied by each spinal root so that an isolated root lesion results in a much smaller area of sensory impairment than the diagram indicates.

36 / Cerebellar syndrome

Record 1

There is nystagmus to the R/L and there is ataxia with the eyes open as shown by impairment of rapid alternate motion on the same side (*dysdiadochokinesis*). The *finger–nose test* is impaired on the R/L with *past pointing* to that side and an *intention tremor* (increases on approaching the target). The *heel–shin test is impaired* on the R/L and the *gait is ataxic* with a tendency to fall to the R/L. There is *ataxic dysarthria* with explosive speech (staccato).

    The patient has a R/L cerebellar lesion.

Causes include

1 Multiple sclerosis (?internuclear ophthalmoplegia, optic neuritis or atrophy, etc.—p. 121).

2 Brainstem vascular lesion.

3 Posterior fossa space-occupying lesion (?papilloedema; e.g. tumour or abscess*).

4 Cerebellar syndrome of malignancy (?clubbing, cachexia, etc.).

5 Alcoholic cerebellar degeneration (nutritional†).

6 Friedreich's ataxia (gl.) (?scoliosis, pes cavus, pyramidal and dorsal column signs, absent ankle jerks, etc.).

Other causes of cerebellar ataxia include

Hypothyroidism (?facies, pulse, reflexes, etc.—p. 251)

Anticonvulsant toxicity (especially phenytoin which can cause gross multidirectional nystagmus)

Ataxia–telangiectasia (recessive; from childhood onwards progressive ataxia, choreoathetosis (gl.) and oculomotor apraxia; later telangiectases on conjunctivae, ears, face and skin creases; low IgA leads to repeated respiratory tract infections; lymphoreticular malignancies common; death usually in second or third decade of life)

Other cerebellar degeneration syndromes.‡

Other cerebellar signs

Ipsilateral hypotonia and reduced power

Ipsilateral pendular knee jerk

Skew deviation of the eyes (ipsilateral down and in, contralateral up and out)

Failure of the displaced ipsilateral arm to find its original posture (ask the patient to hold his arms out in front of him and keep them there. If you push the ipsilateral arm down it will fly past the starting point on release without reflex arrest).

---

*NB Otitis media may underlie a cerebellar abscess. Intracranial abscesses may result from direct spread from the upper respiratory passages (nasal sinuses, middle ear, mastoid). Less often the cause is haematogenous spread (e.g. intrathoracic suppuration), congenital heart disease or fracture of the base of the skull. Abscesses secondary to otitis occur in the temporal lobe about twice as often as they do in the cerebellum.

†Other causes of nutritional deficiency such as pellagra, amoebiasis and protracted vomiting may cause a similar syndrome.

‡The names associated with these other rare hereditary ataxias apart from Friedreich are Charcot, Marie, Déjèrine, Alajouanine, André Thomas, Gowers and Holmes.

Record 2 (vermis lesion)

There is a wide-based *cerebellar ataxia* (ataxic gait and Rombergism more or less the same with eyes open and closed; cf. sensory ataxia (gl.)—worse with eyes closed), but there is little or no abnormality of the limbs when tested separately on the bed. This suggests a lesion of the cerebellar vermis.

Chapter 8
Examine this patient's legs

Possible short cases include

Group 1 (spot)
Paget's disease (p. 99)
Erythema nodosum (p. 233)
Pretibial myxoedema (p. 221)
Diabetic foot (p. 108)
Necrobiosis lipoidica
   diabeticorum (p. 217)
Erythema ab igne (gl.)
Vasculitis (gl.)
Swollen knee (p. 117)
Pemphigus/pemphigoid (p. 223)
Deep venous thrombosis/
   ruptured Baker's cyst (gl.)
Ankle swelling
Vasculitic leg ulcers
Pyoderma gangrenosum (gl.)
Mycosis fungoides (gl.)
Diabetic ischaemia
Ehlers–Danlos syndrome (gl.)
Bilateral below-knee amputation

Group 2 (neurological)
Spastic paraparesis (p. 98)
Peripheral neuropathy (p. 101)
Hemiplegia (p. 103)
Cerebellar syndrome (p. 92)
Cervical myelopathy (p. 106)
Diabetic foot (p. 108)
Motor neurone disease (p. 110)
Old polio (p. 112)
Absent ankle jerks and extensor
   plantars (p. 113)
Friedreich's ataxia (gl.)
Subacute combined degeneration
   of the cord (p. 114)
Charcot–Marie–Tooth disease
   (p. 115)
Polymyositis (gl.)
Lateral popliteal (common
   peroneal) nerve palsy (p. 119)
Tabes dorsalis/taboparesis (gl.)
Diabetic amyotrophy

Examination *routine*

An analysis of the possible short cases shows that they roughly fall into the two broad groups shown above:

Group 1: a spot diagnosis.

Group 2: a neurological diagnosis.

Either way initial clues may be gained by first performing a brief

  1 *visual survey* of the patient as a whole. Look at the head and face for signs such as *enlargement* (Paget's disease), *asymmetry* (hemiparesis), *exophthalmos* with or without *myxoedematous facies* (pretibial myxoedema) or obvious *nystagmus* (cerebellar syndrome). Run your eyes over the patient for other significant signs such as thyroid *acropachy* (pretibial myxoedema), *rheumatoid hands* (swollen knee), nicotine-stained fingers (leg amputations), *wasted hands* (motor neurone disease, Charcot–Marie–Tooth disease, syringomyelia (gl.)) and for muscle *fasciculation* (usually motor neurone disease).

Turning to the legs, look at the skin, joints and general shape and for any

2 obvious lesion, especially from the list of disorders in group 1. If such a lesion is visible a further full examination of the legs will not be required in most cases. You will be able to begin your description and/or diagnosis immediately (see individual short cases). If there is no obvious lesion look again specifically for

3 bowing of the tibia, with or without enlargement of the skull. The changes of vascular insufficiency (absence of hair, shiny skin, cold pulseless feet, peripheral cyanosis, digital gangrene, painful ulcers) should be *briefly* looked for because they will direct you to examine the pulses, etc. rather than the neurological system.

Observing the legs from the neurological point of view, note whether there is

4 pes cavus (Friedreich's ataxia, Charcot–Marie–Tooth disease) or

5 one leg smaller than the other (old polio, infantile hemiplegia). Next note

6 muscle bulk. Bear in mind that some generalized disuse atrophy may occur even in a limb with upper motor neurone weakness (e.g. severe spastic paraparesis). There may be unilateral loss of muscle bulk (old polio), muscle wasting that stops part of the way up the leg (Charcot–Marie–Tooth disease), isolated anterior thigh wasting (e.g. diabetic amyotrophy) or generalized proximal muscle wasting (polymyositis) or muscle wasting confined to one peroneal region (lateral popliteal nerve palsy). Look specifically for

7 fasciculation (nearly always motor neurone disease).

8 Examine the **muscle tone** in each leg by passively moving it at the hip and knee joints (with the patient relaxed roll the leg sideways, backwards and forwards on the bed; lift the knee and let it drop, or bend the knee and partially straighten in an irregular and unexpected rhythm).

9 Test power:*
   (a) 'Lift your leg up; stop me pushing it down' (L1,2)
   (b) 'Bend your knee; don't let me straighten it' (L5,S1,2)
   (c) (Knee still bent) 'Push out straight against my hand' (L3,4)
   (d) 'Bend your foot down; push my hand away' (S1)
   (e) 'Cock up your foot; point your toes at the ceiling. Stop me pushing your foot down' (L4,5).

Move smoothly into testing

10 coordination, take your hand off the foot and run your finger down the patient's shin below the knee saying:

'Put your heel just below your knee then run it smoothly down your shin; now up your shin, now down . . .' etc.†

---

*The screen of instructions from (a) to (e) will identify most legs in which there are abnormalities of motor function. You may wish to embellish these, where necessary, with instructions to test hip extension, hip adduction, hip abduction and hip rotation.

†If there is possible or definite cerebellar disease, you may wish to demonstrate dysdiadochokinesis in the foot by asking the patient to tap his foot quickly on your hand.

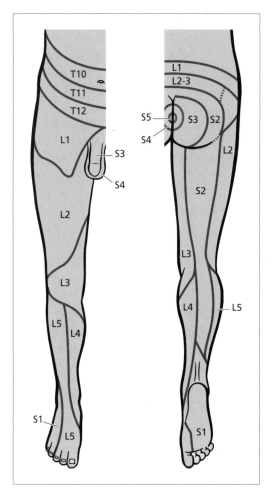

Fig. 8.1 Dermatomes in the lower limb. There is considerable variation and overlap between the cutaneous areas supplied by each spinal root so that an isolated root lesion results in a much smaller area of sensory impairment than the diagram indicates.

11 Check the knee (L3,4) and ankle (S1,2) **jerks*** and if there is any possibility of pyramidal disease try to demonstrate *ankle clonus* (and patellar clonus).

12 Test the **plantar response** remembering that in slight pyramidal lesions an extensor plantar is more easily elicited on the outer part of the sole than the inner.†

13 Turning to **sensation**, dermatomes L2 to S1 on the leg (Fig. 8.1) are tested if you examine *light touch* (dab cotton wool lightly), and *pinprick* once each on the outer thigh (L2), inner thigh (L3), inner calf (L4), outer calf (L5), medial foot (L5) and lateral foot (S1). The most common sensory defect is a

* One study has suggested that the plantar strike technique for examining ankle jerks may be more reliable than the better known tendon strike technique, especially in the elderly (*Lancet* 1994, **344**: 1619–20).

† In slight pyramidal disease the extensor plantar is first elicited on the dorsilateral part of the foot (*Chaddock's manoeuvre*). As the degree of pyramidal involvement increases the area in which a *Babinski's sign* may be elicited increases first to cover the whole sole and then spreads beyond the foot until an *Oppenheim's sign* (extensor response when the inner border of the tibia is pressed heavily; Fig. 8.4b, p. 107) or *Gordon's reflex* (extensor response on pinching the Achilles tendon) can be elicited. In such cases the big toe may be seen to go up as the patient takes his socks off.

peripheral neuropathy with stocking distribution loss. Demonstrate this with light touch (usually the most sensitive indicator) and pinprick:

Test above the sensory level:

'Does the pin feel sharp and prickly'—'Yes'.

Test on the feet:

'Does the pin feel sharp and prickly'—'No'.

'Tell me when it changes'.

Work up the leg to the sensory level and confirm afterwards by demonstrating the same level medially and laterally.* The level of the peripheral neuropathy may be different on the two legs. *Vibration* should be tested on the medial malleoli (and knee, iliac crest, etc., if it is impaired), and *joint position* sense in the great toes (remember to explain to the patient what you mean by 'up' and 'down' in his toes before you get him to close his eyes'; whilst testing the position sense hold the toe by the lateral aspects).

Sometimes the examiner will stop you before you get this far. If the lesion is predominantly motor he may break in before you have tested sensation, and if predominantly sensory he may lead you to test sensation earlier or stop you at this point. You should, however, be sufficiently deft to perform the full examination described above quickly and efficiently, and be prepared to complete it by examining the patient's

14 gait (check the patient can walk by asking for either his or the examiner's permission to examine the gait). First, watch his *ordinary walk* to a defined point and back (see p. 126) and then watch him walk *heel-to-toe* (ataxia) (see Fig. 9.1, p. 125), on his *toes* (see Fig. 9.2, p. 125) and on his *heels* (foot-drop) (see Fig. 9.3, p. 125). Finally perform

15 Romberg's test with the feet together and the arms outstretched (see Fig. 9.4, p. 125). You must be ready to catch the patient if there is any possibility of ataxia. Romberg's test is only positive (sensory ataxia (gl.), e.g. subacute combined degeneration, tabes dorsalis) if the patient is more unsteady (tends to fall) with the eyes closed than open.

For *checklist* see p. 276.

---

* The same method can be used for rapid demonstration of a higher sensory level: normal sensation is demonstrated above the lesion, e.g. on the shoulder or chest. The pin is then rapidly moved up the whole body from the foot until the patient announces that the sensation is changing to normal. That area is then worked over rapidly to detect the actual sensory level.

37 / Spastic paraparesis

Record

The *tone* in the legs is *increased* and they are *weak* (in chronic immobilized cases there may be some disuse atrophy, and in severe cases there may be contractures). There is bilateral *ankle clonus*, patellar clonus and the *plantar responses are extensor*. (?Abdominal reflexes.)

The patient has a spastic paraparesis.* The most likely causes are:

1 Multiple sclerosis (?obvious nystagmus, incoordination or staccato speech from the end of the bed; ?impaired rapid alternate motion of arms when you check at the end of your leg examination—p. 121).

2 Cord compression (?sensory level; root, back or neck pain; no signs above level of lesion. NB Cervical spondylosis—see p. 106).

3 Trauma (?scar or deformity in back).

4 Birth injury (cerebral palsy—Little's disease (gl.)).

5 Motor neurone disease (?no sensory signs, muscle fasciculation, etc.—p. 110).

Other causes

Syringomyelia (gl.) (?kyphoscoliosis, wasted hands, dissociated sensory loss, Horner's syndrome, etc.)

Anterior spinal artery thrombosis (sudden onset, ?dissociated sensory loss up to the level of the lesion)

Friedreich's ataxia (gl.) (?pes cavus, cerebellar signs, kyphoscoliosis, etc.)

Hereditary spastic paraplegia

Subacute combined degeneration of the cord† (?posterior column loss, absent ankle jerks,‡ peripheral neuropathy, anaemia—p. 114)

Parasagittal cranial meningioma (gl.)

Human T-cell lymphotrophic virus type 1 (HTLV-1) infection§ (Afro-Caribbean populations—tropical spastic paraparesis)

Acquired immune deficiency syndrome (AIDS) myelopathy (late phase—direct human immunodeficiency virus (HIV) central nervous system involvement)

General paresis of the insane (gl.) (?dementia, vacant expression, trombone tremor of the tongue, etc.)

Taboparesis (gl.) (?Argyll Robertson pupils, posterior column loss, etc.).

---

* A clue to the underlying cause of spastic paraparesis may be:

Cerebellar signs:	Multiple sclerosis
	Friedreich's ataxia (?pes cavus)
Wasted hands:	Cervical spondylosis (?inverted reflexes)
	Syringomyelia (?Horner's)
	Motor neurone disease (?prominent fasciculation).

† Stocking sensory loss (with or without absent ankle jerks) in association with a spastic paraplegia, i.e. extensor plantars, is strongly suggestive of subacute combined degeneration of the cord.

‡ Absent ankle jerks and upgoing plantars—p. 113.

§ The other main HTLV-1-associated disease is *adult T-cell leukaemia/lymphoma* which is especially found in southern Japan and the Caribbean Islands. The clinical course is often associated with a high white cell count, *hypercalcaemia* and cutaneous involvement. Measurement of HTLV-1 antibodies should always be considered in the patient with unexplained hypercalcaemia. Other HTLV-1-associated diseases include polymyositis (gl.), infective dermatitis—a chronic generalized eczema of the skin—and B-cell chronic lymphocytic leukaemia (gl.).

HTLV-2 has been found in some patients with T-cell hairy cell leukaemia and in parenteral drug abusers but remains a true orphan virus, without, at the time of writing, clear disease association.

38 / Paget's disease

Record

There is (in this elderly patient) *enlargement* of the *skull*. There is also *bowing* of the R/L *tibia* (or femur) which is *warmer* (due to increased vascularity) than the other and the patient is (may be) *kyphotic* (vertebral involvement leads to *loss of height* and kyphosis from disc degeneration and vertebral collapse).

    The diagnosis is Paget's disease. (There may be evidence of complications, e.g. a *hearing aid*—see below.)

Paget's disease occurs in 3% (autopsy series) of the population over the age of 40, rising to 10% over the age of 70, though it is not clinically important in the vast majority of these. Though it is often asymptomatic, patients may have symptoms such as bone pain, headaches, tinnitus and vertigo. Serum *alkaline phosphatase* and *urinary hydroxyproline* are elevated except sometimes in very early disease. Serum calcium and phosphate concentrations are usually normal in mobilized patients but may be increased or decreased. Urinary calcium and hydroxyproline rise in immobilized patients. A high serum uric acid and high erythrocyte sedimentation rate may also occur. There is growing ultrastructural and immunohistochemical evidence that Paget's disease may represent a 'slow' virus infection in susceptible individuals—paramyxoviruses (which include respiratory syncytial virus, measles and distemper) have been implicated. Specific therapies which can be considered if indicated* include bisphosphonates, calcitonin and mithramycin.

Complications

Progressive closure of the skull foramina may lead to:
1 Deafness (also results from Pagetic involvement of the ossicles†)
2 Optic atrophy‡
3 Basilar invagination (platybasia causing brainstem signs).
    Other complications include:
1 High output cardiac failure (?bounding pulse—occurs when more than 30–40% of the skeleton is involved)
2 Pathological fractures
3 Urolithiasis
4 Sarcoma (incidence is probably <1%; increase in pain and swelling may occur; 'explosive rise' in alkaline phosphatase occurs only occasionally).

Causes of 'bowed tibia'

True bowing due to soft bone:
Paget's disease (asymmetrical)
Rickets (bilateral, symmetrical).

Apparent bowing due to thickening of the anterior surface of the tibia secondary to periostitis:
Congenital syphilis (gl.) (?saddle nose, bulldog jaw, rhagades, Hutchinson's teeth, Moon's molars, etc.)
Yaws.

---

* Bisphosphonates are now the first-line treatment with short courses leading to long-term suppression of disease activity and improvement in bone pain, etc. Indications for specific therapy in Paget's disease are: bone pain; osteolytic lesions in weight-bearing bones; neurological complications (except deafness); delayed or non-union of fractures; immobilization hypercalcaemia; before and after orthopaedic surgery.

† Although hearing loss is frequently attributed to compression of the VIIIth cranial nerve in the canal in the temporal bone, this is unlikely to be the major cause because the facial nerve, which follows the same course, is rarely affected.
‡ The other ophthalmological finding which may occur in Paget's disease is angioid streaks in the retina.

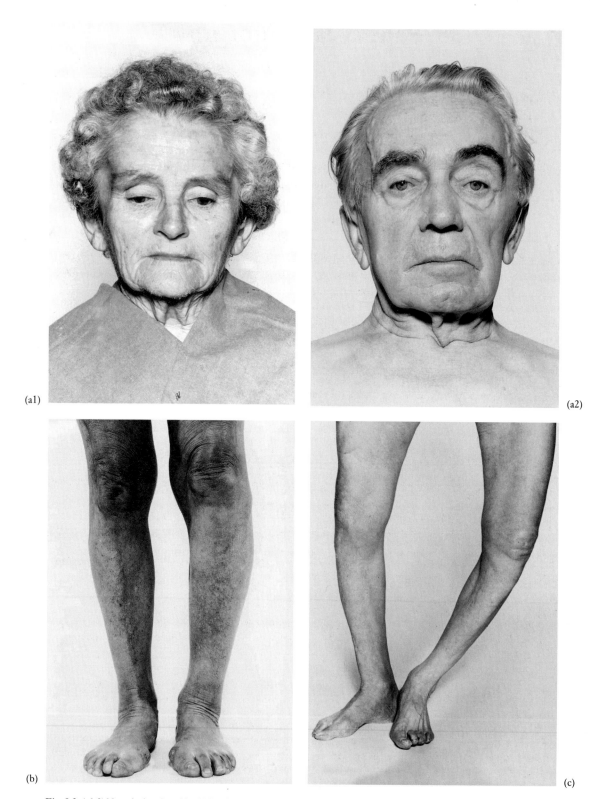

Fig. 8.2 (a1,2) Note the hearing aids. (b) Bowing of the tibiae. (c) Gross deformity.

39 / Peripheral neuropathy

Record

There is *impairment of sensation* to light touch, vibration sense, joint position sense and pinprick over a *stocking* and, to a lesser extent, a *glove distribution* (much less common).

The patient has a peripheral neuropathy.

Most likely causes

1 Diabetes mellitus (?fundi, amyotrophy).
2 Carcinomatous neuropathy (?evidence of primary, cachexia, clubbing).
3 Vitamin B_{12} deficiency (subacute combined degeneration not always present; ?extensor plantars).
4 Vitamin B deficiency (alcoholics*).
5 Drugs (e.g. isoniazid, vincristine, nitrofurantoin, gold, ethambutol, phenytoin, hydrallazine, metronidazole, amiodarone, chloramphenicol, cyclosporin).
6 Idiopathic (in 10–20% of patients with chronic peripheral neuropathy for >1 year, no cause can be found).

There are many rare causes (see below).

Leprosy (gl.) is a cause of major importance worldwide.

Important rare causes

Guillain–Barré syndrome (gl.) (also motor involvement, absent reflexes, ?bilateral lower motor neurone VIIth nerve palsy; ?peak flow rate)

Polyarteritis nodosa (gl.) (?arteritic lesions)

Rheumatoid arthritis and other collagen disease (hands, facies)

Amyloidosis (gl.) (?thick nerves, autonomic involvement)†

AIDS.‡

Causes of predominantly motor neuropathy

Carcinomatous neuropathy (?evidence of primary, cachexia)

Lead (wrists mainly)

Porphyria (gl.)

Diphtheria (gl.)

Charcot–Marie–Tooth disease (?atrophy of peronei, pes cavus, etc. — p. 115).

Other rare causes of peripheral neuropathy

Myxoedema (?facies, pulse, reflexes, etc. — p. 251)

---

* Can also occur with nutritional deficiencies from other causes, e.g. dialysis for chronic renal failure, prison camp victims.

† Neuropathy is a feature of primary and myeloma-associated amyloidosis (it is exceptional in secondary amyloidosis). Carpal tunnel syndrome is not uncommon. Sensory or mixed sensory and motor neuropathy are commonest. Signs of autonomic involvement would be orthostatic hypotension, impotence, impairment of sweating and diarrhoea. The other organs mainly involved in primary and myeloma-associated amyloidosis include heart (cardiomyopathy), tongue (dysarthria), skeletal and visceral muscle and alimentary tract (rectal biopsy). See also footnote on p. 61.

‡ Acute (Guillain–Barré type) or chronic inflammatory neuropathy may be the presenting feature of HIV infection but with a cerebrospinal fluid pleocytosis which is not usually seen in these conditions. A distal sensory neuropathy may also occur in AIDS, sometimes but not always caused by cytomegalovirus infection.

Acromegaly (?facies, hands, etc. — p. 257)

Sarcoidosis (gl.) (?lupus pernio (gl.), chest signs)

Uraemia (?pale brownish-yellow complexion)

Lyme disease (gl.)

Tetanus (gl.)

Botulism (gl.) (can be mistaken for Guillain–Barré, encephalitis, stroke or myasthenia gravis; electromyograph resembles Eaton–Lambert (gl.))

Paraproteinaemia (gl.)

Hereditary ataxias (gl.)

Refsum's disease (gl.) (cerebellar ataxia, pupillary abnormalities, optic atrophy, deafness, retinitis pigmentosa, cardiomyopathy, ichthyosis)

Arsenic poisoning (e.g. pesticides; Mee's transverse white lines may occur on the fingernails and raindrop pigmentation may occur on the skin)

Other chemical poisoning (e.g. tri-ortho-cresyl phosphate).

40 / Hemiplegia

Record

There is a R/L *upper motor neurone* weakness of the facial muscles.* The R/L *arm and leg are weak* (without wasting) with *increased tone* and *hyper-reflexia*. The R/L plantar is *extensor* and the *abdominal reflexes are diminished* on the R/L side.

This is a R/L hemiplegia.

There is also (may be) *hemisensory loss* on the R/L side. Visual field testing reveals (may be) a R/L homonymous hemianopia. The most likely causes are:

1 Cerebrovascular accident due to cerebral
  (a) thrombosis (?hypertension)
  (b) haemorrhage (?hypertension)
  (c) embolism (?atrial fibrillation, murmurs, bruits).
2 Brain tumour (?insidious onset, papilloedema, headaches; ?evidence of primary, e.g. clubbing).

A right-sided hemiplegia associated with dysphasia would suggest (in a right-handed patient) that the causative lesion is affecting the speech centres in the dominant hemisphere (see p. 133) as well as the motor cortex (precentral gyrus) and if there are sensory signs, the sensory cortex (post-central gyrus). If cerebrovascular in origin the causative lesion is likely to be in the *carotid* distribution.

The presence of signs such as nystagmus, ocular palsy, dysphagia (?nasogastric or percutaneous endoscopic gastrostomy (PEG) feeding tube) and cerebellar signs suggest that the hemiparesis is due to a brainstem lesion. If cerebrovascular in origin the lesion is likely to be in the *vertebrobasilar* distribution.

Parietal lobe and related signs†

Agnosia

Though peripheral sensation is intact (tactile, visual, auditory) the patient fails to appreciate the significance of the sensory stimulus without the aid of other senses.

Tactile agnosia or astereognosis (contralateral posterior parietal lobe) — inability to recognize a familiar object placed in the hand (e.g. pen, keys) with the eyes closed. Opening the eyes or hearing the keys rattle may allow recognition

Visual agnosia (parieto-occipital lesions — especially in the left hemisphere of right-handed patients) — the patient is not able to identify the familiar object by sight (e.g. a pen, surroundings) but may do at once when he is allowed to handle it

Auditory agnosia (temporal lobe of dominant hemisphere) — the patient may only be able to recognize the sound of a voice, telephone or music when he is allowed to use the senses of vision or touch

Autotopagnosia (usually a left hemiplegia in a right-handed person) — difficulty in perceiving or identifying the various parts of the body; the patient may be unaware of the left side of his body. It may be associated with anosognosia in which case there is no appreciation of a disability (e.g. hemiplegia, blindness) on the same side.

---

* In an upper motor neurone lesion, the lower face is much weaker than the upper because the muscles frontalis, orbicularis oculi and corrugator superficialis ('raise your eyebrows', 'screw your eyes up tight', 'frown') are bilaterally innervated and are all only minimally impaired. (See also p. 173.)

† **Sensory inattention:** the patient is able to feel the orangestick on both sides when tested independently, but when touched simultaneously on both sides (Fig. 8.3), he ignores one side, usually the left side. Sensory inattention indicates a parietal lobe lesion, usually of the non-dominant side (right parietal lobe).

Apraxia

Whereas in agnosia the difficulty is in recognition, in apraxia it is in execution. Though power, sensation and coordination are all normal, the patient is unable to perform certain familiar activities. It may affect:

The upper limbs—e.g. difficulty using a pen, comb or toothbrush, winding a watch, dressing or undressing ('dressing apraxia'‡)

The lower limbs—may mimic ataxia or weakness§—the patient may appear unable to lift one foot in front of the other (gait apraxia)

The trunk—the patient may have difficulty seating himself on a chair or lavatory seat, getting on to his bed, or in turning over in bed

The face—the patient may be unable to whistle, put out his tongue or close his eyes.

The lesions (tumours or atrophy) tend to be in the corpus callosum, parietal lobes and pre-motor areas. Dominant lobe lesions may produce bilateral apraxia. Unilateral left-sided apraxia may be caused by a lesion in the right posterior parietal region or in the corpus collosum of a right-handed patient. The lesion in 'dressing apraxia' is usually in the right parieto-occipital region. In 'constructional apraxia' (most often seen in patients with hepatic encephalopathy) the patient is unable to construct simple figures such as triangles, squares or crosses from matchsticks.

Dyslexia (impairment of reading ability), **dysgraphia** (impairment of writing ability) and **dyscalculia** (difficulty with calculating) usually represent lesions in the posterior parietal lobe.

---

‡ Some authorities consider this to be a visuospatial right hemisphere disorder and not a true apraxia.
§ A parietal lobe lesion may cause ataxia, hemiparesis or marked astereognosis. In hemiparesis of parietal origin, the limbs are often hypotonic with an absent plantar response, rather than spastic. The limb muscles may even waste (like a lower motor neurone lesion). Often the patient is disinclined to move the limb rather than being actually paralysed.

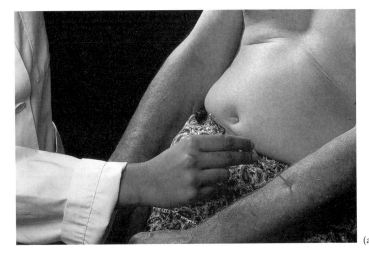

(a)

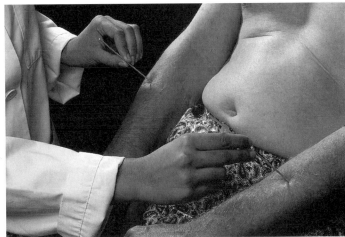

(b)

Fig. 8.3 Testing for sensory inattention. (a) The patient feels the touch when tested on each arm individually, but (b) only feels on the right arm and ignores the left when tested simultaneously (right parietal lobe lesion).

41 / Cervical myelopathy

Note: a cervical collar may be a clue.

Record

The legs (of this middle-aged or elderly patient) show *spastic weakness,** the *tone* being *increased,* the *reflexes brisk* (?clonus) and the *plantar responses extensor. Vibration* and joint position senses are (may be) lost in the lower limbs (spinothalamic loss may also occur but is less common). In the upper limbs† there is (often asymmetrical) *inversion‡* of the biceps and supinator jerks.

These features suggest cervical myelopathy as the cause of the spastic paraparesis. *Cervical spondylosis* is the commonest cause though a *spinal cord tumour* cannot be excluded clinically.

In the upper limbs there may be segmental muscle wasting and weakness particularly if there is an associated radiculopathy. Gross wasting of the small muscles of the hand due to cervical spondylosis is uncommon because the latter usually affects C5/6 or C6/7 and the small muscles are supplied by C8/T1. Mild wasting of the small muscles does sometimes occur, probably due to vascular changes in the cord below the lesion.

There is often no sensory loss in the hand. Sometimes in the elderly a complaint of numb, useless hands may be accompanied by constant unpleasant paraes-

thesiae and writhing ('sensory wandering' or 'pseudo-athetosis') of the fingers when the eyes are closed. Position and vibration senses are lost in such hands.

Neck pain is surprisingly rare in cervical spondylosis causing cervical myelopathy, and sphincter function is seldom disturbed. Among patients with cervical spondylosis (which is very common) those with a narrow cervical canal are most likely to develop cervical myelopathy. Lhermitte's phenomenon may occur (see p. 114).

---

*In this condition signs often exceed symptoms and spasticity often exceeds weakness.

† The myelopathy hand sign may be present; see footnote, p. 89.

‡ When attempts are made to elicit the normal biceps and supinator tendon reflexes, there is a brisk finger flexion despite little or no response of the biceps and supinator jerks

themselves. This is because the lower motor neurones and pyramidal tracts are damaged at the C5/6 level producing lower motor neurone signs at that level and upper motor neurone signs below. The combination of inverted biceps and supinator jerks (the C5/6 jerks) and a brisk triceps jerk (C7/8) is termed the 'mid-cervical reflex pattern'.

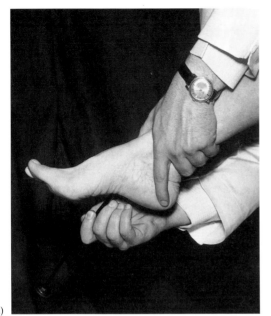

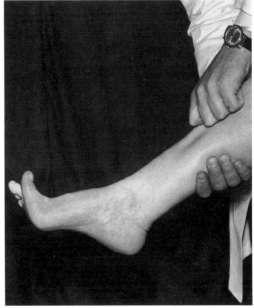

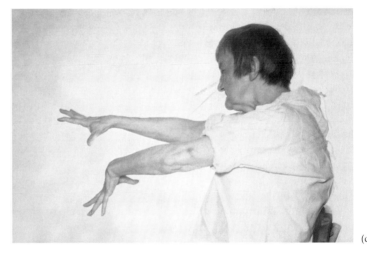

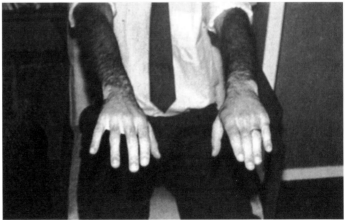

Fig. 8.4 (a) Babinski's sign.
(b) Oppenheim's sign (see p. 96).
(c) Pseudoathetosis. (d) The
myelopathy hand sign (in the right
arm).

42 / Diabetic foot

Record 1

There is an *ulcer* on the sole of the R/L foot (most commonly at the site of the pressure point under the head of the first metatarsal) and two of the toes have previously been amputated. There is thick *callous* formation over the pressure points of the feet, and the normal concavity of the transverse arch at the head of the metatarsals is lost. There is *loss of sensation* to light touch, vibration and pinprick in a *stocking distribution*. The feet are *cold*, the foot pulses are not palpable* and there is *loss of hair* on the lower legs which are *shiny*.

This patient has *peripheral neuropathy*, a *neuropathic ulcer* on the sole of his foot and evidence of *peripheral vascular disease*. It is likely that he has underlying diabetes mellitus (?fundi).

Factors which may contribute to the production of the diabetic foot lesions

Injury—always a provocative factor

Neuropathy—trivial injury is not noticed

Consequent formation of callosities at repeatedly traumatized pressure points

Small vessel disease

Large vessel disease producing ischaemia and gangrene of the foot

Increased susceptibility to infection

Maldistributed pressure and foot deformity leading to increased likelihood of friction and trauma.

From the list of the other causes of peripheral neuropathy (p. 101) **neuropathic ulcers** are particularly associated with:

1 Tabes dorsalis (gl.) (?facies, pupils, etc.)
2 Leprosy (gl.)
3 Porphyria (gl.) (?vesicles, crusts)
4 Amyloidosis (gl.)
5 Progressive sensory neuropathy (both familial and cryptogenic)

and rarely as a late manifestation of

6 Charcot–Marie–Tooth disease (distal muscle wasting, pes cavus, etc.—p. 115).

Record 2 (Charcot's joint)

As relevant from *record* 1 plus: the ankle joint is greatly *deformed* and *swollen*, and there is loud *crepitus* accompanying *movement* which is of an *abnormal range*.

This is a Charcot's joint (gl.) (neuropathic arthropathy—gross osteoarthrosis and new bone formation from repeated minor trauma without the normal protective responses which accompany pain sensation; the joint is painlessly destroyed).

Main causes of a Charcot's joint

Diabetes mellitus (toes—common; ankles—rare)

Tabes dorsalis (especially hip and knee;—?facies, pupils, etc.)

Syringomyelia (gl.) (elbow and shoulder;—?Horner's, wasted hand muscles, dissociated sensory loss, etc.)

Leprosy (important on a worldwide basis).

Other rare causes include yaws, progressive sensory neuropathy (familial and cryptogenic), other hereditary neuropathies (e.g. Charcot–Marie–Tooth) and neurofibromatosis (pressure on sensory nerve roots), though any cause of loss of sensation in a joint may render it liable to the development of a neuropathic arthropathy.

---

*NB In the predominantly neuropathic foot the pulses may be present or even bounding, and the veins may be prominent—autonomic denervation opens up arteriovenous shunts; as a consequence blood passes down the arteries, through the shunts and back up the veins, missing out the nutrient capillaries on the way—this contributes to the poor healing.

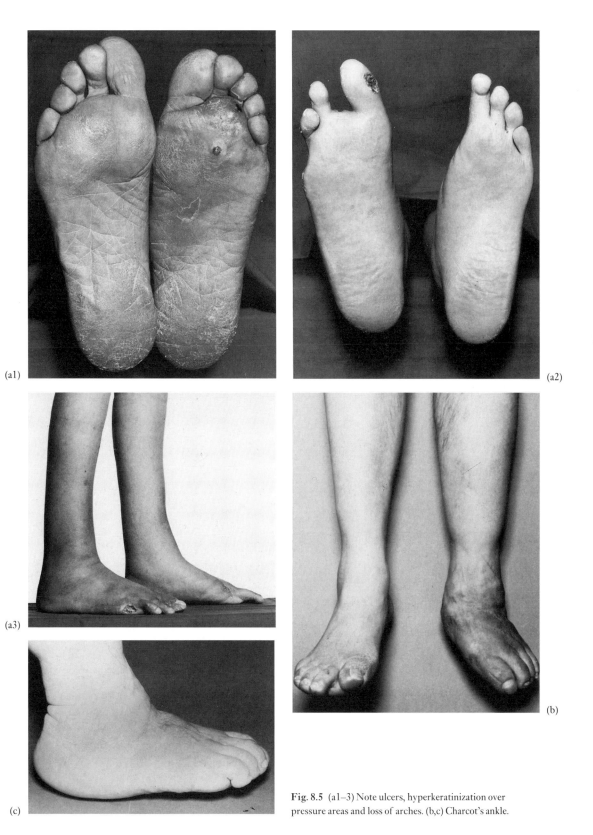

Fig. 8.5 (a1–3) Note ulcers, hyperkeratinization over pressure areas and loss of arches. (b,c) Charcot's ankle.

(a1)

(a2)

(a3)

(b)

(c)

43 / Motor neurone disease

Record

This patient has *weakness, wasting* and *fasciculation* of the muscles of the hand (p. 192), arms and shoulder girdle (*progressive muscular atrophy* in its pure form is characterized by minimal pyramidal signs), but the upper limb reflexes are exaggerated (reflexes in motor neurone disease may be increased, decreased or absent depending on which lesion is predominant). There is upper motor neurone *spastic weakness* with *exaggerated reflexes* in the legs (*amyotrophic lateral sclerosis**). There is ankle clonus and the patient has bilateral *extensor plantar responses*. The patient also has (may have) indistinct *nasal speech*, a *wasted fasciculating tongue* and *palatal paralysis* (*progressive bulbar palsy* — p. 85). There are *no sensory signs*.

The diagnosis is motor neurone disease.

Other conditions in which fasciculation may occur

Cervical spondylosis (see below)

Syringomyelia (gl.) (fasciculation less apparent, dissociated sensory loss, etc.)

Charcot–Marie–Tooth disease (fasciculation less apparent, atrophy which stops abruptly part of the way up the legs, pes cavus, sometimes palpable lateral popliteal and ulnar nerves, etc. — p. 115)

Acute stages of poliomyelitis (and rarely also in old polio; see below)

Neuralgic amyotrophy (pain, wasting and weakness of a group of muscles in a limb, sometimes following a viral infection; usually C5, C6 innervated muscles — shoulder)

Thyrotoxic myopathy (tachycardia, tremor, sweating, goitre with bruit, lid lag, etc. — p. 155)

Syphilitic amyotrophy (see below)

Chronic asymmetrical spinal muscular atrophy (see below)

After exercise in fit adults

After edrophonium test dose (p. 162)

Benign giant fasciculation.

Differential diagnosis of motor neurone disease

Cervical cord compression (p. 106) is the most important condition to be excluded in the diagnosis of motor neurone disease. Bulbar palsy and sensory signs should be carefully sought but a cervical MRI scan is often required to exclude it. *Syphilitic amyotrophy* (slowly progressing wasting of the muscles of the shoulder girdle and upper arm with loss of reflexes and no sensory loss; fasciculation of the tongue may occur) should always be excluded in the investigation of motor neurone disease as it is amenable to treatment. Occasionally patients with *old polio*, after many years, develop a progressive wasting disease (with prominent fasciculation) which is indistinguishable from progressive muscular atrophy motor neurone disease. Also, in immunologically incompetent patients (carcinoma, lymphoma (gl.), steroid therapy) a pure amyotrophy may develop that progresses over several months and is found at autopsy to be chronic poliomyelitis. The diagnosis of *chronic asymmetrical spinal muscular atrophy* (CASMA), a condition which appears to be distinct from classic motor neurone disease, is favoured by age of onset under 40 years, absence of pyramidal or bulbar involvement after 3 or more years of symptoms, and depressed or absent reflexes. CASMA is only slowly progressive and carries a considerably better prognosis than classic motor neurone disease. CASMA may be inherited and there are reports of patients with this condition having relatives with Werdnig–Hoffmann disease (gl.) — a fatal early infantile form of spinal and bulbar muscular atrophy that appears to be a single genetic entity.

---

* Glutamate toxicity has been implicated as a factor leading to neuronal damage in amyotrophic lateral sclerosis. Trials suggest riluzole may retard progression and lengthen survival.

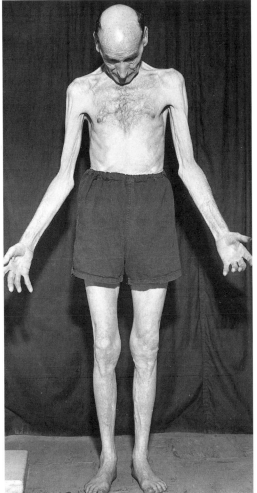

(a1)

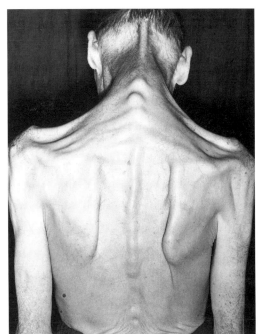

(a2)

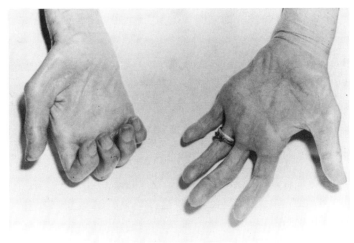

(b)

Fig. 8.6 (a1,2) Generalized muscle wasting (note weakness of the extensors of the neck). (b) Wasting of the small muscles of the hand.

44 / Old polio

Record

The R/L leg is *short*, *wasted*, *weak* and *flaccid* with *reduced* (*or absent*) *reflexes* and a normal plantar response. There is *no sensory defect*. The disparity in the length of the limbs suggests growth impairment in the affected limb since early childhood. The complete absence of sensory and pyramidal signs point to a condition affecting only lower motor neurones.*

The diagnosis is old polio affecting the R/L leg.

If you see one limb smaller than the other a possible differential diagnosis to consider is infantile hemiplegia. In this there is usually hemi-smallness of the whole of that side of the body and the neurological signs will reflect a contralateral hemisphere lesion (i.e. upper motor neurone).

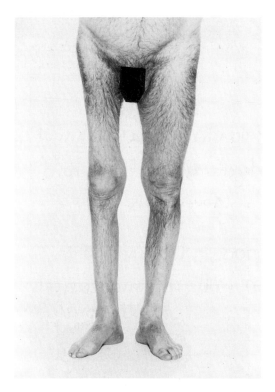

Fig. 8.7 Generalized wasting of the right lower limb due to old poliomyelitis.

*Fasciculation is only occasionally seen in old polio. Very rarely patients with old polio for many years develop a progressive wasting disease (with prominent fasciculation) which is indistinguishable from progressive muscular atrophy motor neurone disease or chronic asymmetrical spinal muscular atrophy (see p. 110).

45 / Absent ankle jerks and extensor plantars

Record
The knee and *ankle jerks are absent* and the *plantar responses are extensor*.

Possible causes

Vitamin B12 deficiency

1 Subacute combined degeneration of the cord (?posterior column signs, positive Romberg's sign, clinical anaemia, splenomegaly, etc. — p. 114).

2 Syphilitic taboparesis (gl.) (?Argyll Robertson pupils, ptosis and wrinkled forehead, posterior column signs, positive Romberg's sign, etc.).

3 Multisystem degeneration, e.g. Friedreich's ataxia (gl.) (?pes cavus, (kypho)scoliosis, nystagmus, cerebellar ataxia, scanning speech, etc.).

4 Motor neurone disease (?fasciculation, absence of sensory signs, etc. — p. 110).

5 Common conditions in combination* (e.g. an elderly person with diabetes and cervical myelopathy or cervical and lumbar spondylosis causing a mixture of upper and lower motor neurone signs in the legs).

MAST : MND, Friedreich's ataxia, subacute combined degeneration of the cord (Vit B12 deficiency), taboparesis

or common conditions in combination
e.g. elderly person with DM and cervical myelopathy

* Whilst the above order in which the possible causes are listed represents the traditional order in which the conditions are presented, in practice number 5 is by far the commonest.

46 / Subacute combined degeneration of the cord

Record

There is (in this patient who may complain of burning paraesthesiae in the feet) loss of *light touch*, *vibration* and *joint position* sensation over the feet (*stocking*, may also be *glove*), and *Romberg's sign* is positive. The legs are (may be) weak, and though the knee (may be brisk) and *ankle jerks are lost* (due to peripheral neuropathy) the *plantar responses are extensor*.

The pupils are normal, there are no cerebellar signs or pes cavus (p. 113) and though the patient is not (may not be) clinically anaemic* (having checked conjunctival mucous membranes) and the tongue and complexion are normal (glossitis and classic 'lemon yellow' pallor are now rarely seen in subacute combined degeneration of the cord—SACD), these findings suggest the diagnosis of SACD. (Findings in the abdomen might be splenomegaly, carcinoma of the stomach as this is commoner in pernicious anaemia, or a laparotomy scar from a previous gastrectomy.)

Though vitamin B_{12} neuropathy usually starts with peripheral neuropathy followed by posterior column signs, and signs of pyramidal disturbances are seldom marked in the early stages (progressive spasticity may occur), vitamin B_{12} deficiency should always be excluded in a patient in whom any of the following are unexplained:
Peripheral sensory neuropathy
Spinal cord disease
Optic atrophy (rare)
Dementia (frank dementia rare; progressive enfeeblement of intellect and memory, or episodes of confusion or paranoia may be seen; more commonly the patient is simply difficult and uncooperative).

Causes of severe vitamin B_{12} deficiency

Addisonian pernicious anaemia (NB associated organ-specific autoimmune diseases especially autoimmune thyroid disease, diabetes mellitus, Addison's, vitiligo and hypoparathyroidism (gl.)—see also p. 214)
Partial or total gastrectomy
Stagnant loop syndrome
Ileal resection or Crohn's disease
Vegan diet
Fish tapeworm
Chronic tropical sprue
Congenital intrinsic factor deficiency.

Lhermitte's phenomenon

The patient describes a 'tingling', 'electric feeling' or 'funny sensation' which passes down his spine, and perhaps into the lower limbs, when he bends his head forward.†The most common cause is multiple sclerosis but it can also occur in cervical cord tumour, cervical spondylosis and SACD.

---

* Though the patient may be anaemic, vitamin B_{12} neuropathy may develop without anaemia and with normal blood film and bone marrow. A serum vitamin B_{12} level may be required to confirm the diagnosis.

† A similar sensation provoked by neck *extension* is termed 'reversed Lhermitte's phenomenon' and strongly suggests cervical spondylosis.

47 / Charcot–Marie–Tooth disease

Motor

6 Obeys commands
5 Localizing response to pain
4 Withdraws to pain
3 Flexor posturing
2 Extensor posturing
1 None

~~Again~~ Verbal
5 ~~spontaneously~~ orientated
4 ~~Towards~~ confused convers.
3 ~~to form~~ inapprop speech
2 Incomprehensible speech
1 none

~~Newborn~~ Eyes
4 spontaneous
3 in response to speech
2 in response to pain
1 None

~~VMGVSM~~4 $M_6 V_5 E_4$

iscles with relatively well-preserved
nd clawing of the toes, and there is
feet. The *ankle jerks are absent* and
here is only slight *distal involvement*
gh occasionally marked sensory loss
The lateral popliteal (?and ulnar)
ly). The patient has a *steppage gait*
sting *of the small muscles of the hand.*
ophy.†

also found in the dorsal roots and dorsal
d slight pyramidal tract degeneration is
however, in classic cases extensor plantars
nd). The condition usually becomes
nid-life. Other members of the patient's
have a *formes fruste* and show just minor
pes cavus and absent ankle jerks only.

f the way up the leg. In practice it is not usually
d can be considered to be an example of
gy.
arie–Tooth disease is now called *hereditary*
ory neuropathy (HMSN) and is subdivided into
(the hypertrophic form of Charcot–Marie–
), HMSN type II (the neuronal form of
ie–Tooth disease) and HMSN type III
lled Déjérine–Scotas disease).

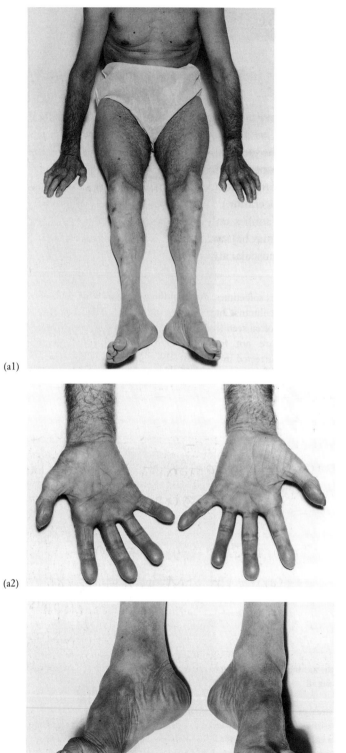

(a1)

(a2)

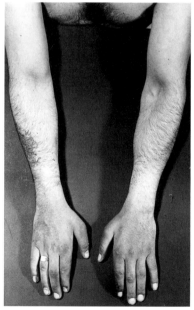

(b)

(a3)

Fig. 8.8 (a1–3) Note that the muscle wasting stops in the thighs; foot-drop, pes cavus and wasting of the small muscles of the hand all in the same patient. (b) Distal wasting in the upper limbs.

48 / Swollen knee

Record

There is generalized *swelling* of the R/L *knee joint* obscuring the lateral dimples. The *patellar tap sign* is positive* suggesting the presence of fluid in the synovial cavity. The swelling does not extend to the back in the popliteal fossa (always check).† The joint is *painful* to move and it is *warm*.

There is an *effusion* in the knee joint. (Now look at the hands for evidence of rheumatoid arthritis — p. 189.)

Causes of a swollen knee

Rheumatoid arthritis (the swelling may be due to synovial thickening—synovium palpable as boggy tissue around the joint margin)

Osteoarthritis (osteophytes on X-ray)

Rupture of a Baker's cyst (gl.) (?rheumatoid arthritis)

Pseudogout (calcified menisci; birefringent calcium pyrophosphate crystals; associated with a large variety of conditions including hyperparathyroidism, haemochromatosis (gl.), acromegaly,

diabetes mellitus, Wilson's disease (gl.), hypothyroidism, alkaptonuria and gout; there are also idiopathic and hereditary varieties)

Septic arthritis (purulent fluid, organisms in a smear)

Gout (urate crystals)

Trauma

Charcot's knee (gl.) (painless, ?tabes dorsalis)

Haemarthrosis of haemophilia (gl.)

Oedematous states (congestive cardiac failure, nephrotic syndrome (gl.)).

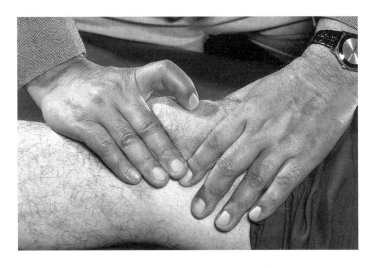

Fig. 8.9 Patellar tap.

* With one hand above the knee joint, exert pressure to drive fluid from the suprapatellar pouch into the knee joint proper. With the index finger of the other hand, depress the patella with a sharp jerky movement (Fig. 8.9). If the patella rebounds this is definite evidence of fluid in the knee joint. The sign may not be positive if there is too much or too little fluid. To test for a small amount of fluid in the knee joint, displace fluid by depressing one of the obliterated hollows on either side of the ligamentum patellae. The hollow will slowly refill. This can be felt by one finger while gentle pressure is applied by the other finger on the other side of the patella.

† Swelling in the popliteal fossa extending down to the upper third of the calf in cases of ruptured Baker's cyst.

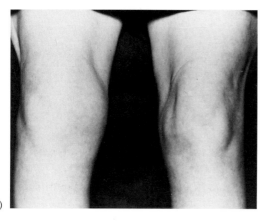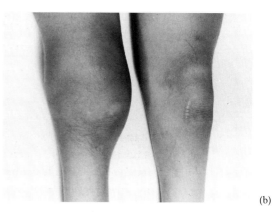

(a)

(b)

Fig. 8.10 (a) Osteoarthrosis with effusion of the knee joint.
(b) Charcot's knee (spina bifida).

49 / Lateral popliteal (common peroneal) nerve palsy

Record

There is *wasting of the anterior tibial* and *peroneal* group of *muscles*, the patient *cannot dorsiflex* or *evert* the R/L foot, and there is *impairment of sensation* over the *outer side of the calf*. He cannot stand on the R/L heel and the gait is altered as a result of *foot-drop* (there is an audible 'clop' of the foot as he walks).

The diagnosis is lateral popliteal (common peroneal) nerve palsy.

Injury to the nerve is usually at the head of the fibula where it can be involved in fractures or compressed by splints, tourniquets or bandages. Some individuals are particularly susceptible to temporary pressure palsy of this nerve (and in some cases other nerves such as the radial and ulnar as well), experiencing symptoms induced by crossing knees, squatting (strawberry picker's palsy) or unusual physical activity.

The nerve has two branches—the superficial and deep peroneal nerves. The superficial supplies sensation to the lateral calf and dorsum of the foot supplying the peroneus longus and brevis muscles. The deep branch supplies sensation to a triangular area of skin between the first and second toes dorsally and it innervates the anterior tibial muscles, the long extensors of the toes and the peroneus tertius muscle.

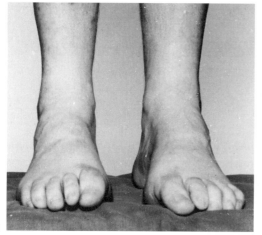

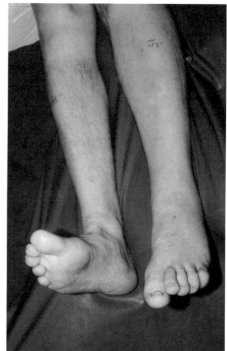

Fig. 8.11 (a) Right common peroneal nerve palsy. Note
failure of eversion. (b) Left common peroneal nerve palsy.
Note failure of eversion and dorsiflexion on the left side.

50 / Multiple sclerosis

Record 1

The patient (?a young adult) has *ataxic nystagmus* (p. 159), *internuclear ophthalmoplegia* (p. 156), *temporal pallor of the discs* (p. 145), and *slurred speech* (p. 133) with *ataxia* (p. 126) and widespread *cerebellar* signs (p. 92). There are *pyramidal* signs and *dorsal column* signs.

In view of these multiple lesions *involving different sites in the brain*, the likely diagnosis is demyelinating disease* (a useful euphemism for multiple sclerosis).

Record 2

The legs of this (?middle-aged) patient have increased tone, they are bilaterally spastic and weak. There is bilateral *ankle clonus* and patellar clonus and the *plantars are extensor*. The *abdominal reflexes* are absent. The heel–shin test suggests some *ataxia* in the legs and there is slight *impairment of rapid alternate motion* in the upper limbs.

These features (of *cerebellar dysfunction*) suggest that this *spastic paraplegia* is due to demyelinating disease. An examination of the fundi may show pale discs (p. 145).†

Male to female ratio is 2:3.

Features of multiple sclerosis

Rare in tropical climates

Euphoria despite severe disability (not invariable—the patient may be depressed)

Unpredictable course

May present acutely, subacutely, remittently or insidiously

Relapses and remissions (occurring in two-thirds of patients) are often a useful diagnostic pointer

May very closely imitate other neurological conditions (including neurosis)

Fatigue or a rise in temperature may exacerbate symptoms (the patient may be able to get into, but not out of, a hot bath)

Paroxysmal symptoms (e.g. trigeminal neuralgia) may occur and may respond to carbamazepine

Lhermitte's phenomenon may occur (see p. 114)

Benign course is more likely if there is:
an early age of onset,
relapses and remissions,
onset with optic neuritis, or sensory or motor symptoms—in contrast to those of brainstem or cerebellar lesions

The visual evoked response (VER) test is useful in a patient with an isolated lesion which may be due to multiple sclerosis—e.g. spastic paraparesis,† VIth nerve palsy, trigeminal neuralgia, facial palsy, postural vertigo

Cerebrospinal fluid examination may show an increase in total protein of up to $1\,g\,l^{-1}$ or an increase in lym-

---

* The features in this *record* are some of those which are commonly seen in a case of multiple sclerosis. There are, of course, few neurological signs which it may not produce.
† Multiple sclerosis (MS) may present in middle age with insidious spastic paraplegia mimicking cord compression. Signs above the level of the cord lesion may point clinically to demyelination as the cause. In this case the slight cerebellar

signs are highly suggestive of MS. However, syringomyelia (gl.) or a tumour at the foramen magnum could also be the cause. If the diagnosis is of a tumour there may be papilloedema. If the diagnosis is MS the discs may show global or temporal pallor (and the VERs may be delayed — even if, as is often the case, the discs are normal).

phocytes of up to 50 cells mm^{-3} in 50% of patients. The IgG proportion of the total protein is increased in two-thirds of patients. Oligoclonal bands in the gamma region on agarose or polyacrylamide gel electrophoresis are seen in 90% of patients including some with normal IgG. Myelin basic protein can be detected by radioimmunoassay and can be used as an index of disease activity

MRI scans often detect many more multiple sclerosis lesions than are suspected clinically (computerized tomography (CT) scans can also detect lesions but are much less sensitive than MRI).

Chapter 9
Examine this patient's gait

Possible short cases include

Ataxia

Spastic paraparesis (p. 98)

Parkinson's disease (p. 260)

Charcot–Marie–Tooth disease (p. 115)

Ankylosing spondylitis (p. 268).

Examination *routine*

As you approach the patient perform

1 a *quick visual survey* noting any *cerebellar signs* (nystagmus, intention tremor) or obvious signs of conditions such as *Parkinson's* disease (facies, tremor), *Charcot–Marie–Tooth* disease (peroneal wasting, pes cavus, etc.) or *ankylosing spondylitis*. Introduce yourself to the patient and ask him

2 **whether he can walk** without help (*cerebellar dysarthria* heard during his reply may be a useful clue). If he reports difficulty reassure him that you will stay with him in case of any problems.

3 **Ask him to walk** to a defined point and back whilst you look for any of the classic abnormal gaits (see p. 126), particularly ataxic (cerebellar or sensory), spastic, steppage (Charcot–Marie–Tooth) or parkinsonian (?pill-rolling tremor). As the patient walks make sure you note specifically

4 the **arm swing** (Parkinson's) and

5 any *clumsiness* on **the turns** (ataxia, Parkinson's). Next test

6 **heel-to-toe gait** (Fig. 9.1) (demonstrate as you ask the patient to do this) which will *exacerbate* ataxia (note the side to which the patient tends to fall). Ask the patient to walk

7 **on his toes** (Fig. 9.2) (S1) and then

8 **on his heels** (Fig. 9.3) (L5; foot-drop—lateral popliteal nerve palsy, Charcot–Marie–Tooth disease). If he has a spastic gait or a hemiparesis he may find both these tests difficult to perform.

9 Now ask him to stand with his *feet together, arms out* in front; when you are satisfied with the degree of steadiness with the eyes open, ask him to *close his eyes* (you should be standing nearby to catch him if he shows a tendency to fall—Fig. 9.4). **Romberg's test** is only positive (*sensory ataxia* (gl.)) if the patient is more unsteady (tends to fall) with the eyes closed than with them open (dorsal column disease, e.g. subacute combined degeneration, tabes dorsalis (gl.), etc.).

10 If you suspect sensory ataxia a further test is to ask the patient to **close his eyes while walking** (he will become *more* ataxic). Again you should be ready to catch the patient should he fall. As always be ready to look for

11 **additional features** of the conditions on the list if appropriate (see individual short cases, and consider what you would do with each).

For *checklist* see p. 276.

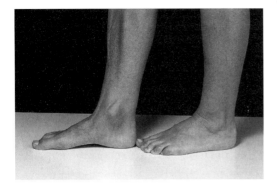

Fig. 9.1 Walking heel to toe.

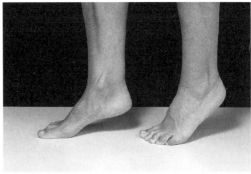

Fig. 9.2 Walking on the toes.

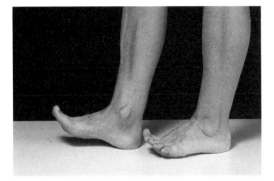

Fig. 9.3 Walking on the heels.

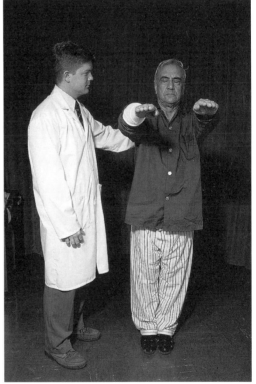

Fig. 9.4 Romberg's test.

51 / Abnormal gait

Record 1

The gait is *wide-based* and the arms are held wide (both upper and lower limbs tend to tremble and shake). The patient is *ataxic* and tends to fall to the R/L, especially during the *heel-to-toe* test which he is unable to perform. Romberg's test is negative.

This suggests *cerebellar disease* which is predominantly R/L sided. (Now, if allowed, examine for other cerebellar signs: finger–nose, rapid alternate motion, nystagmus, staccato dysarthria, etc.—p. 92)

Possible causes

1 Demyelinating disease (?pale discs, pyramidal signs, etc.—p. 121).
2 Tumour (primary or secondary—?evidence of primary, e.g. bronchus, breast, etc.).
3 Non-metastatic syndrome of malignancy (?evidence of primary especially bronchus—clubbing, cachexia, etc.).
4 Alcoholic cerebellar degeneration.
5 Other cerebellar degenerations (?pes cavus, kyphoscoliosis, absent ankle jerks and extensor plantars, etc. of Friedreich's ataxia (gl.)).

Record 2

The patient has a *stiff*, awkward 'scissors' or 'wading through mud' gait.

This suggests *spastic paraplegia*. (Now, if allowed, examine tone, reflexes, plantars, sensation, etc.—p. 98.)

Possible causes

1 Demyelinating disease (?impaired rapid alternate motion in arms, pale discs etc.—p. 121).
2 Cord compression (?sensory level with no signs above).
3 Hereditary spastic paraplegia (rare).
4 Cerebral diplegia (rare).

Record 3

The gait is ataxic and *stamping* (his feet tend to 'throw'; both the heels and the toes slap on the ground). The patient walks on a wide base, *watching his feet and the ground* (to some extent he can compensate for lack of sensory information from the muscles and joints by visual attention). He has difficulty walking heel to toe and the ataxia becomes much worse when he closes his eyes; *Romberg's test is positive.*

He has *sensory ataxia* (now look for Argyll Robertson pupils and for clinical anaemia).

Possible causes

1 Subacute combined degeneration of the cord (?pyramidal signs, absent ankle jerks plus peripheral neuropathy; anaemia, spleen, etc.; no Argyll Robertson pupils — p. 114).

2 Tabes dorsalis (gl.) (?facies, pupils, pyramidal signs if taboparesis (gl.), etc.).

3 Cervical myelopathy (?mid-cervical reflex pattern in the arms; pyramidal signs in the legs — p. 106).

4 Diabetic pseudotabes (?fundi).

5 Friedreich's ataxia (pes cavus, scoliosis, cerebellar signs, etc.).

6 Demyelinating disease (ataxia in multiple sclerosis is usually mainly cerebellar).

Record 4

This (depressed, expressionless, unblinking and stiff) patient *stoops* and his gait, initially *hesitant*, is *shuffling* and has lost its spring. The *arms* are held flexed and *do not swing*. The hands show a *pill-rolling tremor*. His gait is *festinant*, i.e. he appears to be continually about to fall forward as if chasing his own centre of gravity.

He has *Parkinson's disease*.* (Now examine the wrists for cog-wheel rigidity, elbows for lead-pipe rigidity, and for the glabellar tap sign, etc. — p. 260.)

Record 5

The patient has a *steppage* gait. He lifts his R/L foot high to avoid scraping the toe because he has a R/L *foot-drop*. He is unable to walk on his R/L heel.

Possible causes

1 Lateral popliteal nerve palsy (?evidence of injury just below and lateral to the knee — p. 119).

2 Charcot–Marie–Tooth disease (?pes cavus, atrophy which stops abruptly part of the way up the leg, wasting of the small muscles of the hand, palpable lateral popliteal ± ulnar nerve — p. 115).

3 Old polio (?affected leg short due to polio in childhood — p. 112).

4 Heavy metal poisoning such as lead (rare).

Record 6

The R/L leg is stiff and with each step he tilts the pelvis to the other side trying to keep the toe off the ground; the R/L leg describes a *semicircle* with the toe scraping the floor and the forefoot flops to the ground before the heel. The R/L arm is flexed and held tightly to his side and his fist is clenched.†

The patient has a *hemiplegic gait*.

---

* In a mild case, tell-tale signs are: (i) the lesser swing of one arm compared to the other; and (ii) the tremor which is often unilateral.

† Should not be seen these days with good physiotherapy care!

Record 7

The patient has a lumbar lordosis and walks on a wide base with a *waddling gait*, his trunk moving from side to side and his pelvis dropping on each side as his leg leaves the ground. At each step his toes touch the ground before his heel. (This is a description of the typical gait of a patient with Duchenne muscular dystrophy — the commonest cause of a waddling gait. Other conditions causing wasting or weakness of the proximal lower limb and pelvic girdle muscles also cause it — e.g. polymyositis (gl.), rickets/osteomalacia.)

Record 8

The patient (an elderly person) walks with a broad-based gait, taking short steps and placing his feet flat on the ground like a person 'walking on ice'. (There is a tendency to retropulsion which increases the danger of falling.) The patient cannot hop on one foot.

This is *gait apraxia* (a common but little recognized disorder of the elderly; frontal lobe signs including dementia and grasp and suck reflexes will confirm the diagnosis). The commonest cause is a degenerative process similar to Alzheimer's disease (gl.). Other causes include subdural haematoma, tumour, normal pressure hydrocephalus, or a lacunar state. (Treatments include: small doses of L-dopa, mild stimulants, balancing exercises, use of a cane, daily walking.)

Chapter 10
Ask this patient some questions

Possible short cases include
Dysphasia (p. 133)
Cerebellar **dysarthria** (p. 132)
Raynaud's phenomenon (gl.)
Systemic sclerosis/CRST syndrome (p. 176)
Pseudobulbar palsy (p. 87)
Myxoedema (p. 251)
Graves' disease (p. 247)
Senile dementia
Parkinson's disease (p. 260)

Examination *routine*
Inspection of the above list reveals that the cases fall roughly into four groups, each with a very different reason for the given instruction:
Group 1: to spot the diagnosis and confirm it by eliciting *revealing answers*.
Group 2: to demonstrate and diagnose the type of a dysarthria.
Group 3: to diagnose a dysphasia.
Group 4: to assess higher mental function.

With the group 1 patients you may have been given a lead such as 'Look at the hands' (Raynaud's) or 'Look at the face' (systemic sclerosis, myxoedema, etc.) before the instruction 'Ask this patient some questions'. At any rate you should start your examination as usual with

1 a *visual survey* of the patient from head to foot, particularly looking for evidence of: (i) the spot diagnosis in group 1 patients (Raynaud's, systemic sclerosis/CRST, hypo- or hyperthyroidism); (ii) a *hemiplegia* which may be associated with dysphasia; or (iii) any of the conditions associated with dysarthria (see p. 132) especially *nystagmus* or *intention tremor* (which may be revealed by even minor movements) in cerebellar disease, *pes cavus* in Friedreich's ataxia (gl.) and the *facies/tremor* of Parkinson's disease.

In the group 1 patients once you are on to the diagnosis, the sort of

2 **specific questions** the examiners are looking for (see also the individual short cases) are:

Raynaud's:
  'Do your fingers change colour in the cold?'
  'What colour do they go?' ('Is there a particular sequence of colours?')
  'How long have you had the trouble?'

'What is your job?' (vibrating tools, etc.)
and if there is any possibility of connective tissue disease
'Do you have any difficulty with swallowing?' etc.

Systemic sclerosis:

'Do you have any difficulty with swallowing?'

'Do your fingers change colour in the cold?'

'Do you get short of breath?' (on hills? on the flat? etc.)

We leave you to work out the straightforward questions you would ask the slow, croaking patient with *myxoedematous facies* (hypothyroidism), the patient with *exophthalmos*, or the one who has *lid retraction* and is *fidgety* (hyperthyroidism), or the patient who has *multiple scars* and *sinuses* on his abdomen (Crohn's disease). In a young patient who may have nephrotic syndrome (gl.) you would be looking for a history of a sore throat.

If there are no features suggesting a group 1 patient, it is likely that the problem is either a dysarthria or dysphasia, and, as already mentioned, there may be clues pointing to one of these. You need to ask the patient

3 some **general questions** to get him *talking*:

'My name is . . . Please could you tell me your name?'

'What is your address?'

If you need to hear a patient speak further ask

4 **more questions** which require *long answers* such as

'Please could you tell me all the things you ate for breakfast/lunch'.

5 To test **articulation** ask the patient to repeat traditional words and phrases such as 'British Constitution', 'West Register Street', 'biblical criticism' and 'artillery'. As well as testing articulation such

6 **repetition** is useful for assessing speech when the patient only gives one word answers to questions. If necessary ask the patient to repeat long sentences after you. Information gained from repetition may also be useful in your assessment of dysphasia (see below).

If the problem is *dysarthria*, it is really a spot diagnosis to test your ability to recognize and demonstrate the features of the different types (see p. 132). It is recommended that you find as many patients as possible with the conditions causing the various types of dysarthria and listen to them speak so that, as with murmurs, the diagnosis is a question of instant recognition. This is particularly true of the ataxic dysarthria of cerebellar disease. When you have heard enough to make the diagnosis, you should either describe the speech (p. 132) and, with supporting signs seen on inspection, give the diagnosis, or proceed to look for

7 **additional signs** (in the same way as you might do after the 'What is the diagnosis' instruction).

If the patient has a *dysphasia* (see p. 133) you may wish to demonstrate that

8 **comprehension** is good (expressive dysphasia) or impaired (receptive dysphasia). Perform a few simple commands *without gesturing*, e.g.

'Please put your tongue out'.

'Shut your eyes'.

'Touch your nose', etc.

Assuming these are performed adequately proceed to look for expressive dysphasia by asking the patient to name some everyday items, e.g. a comb, pen, coins. If the patient is unable to name the objects, test for

9 nominal dysphasia. Hold up your keys:

'What is this?' — patient does not answer.

'Is this a spoon' — 'No'.

'Is it a pen' — 'No'.

'Is it keys' — 'Yes'.

If the patient is able to name objects, test the ability to form sentences by asking the patient to describe something in more detail, e.g.

'Could you tell me where you live and how you would get home from here?'

'Could you tell me the name of as many objects in this room as possible?'

If there are expressive problems you should check to see if the problem is true expressive dysphasia or whether there is

10 orofacial dyspraxia.* Ask the patient to perform various orofacial movements (assuming there is no receptive dysphasia). These should be tested first by command *without gesture*, e.g.

'Please show me your teeth'.

'Move your tongue from side to side'.

Subsequently ask the patient to obey the same commands but *with gesture*, i.e. so the patient can mimic. This should give some idea as to whether the patient has either ideational or ideomotor dyspraxia.†

It is extremely rare for students to be asked to assess

11 higher mental functions. This is, however, an assessment which every student should be equipped to make. The following is the 'abbreviated mental test' (AMT) — more than four of the questions wrong suggests a well-established dementia:

1 Age.

2 Time (to nearest hour).

3 Address for recall at end of test — this should be repeated by the patient to ensure it has been heard correctly: 42 West Street.

4 Year.

5 Name of this place.

6 Recognition of two persons (doctor, nurse, etc.).

7 Date of birth (day and month sufficient).

8 Year of First World War.

9 Name of present Monarch.

10 Count backwards from 20 to 1.

Agnosia, apraxia, dyslexia, dysgraphia and dyscalculia are considered on p. 103.

For *checklist* see p. 277.

---

* It is important to make this distinction so that the type of speech therapy is appropriate — in orofacial dyspraxia the therapist needs to work on mouth movements rather than concentrating only on linguistic problems. It has recently been established that the lesion which leads to orofacial dyspraxia is in the operculum.

† Again it is relevant to therapy to establish if patients can make movements when aided by gesture.

52 / Dysarthria

Record

There is dysarthria with *slurred, jerky* and *explosive* (slow, lalling, staccato, scanning) speech. (There may be inspiratory whoops indicating a lack of coordination between respiration and phonation.)

    This suggests cerebellar disease (?nystagmus, dysdiadochokinesis, finger–nose test, etc. —p. 92).

Other varieties of dysarthria

Spastic dysarthria

Conditions in which all or some of the articulatory parts are rigid or spastic:

Pseudobulbar palsy (indistinct, suppressed, without modulations, high-pitched, 'hot potato', 'Donald Duck' speech due to a tight, immobile tongue — ?bilateral spasticity with extensor plantars —p. 87)

Parkinson's disease (monotonous without accents or emphasis, somewhat slurred speech—?expressionless unblinking face, glabellar tap sign, tremor, etc. — p. 260)

Dystrophia myotonica (slurred and suppressed speech—?ptosis, frontal balding, etc.—p. 209)

Huntington's chorea (gl.) (slurred and monotonous— ?chorea, dementia)

General paresis of the insane (gl.)—very rare (slurred, hesitant or feeble voice—?dementia, vacant expression, trombone tremor of tongue, brisk reflexes, extensor plantars, etc.).

Flaccid dysarthria

Bulbar palsy (nasal, decreased modulation, slurring of labial and lingual consonants—?lingual atrophy, fasciculations, etc. —p. 85)

Paralysis of the VIIth, IXth, Xth or XIIth nerves (cerebrovascular accident).

Myopathic dysarthria

Myasthenia gravis (weak hoarse voice with a nasal quality, pitch unsustained, soft accents—?ptosis, variable strabismus, facial and proximal muscle weakness all of which worsen with repetition, etc. — p. 162).

Variegated dysarthria

Hypothyroidism (low-pitched, catarrhal, hoarse, croaking, gutteral voice as if the tongue is too large for the mouth —?facies, pulse, ankle jerks, etc. —p. 251)

Amyloidosis (gl.)—large tongue (rolling and hollow, hardly modulated)

Multiple ulcers or thrush in the mouth (some parts of the speech indistinct)

Parotitis or temporomandibular arthritis (monotonous, suppressed, badly modulated).

53 / Dysphasia

Record 1

The patient's speech *lacks fluency*. He has *difficulty finding certain words* and sometimes produces the *wrong word* and makes grammatical errors. *Comprehension*, however, is *well preserved* (as are the higher cerebral functions and general intellect—the prognosis for eventual adaptation of the patient to his disability is good). His ability to repeat and to name objects is impaired.

The patient has Broca's (*expressive*, motor, non-fluent) *dysphasia* (?associated *right hemiplegia*). The brain damage causing this condition is believed to disconnect the dominant* inferior frontal gyrus (Broca's area) (Fig. 10.1).

Record 2

Though the patient *speaks fluently* (often rapidly) with normal intonation, his speech is completely *unintelligible*. He puts words together in the wrong order and mixes them with non-existent words† and phrases (*jargon dysphasia*). Attempts to repeat result in paraphasic† distortions and irrelevant insertions. *Comprehension* is severely *impaired* (and the patient may seem unaware of his dysphasia).

The patient has Wernicke's (*receptive*, fluent) *dysphasia* (?associated *homonymous visual field defect* and/or *sensory diminution* down the right side of the body). The brain damage causing this condition is believed to disconnect the posterior part of the dominant* superior temporal gyrus (Wernicke's area) (Figs 10.1 and 10.2).

Record 3

The patient shows combined expressive and receptive dysphasia. There is marked disturbance in comprehension (and inability to read or write).

The patient has *global dysphasia*‡ (?dense right hemiplegia with sensory loss, homonymous visual field defect and general intellectual deterioration). The common cause of this is infarction of the territory supplied by the left middle cerebral artery. The prognosis for recovery is poor.

Record 4

The patient has difficulty naming objects though he knows what they are (e.g. hold up some keys: 'What is

---

* The left hemisphere is dominant in right-handed and in 50% of left-handed people.

† **Paraphasia:** an incorrect syllable in a word (usually there is some phonemic relationship to the original word, e.g. 'tooth spooth' for 'toothbrush') or an incorrect word in a phrase (often with a semantic relationship to the correct word, e.g. 'hand' for 'foot').

Neologism: paraphasia with slight or no relationship to the original syllable/word.

‡ Global dysphasia is sometimes confused with Broca's dysphasia but the speech defects are severe in this condition affecting fluency, repetition, naming and comprehension. Some stereotypes may be preserved and the patient may be able to recite automatic sequences of prayer or popular songs (*speech automatism*).

this?'—Patient does not answer. 'Is this a spoon?'—'No'. 'Is it a pen?'—'No'. 'Is it keys?'—'Yes'). Despite this, comprehension and other aspects of speech production are relatively normal.

This is *nominal dysphasia* (uncommon in its pure form—usually it is part of a wider dysphasia). The underlying brain damage is believed to be in the most posterior part of the superior temporal gyrus and the adjacent inferior parietal lobule.

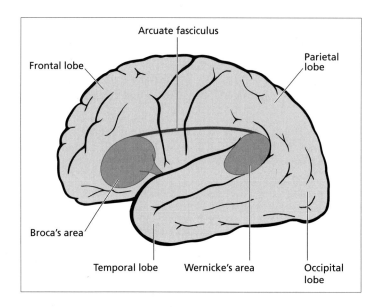

Fig. 10.1 The major speech centres (reproduced with permission from A. Mir, *Atlas of Clinical Skills*, 1997, Saunders).

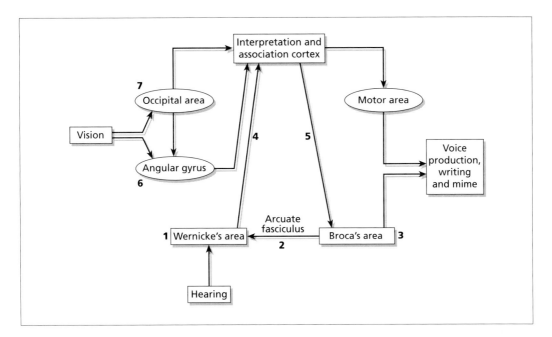

Fig. 10.2 Speech pathways—written and spoken information is processed in the association cortex, passed on to Broca's area and from there to the opposite motor area for execution (speaking/writing). Lesions at: 1, Wernicke's aphasia: poor comprehension, meaningless words, no repetition; 2, conduction aphasia: comprehension intact, repetition lost; 3, Broca's aphasia: comprehension preserved, non-fluent speech, no repetition; 4, transcortical sensory aphasia: as in (1) but with repetition preserved; 5, transcortical motor aphasia: as in (3) but with repetition preserved; 6, alexia with agraphia: can neither read nor write; 7, alexia, unable to comprehend written words, can spell and write but unable to read own writing. (Reproduced with permission from A. Mir, *Atlas of Clinical Skills*, 1997, Saunders.)

Chapter 11
Examine this patient's fundi

Possible short cases include
Diabetic retinopathy (p. 139)
Optic atrophy (p. 145)
Hypertensive retinopathy (p. 143)
Retinitis pigmentosa (p. 149)
Papilloedema (p. 147)
Cataracts (p. 168)
Choroidoretinitis
Retinal vein thrombosis (gl.)
Myelinated nerve fibres
Retinal artery occlusion

Special note

Many finals candidates receive this instruction. Though there are only a limited number of possibilities, it is clear that a lot of students experience more difficulty with a fundus than with any other short case. After exams, students commonly say such things as: 'I said optic atrophy . . .', or 'I said diabetic retinopathy . . . but I hadn't got a clue what it was'. Clearly there is not a lot that a book like this can do to help other than to warn you in advance of the problem, to provide you with a list of the likely conditions and to describe them (see individual short cases). Other than this the art of fundoscopy and fundal diagnosis is like driving in heavy traffic and can only be acquired with practise. With a moderate degree of clinical expertise and common sense most students ought to be able to overcome this hurdle.

Examination *routine*

Almost invariably if you are asked to look at the fundus the diagnosis must be in the fundus. However, it is a good practice to precede fundoscopy with
1 a **quick general look** at the patient (this will rarely help but the occasional diabetic in the examination may also have *foot ulcers* or *necrobiosis lipoidica* or may be wearing a *medic-alert* bracelet or neck chain), at his eyes (*arcus lipidus* at an inappropriately young age may suggest diabetes) and at his pupils (usually, but not always, dilated for the examination).

Turning to ophthalmoscopy, it may be your practice to focus immediately on the fundus and, in the vast majority of cases, this will provide the diagnosis. However, it would be preferable to cultivate the habit (if you can gain sufficient expertise to do it quickly and efficiently) of looking first at

2 the structures in front of the fundus, particularly the **lens** (diabetics will often reward you with early *cataract* formation; your examiner will sometimes not have noticed it, but as long as you are right when he checks you may score points). Adjust the lenses of the ophthalmoscope so that you move down through

3 the **vitreous** noting any *opacities* (e.g. asteroid hyalinosis (gl.)), *haemorrhages, fibrous tissue* or *new vessel formation* (diabetes) until you get to

4 the **fundus**. Localize the disc and examine it and its margins for *optic atrophy* (p. 145),* *papillitis* (p. 147) or *papilloedema* (p. 147) and for *myelinated nerve fibres*. Are there any new vessels (diabetes)? Trace the

5 **arterioles** and **venules** out from the disc noting particularly their calibre, light reflex (*silver wiring*) and arteriovenous (AV) crossing points (*AV nipping*, see p. 143).

6 Examine **each quadrant** of the fundus and especially the **macular area** and its temporal aspect.† You are looking particularly for *haemorrhages* (dot, blot, flame-shaped), *microaneurysms, exudates* both hard (well-defined edges; increased light reflex) and soft (fluffy with ill-defined edges; *cotton-wool spots*). If hard exudates are present see if these form a ring (*circinates* in diabetes).

If you see haemorrhages you must look specifically for:

(a) dot haemorrhages/microaneurysms,

(b) new vessel formation, and

(c) photocoagulation scars.

If you diagnose diabetic retinopathy your examiner will expect you to be able to comment on the presence or absence of all of these. If you cannot find these diagnostic clues you may have noted features that suggest hypertensive rather than diabetic retinopathy (silver wiring, AV nipping, more soft exudates than hard, haemorrhages which are mainly flame-shaped, early disc swelling with loss of venous pulsation‡ or frank papilloedema).

In the patient with diabetic retinopathy, it is of particular clinical significance to assess whether lesions (especially haemorrhages and hard exudates) involve or threaten (i.e. are near to) the macula.§

It would be useful if you knew that the patient was a diabetic, but if you remain in doubt remember that diabetes and hypertension often coexist in a

---

* There are normal variations in disc colour; in both infancy and old age it is naturally pale, as is the enlarged disc of a myopic eye. The advice of a well-known neurologist and experienced teacher to his students was: 'Don't diagnose optic atrophy unless it is a "barn door" optic atrophy'. It is well worth bearing this advice in mind. Temporal pallor of the disc due to a lesion in the papillomacular bundle is often seen in multiple sclerosis. However, temporal pallor is not always pathological.

† The macula will come into view if you ask the patient with a dilated pupil to look at the ophthalmoscopic light. Ideally, you should use the dot light for this, if it is available in your ophthalmoscope.

‡ Observation of venous pulsation is an expertise which comes with much practise of looking at normal as well as abnormal fundi. Though it could be useful if you have acquired this expertise (and some medical students certainly have) before the examination, do not get bogged down studying the venous pulsation for too long if you are not used to it.

§ European diabetic retinopathy screening guidelines suggest that patients with haemorrhages or hard exudate within one disc diameter of the macula should be considered for referral to an ophthalmologist (p. 140).

patient, and that it is more important that you have checked comprehensively for the above features, and report your findings honestly (mentioning the features in favour of one diagnosis or the other), than to guess or make up findings.*

We leave you to master the findings of the other fundal short cases and to ensure that you would recognize each (see individual short cases). The final point in this important *routine* is to

7 stay examining until you have finished and are **ready** to present your findings. Do not be put off by the impatient words or mumblings of your examiner; these will be forgotten when you present accurate findings and get the diagnosis right. Conversely, it is too late to go back and check if the examiner asks whether you saw a . . . and you are not sure. You need to be able to give a clear and unequivocal 'Yes' or 'No'. Thus, the best tip we can offer as you look around the fundus is to stop at the disc, the macula, and in each quadrant of each eye and ask yourself the question: 'Are there any abnormalities? What are they?' before moving on to the next area.

For *checklist* see p. 277.

---

* Making up findings is strictly inadvisable and can result in failure whereas missing one short case need not fail you.

54 / Diabetic retinopathy

Note: this is one of the commonest short cases; it is also one of the easiest to fail. Some students who see haemorrhages fail to note whether there are also microaneurysms. The uninitiated fail to recognize photocoagulation scars. The commonest forms of retinopathy in the examination setting are background diabetic retinopathy and proliferative retinopathy treated with photocoagulation. Most of the rest are fundi with untreated proliferative retinopathy. Advanced diabetic eye disease is only rarely seen.

Record 1

There are *microaneurysms, blot haemorrhages* and *hard exudates* (due to lipid deposition in the retina).*

The patient has background diabetic retinopathy.

Record 2

The above plus: in the R/L eye there is a *circinate formation of hard exudates* (indicating oedema) *near*† the R/L *macula* suggesting that macular oedema is present or imminent. It would be important to assess the patient's visual acuity.

Record 3

Any of the above plus: there are *cotton-wool spots, flame-shaped haemorrhages* (both indicating ischaemia), and leashes of *new vessels* (say where). *Photocoagulation scars* are seen (say where).

The patient has proliferative diabetic retinopathy treated by photocoagulation.

Record 4

Any of the above plus: *vitreous haemorrhage/vitreous scar/retinal detachment* (widespread and impairing vision) indicate advanced diabetic eye disease.

NB With diabetic retinopathy there may also be:

1 Cataracts (p. 168).

2 AV nipping (indicating either coexistent hypertension or arteriosclerosis).

Indications for photocoagulation are the sight-threatening forms of retinopathy:

Maculopathy (especially type II = non-insulin-dependent diabetes): warning signs are hard exudates often in rings (indicating oedema) encroaching on the macula, sometimes with multiple haemor-

---

* Say where the lesions are; particularly in relation to the macula — see criteria for referral to an ophthalmologist.
† If you use the tiny spotlight of the ophthalmoscope and ask the patient to *look at* the light while you look in, you will be looking at the macula and this may help you assess whether there are hard exudates or haemorrhages involving the macula.

rhages (indicating ischaemia). Macular oedema itself is difficult to recognize with the direct ophthalmoscope though signs of an abnormal greyish reflection or discoloration at the macula are suggestive. Even slight visual deterioration is highly significant if there is any suspicion of maculopathy

Preproliferative and proliferative retinopathy (commonly type I = insulin-dependent diabetes): preproliferative lesions suggesting that neovascularization is imminent are:

Multiple cotton-wool spots
Multiple large blot haemorrhages
Venous beading
Venous loops
Arterial sheathing
Atrophic-looking retina.

Criteria for referral to an ophthalmologist (according to European diabetic retinopathy screening guidelines):

Proliferative retinopathy (new vessels on disc or elsewhere; preretinal haemorrhage; fibrous tissue)

Advanced diabetic eye disease (vitreous haemorrhage; fibrous tissue; recent retinal detachment; rubeosis iridis)

Preproliferative retinopathy (venous irregularities—beading, reduplication, loops; multiple haemorrhages; multiple cotton-wool spots; intraretinal microvascular abnormalities (IRMA))

Non-proliferative retinopathy with macular involvement (reduced visual acuity not corrected by pinhole, i.e. suggesting macular oedema; haemorrhages and/or hard exudates within one disc diameter of the macula, with or without visual loss

Non-proliferative retinopathy without macular involvement (large circinate or plaque of hard exudates within the major temporal vasular arcades).

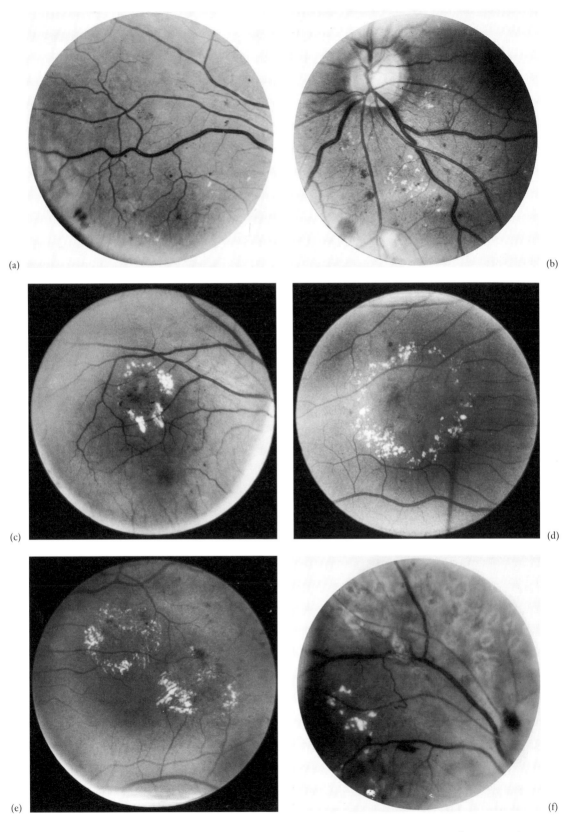

(a)

(b)

(c)

(d)

(e)

(f)

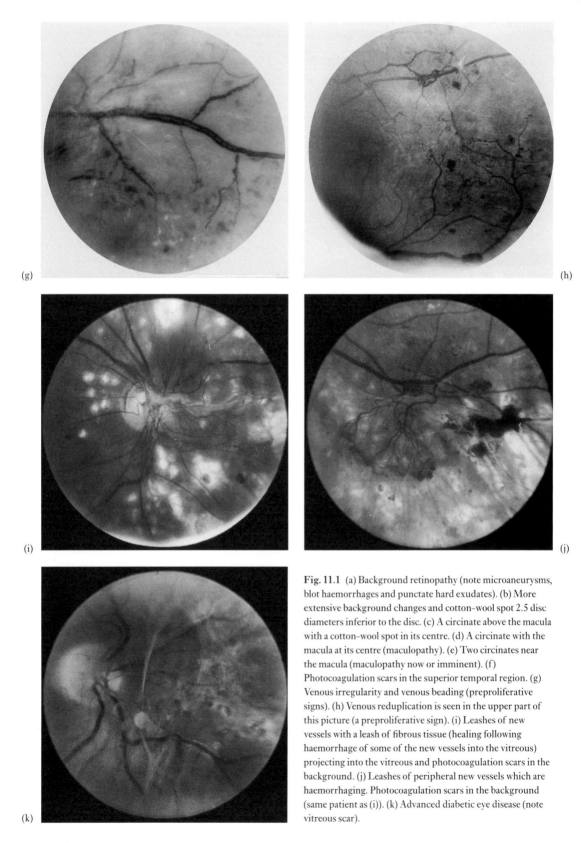

(g)

(h)

(i)

(j)

Fig. 11.1 (a) Background retinopathy (note microaneurysms, blot haemorrhages and punctate hard exudates). (b) More extensive background changes and cotton-wool spot 2.5 disc diameters inferior to the disc. (c) A circinate above the macula with a cotton-wool spot in its centre. (d) A circinate with the macula at its centre (maculopathy). (e) Two circinates near the macula (maculopathy now or imminent). (f) Photocoagulation scars in the superior temporal region. (g) Venous irregularity and venous beading (preproliferative signs). (h) Venous reduplication is seen in the upper part of this picture (a preproliferative sign). (i) Leashes of new vessels with a leash of fibrous tissue (healing following haemorrhage of some of the new vessels into the vitreous) projecting into the vitreous and photocoagulation scars in the background. (j) Leashes of peripheral new vessels which are haemorrhaging. Photocoagulation scars in the background (same patient as (i)). (k) Advanced diabetic eye disease (note vitreous scar).

(k)

55 / Hypertensive retinopathy

Record

The retinal arterioles are *narrow* (normal ratio of vein to artery is 1.1 : 1), they are (may be) tortuous and (may) vary in calibre (localized constriction followed by segments of arteriolar dilatation) with increased light reflex (copper or *silver wiring*) and *AV nipping* (these changes all occurring with ageing and arteriosclerosis as well as with hypertension). There are *flame-shaped* and (less frequently) *blot haemorrhages, cotton-wool exudates* (all indicating grade 3 retinopathy and a diagnosis of malignant (accelerated) hypertension *even without* papilloedema) and there is *papilloedema* (indicating cerebral oedema; papilloedema may occur in malignant hypertension even without haemorrhages and exudates).

This is grade 4 hypertensive retinopathy.

Causes of hypertension

Essential — 94% (cause unknown)

Renal — 4% (renal artery stenosis — ?*bruit*, acute nephritis, pyelonephritis, glomerulonephritis, polycystic disease, systemic sclerosis, systemic lupus erythematosus (SLE), hydronephrosis, renin-secreting tumour and renoprival — after bilateral nephrectomy)

Endocrine — 1%* (Cushing's, Conn's, phaeochromo-cytoma (gl.),† acromegaly, hyperparathyroidism (gl.), hypothyroidism and oral contraceptive use)

Miscellaneous — <1% (coarctation of the aorta — ?*radiofemoral delay*, polycythaemia (gl.), acute porphyria (gl.), pre-eclampsia).

NB Cerebral tumour or raised intracranial pressure from any cause may lead to secondary hypertension (Cushing's reflex).

---

* The figure 1% does not include hypertension due to oral contraceptive use.

† All patients with phaeochromocytomata should be screened for multiple endocrine neoplasia (MEN) type II (p. 241) and von Hippel–Lindau disease (p. 64) to avert further morbidity and mortality in the patients and their families. All patients in families with MEN-II or von Hippel–Lindau disease should be screened for phaeochromocytoma even if they are asymptomatic.

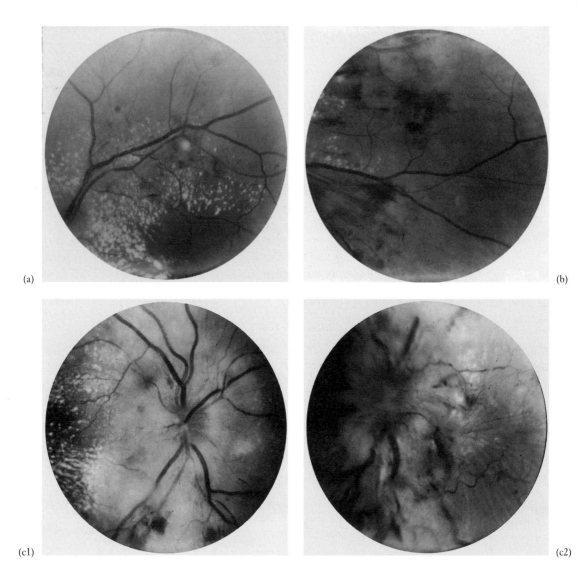

Fig. 11.2 (a) Thin, irregular arterioles, AV nipping, haemorrhages and exudates forming a macular star in hypertension. (b) Flame-shaped haemorrhages in hypertension. (c1,2) Papilloedema — hypertension.

56 / Optic atrophy

Record

The disc is *pale* and *clearly delineated* and (in the severe case) the *pupil reacts consensually* to light but *not directly*.* Field testing with the head of a hat pin (maybe) reveals a *central scotoma*.

The diagnosis is optic atrophy. The well-defined disc edge suggests that it is not secondary to papilloedema† (yellow–grey disc with blurred margins). Common causes of primary optic atrophy are:

1 Multiple sclerosis (may be temporal pallor only; ?nystagmus, scanning speech, cerebellar ataxia, etc. — p. 121).
2 Compression of the optic nerve by:
    (a) tumour (e.g. pituitary — ?bitemporal hemianopia),
    (b) aneurysm.
3 Glaucoma (gl.) (?pathological cupping).

Other causes

Ischaemic optic neuropathy (abrupt onset of visual loss in an elderly patient; may be painful; thrombosis or embolus of posterior ciliary artery; temporal arteritis is sometimes the cause)

Leber's optic atrophy (gl.) (males : females = 6 : 1)

Retinal artery occlusion

Toxic amblyopia (lead, methyl alcohol, arsenic, insecticides, quinine)

Nutritional amblyopia (famine, etc., tobacco–alcohol amblyopia, vitamin B_{12} deficiency, diabetes mellitus‡)

Friedreich's ataxia (gl.) (?cerebellar signs, pes cavus, scoliosis, etc.)

Tabes dorsalis (gl.) (?Argyll Robertson pupils, etc.)

Paget's disease (?large skull, bowed tibia, etc. — p. 99)

Consecutive optic atrophy.†

---

* In early unilateral optic neuritis before the direct reflex is lost, it may simply become more sluggish than the consensual reflex. In this situation it may be possible to demonstrate the *Marcus Gunn* phenomenon. In this the direct reflex may at first appear to be brisk. However, when the light is alternated from one side to the other, the pupil on the affected side may be seen to dilate slowly when exposed to the light. The mechanism is as follows: when the light shines in the healthy eye a rapid constriction occurs in both eyes. As the light then moves to the affected eye, this fails to transmit the message to continue constriction as quickly as normal. As a result the pupils have time to recover and dilate, despite the light shining on the abnormal eye.

† Optic atrophy can be divided into primary, secondary and consecutive. Consecutive optic atrophy follows damage to the parent ganglion cells of the retina as in widespread choroidoretinitis, retinitis pigmentosa and retinal artery occlusion.

‡ Optic atrophy in diabetes mellitus may also occur in the DIDMOAD syndrome — with diabetes insipidus (gl.), diabetes mellitus and deafness. It is a rare, recessively inherited disorder.

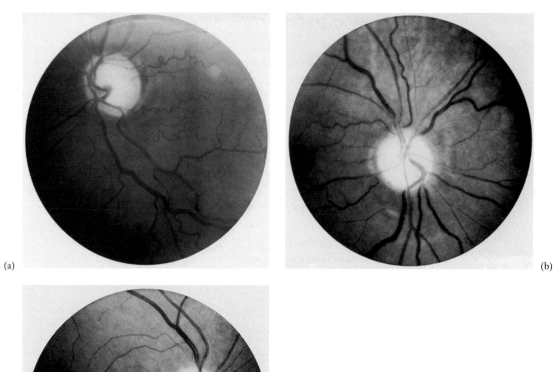

(a)

(b)

(c)

Fig. 11.3 (a–c) Optic atrophy.

57 / Papilloedema

Record

There is bilateral papilloedema* (search carefully for haemorrhages, exudates and AV nipping).

Possible causes

1 These include:

(a) an *intracranial space-occupying lesion* (?localizing neurological signs†),

(b) tumour (infratentorial more often than supratentorial),

(c) abscess (fever not always present, ?underlying middle ear infection, underlying suppuration elsewhere—e.g. bronchiectasis or empyema),

(d) haematoma.

2 *Malignant hypertension* (check blood pressure—haemorrhages and exudates are not always present; ?narrow tortuous arterioles that vary in calibre, AV nipping—p. 143).

3 *Benign intracranial hypertension*‡ (?obese female aged 15–45, no localizing neurological signs).

---

* The disc oedema of papillitis (disc usually pink due to hyperaemia) must be differentiated from developing papilloedema due to raised intracranial pressure. Papilloedema causes enlargement of the blind spot and constriction of the peripheral field, but visual acuity is unaffected. Papillitis (optic neuritis affecting the intraorbital portion of the optic nerve) causes central scotoma, diminished visual acuity, and sometimes tenderness and pain on eye movement during an acute attack. Furthermore, in papillitis there may be a pupillary reflex defect, loss of the central cup and cells may be present in the vitreous over the disc.

† VIth nerve palsy in the presence of papilloedema may be a false localizing sign due to raised intracranial pressure stretching the nerve during its long intracranial course. A localizing sign may occasionally be rapidly apparent in the case of contralateral optic atrophy—the *Foster–Kennedy syndrome* (gl.) (a frontal tumour pressing on the optic nerve to cause atrophy and at the same time raising intracranial pressure to cause papilloedema in the other eye). It must be remembered that tumours in and around the frontal lobes can present simply with dementia in the absence of signs and symptoms of raised intracranial pressure (i.e. without papilloedema). A classic lesion to present in this manner is a subfrontal olfactory groove meningioma (gl.). These may grow to considerable size, initially causing only memory impairment and marked apathy. On examination and upon closer questioning there is usually a history of diminished or absent sense of smell. Loss of urinary control associated with dementia should be regarded as indicating organic pathology until proven otherwise. A much shorter history of dementia and urinary incontinence together with increasingly severe headache may indicate an underlying malignant glioma of the corpus callosum or of one or other frontal lobe.

‡ This syndrome (also called pseudotumour cerebri, serous meningitis or otitic hydrocephalus) is known to have occurred following a middle ear infection which caused lateral sinus thrombosis. It may be that thrombosis of the venous sinuses is the aetiological factor in many other cases. The condition has been associated with the contraceptive pill, long-term tetracycline treatment for acne, corticosteroids (often reduction in dose during long-term therapy), head injury and times of female physiological hormone disturbance such as menarche, pregnancy and puerperium. The cerebrospinal fluid pressure is high, frequently above 300 mm, but the composition of the fluid is normal; the protein content is usually low normal, below 20 mg dl^{-1}.

The first sign of raised intracranial pressure is loss of venous pulsation, but recognition of this sign requires much practise and experience (see p. 137). If there is doubt about the normality of the disc, the presence of venous pulsation makes papilloedema and raised intracranial pressure unlikely.

Other causes of papilloedema

Meningitis (especially tuberculous)

Hypercapnoea (cyanosis, flapping tremor of the hands)

Central retinal vein thrombosis (gl.) (sight affected, usually unilateral, dilated veins, widespread haemorrhages)

(Graves') congestive ophthalmopathy (= malignant exophthalmos though exophthalmos is not always present; prominent eyes, eyelids and conjunctivae swollen and inflamed, marked ophthalmoplegia, often pain)

Cavernous sinus thrombosis (usually becomes bilateral, follows infection of orbit, nose and face; eyeball(s) protrudes, is painful, immobile and there is extreme venous congestion)

Hypoparathyroidism (gl.) (tetany, epilepsy, cataracts, etc.)

Severe anaemia especially due to massive blood loss and leukaemia (there may be haemorrhages and cotton-wool spots as well)

Guillain–Barré syndrome (gl.) (papilloedema possibly due to impaired cerebrospinal fluid resorption because of the elevated protein content)

Paget's disease (large head, bowed tibiae)

Hurler's syndrome (gl.) (dwarf, large head, coarse features, hepatosplenomegaly, heart murmurs)

Poisoning with vitamin A, lead, tetracyclines or naladixic acid

Ocular toxoplasmosis.

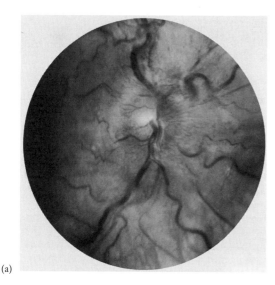 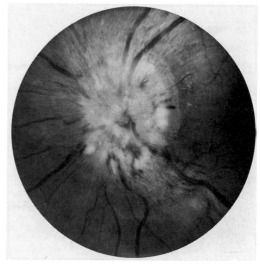

(a)

(b)

Fig. 11.4 (a,b) Papilloedema.

58 / Retinitis pigmentosa

Record

There is *widespread* scattering of *black pigment* in a pattern resembling *bone corpuscles*. The macula is spared. There is *tunnel vision*.*

The diagnosis is retinitis pigmentosa.

The patient may well have presented with night blindness. The condition progresses remorselessly with increasing retinal pigmentation, deepening disc pallor of consecutive optic atrophy as the ganglion cells die, and increasing constriction of the visual field. It may occur on its own although it is often associated with other abnormalities such as cataracts,† deaf–mutism and mental deficiency. Pigmentary degeneration of the retina may also occur in many conditions such as:

Laurence–Moon–Biedl syndrome (gl.) (autosomal recessive; ?obesity, hypogonadism, dwarfism, mental retardation and polydactyly)

Refsum's disease (gl.) (autosomal recessive; ?pupillary abnormalities, cerebellar ataxia, deafness, peripheral neuropathy, cardiomyopathy and icthyosis)

As well as some of the:

Hereditary ataxias (gl.)

Familial neuropathies

Neuronal lipidoses (ceroid lipofuscinosis).

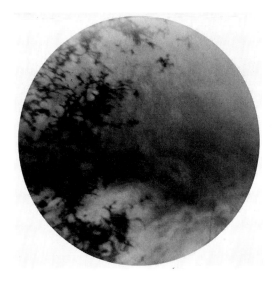

Fig. 11.5 Peripheral pigmentation resembling bone corpuscles.

*The examiner may ask you to demonstrate this either before, after or instead of asking you to examine the fundi. Make sure that you test the visual acuity (the patient may be blind in one or both eyes) before proceeding to test the visual fields. The examiners often suspect that such a patient may be known to students and they therefore alter the instruction and/or seating arrangement after each batch of students!

† Visual acuity may sometimes be considerably improved by cataract removal.

Chapter 12
Examine this patient's eyes

Possible short cases include
Exophthalmos (p. 152)
Ocular palsy (p. 155)
Nystagmus (p. 159)
Diabetic retinopathy (p. 139)
Optic atrophy (p. 145)
Myasthenia gravis (p. 162)
Visual field defect (p. 76)
Ptosis (p. 165)
Retinitis pigmentosa (p. 149)
Horner's syndrome (p. 180)
Holmes–Adie pupil (gl.)
Argyll Robertson pupils (p. 170)
Cataracts (p. 168)
Papilloedema (p. 147)

Examination *routine*

The examination of the eyes is basically going to be a part of your cranial nerves *routine* (p. 79) but carried out in slightly more detail. It should be your habit to commence all examination *routines* by *scanning* the whole patient. The patient with nystagmus due to cerebellar disease (p. 92) may have an *intention tremor* which will occasionally be noticeable even with minor movements. The patient with exophthalmos may have *pretibial myxoedema* or *thyroid acropachy* (gl.). A number of other conditions with stigmata elsewhere on the body may cause eye signs. These conditions should be borne in mind as you complete this *visual survey*: face and hands of acromegaly, foot ulcers in diabetes, pes cavus in Friedreich's ataxia (gl.), the long, lean look of dystrophia myotonica, etc. As you finish your *visual survey* briefly look again at

1 the **face** (e.g. myasthenic facies, tabetic facies, facial asymmetry in hemiparesis), and then concentrate on

2 the **eyes**. Ask yourself if there is:

   (a) exophthalmos,

   (b) strabismus,

   (c) ptosis, or

   (d) other abnormalities such as xanthelasma or arcus senilis.

Look at

3 the **pupils** for inequality of size and shape; whether one or both are small

(Argyll Robertson, Horner's) or large (Holmes–Adie, IIIrd nerve palsy). Next, it is traditional to check

4 the **visual acuity** by asking the patient to read a newspaper or other print which you hold up, and by asking him to look at the clock on the wall (see p. 80); alternatively it would be preferable to pull out a pocket-sized Snellen's chart.* In the traditional *routine* you should next test

5 the **visual fields** (see p. 74). However, in the majority of cases the important findings are on testing

6 the **eye movements** (see p. 81). We leave you to decide if you wish to follow the traditional *routine* or check eye movements before acuity and visual fields. You are looking for:

  (a) ocular palsy (p. 155),
  (b) diplopia,
  (c) nystagmus, or
  (d) lid lag.

In order to test

7 the **pupillary light reflex**, take out your pen torch and shine the light twice (*direct* and *consensual*) in each eye. Then test

8 the **accommodation–convergence reflex** — hold your finger close to the patient's nose:

  'Look into the distance'

then suddenly

  'Now look at my finger'.†

Finally, examine

9 the **fundi**.

   As usual, when you have the diagnosis, think what else you could look for (e.g. cerebellar signs in a patient with nystagmus; sympathectomy scar over the clavicle in a patient with Horner's syndrome; absent limb reflexes in Holmes–Adie pupil) before shouting out the diagnosis even if it is obvious (e.g. exophthalmos).

For *checklist* see p. 277.

---

* We advise you to take a pocket-sized Snellen's chart (like the one provided in Appendix 4). It will enable you to put an approximate value on the patient's visual acuity while taking no extra time.

† Some neurologists believe that as this traditional method of examining the accommodation–convergence reflex may involve a change in optical axis and luminance, it is better to get the patient to follow a target down the optical axis over 2 m.

59 / Exophthalmos

Record 1

There is (may be) bilateral *swelling* of the *medial caruncle* and *vascular congestion of the lateral canthus* with exophthalmos (protrusion of the eye revealing the *sclera above the lower lid* in the position of forward gaze) which is greater on the R/L side. Likely causes include:

1 Hyperthyroid Graves' disease* (?lid retraction or lag, tachycardia, bruit over the goitre; exophthalmos usually symmetrical).

2 Euthyroid Graves' disease (?no lid lag, *normal* pulse rate, no sweating or tremor, etc.).

3 Hypothyroid Graves' disease (?facies, scar of thyroidectomy, hoarse voice, slow pulse, ankle jerks, etc.).

Record 2

There is severe exophthalmos, *chemosis*, *corneal ulceration* and *ophthalmoplegia†* which is reducing the upward and lateral gaze most and which is responsible for the *diplopia*. Convergence (check for this) is also impaired. Testing the eye movements caused the patient discomfort (or pain).

The diagnosis is Graves' malignant exophthalmos (patient may be hyper-, eu- or hypothyroid).

Graves' malignant exophthalmos (congestive ophthalmopathy) can cause severe pain and the patient is at risk of blindness due to pressure on the optic nerve, if not treated. The condition may require large doses of systemic steroids and sometimes *tarsorrhaphy* (which may be in evidence in the examination patient) or even orbital decompression may be necessary. Radiotherapy has also been successfully used.

Other causes of exophthalmos

Bilateral (though asymmetrical) with conjunctival oedema:

Cavernous sinus thrombosis (follows infection of the orbit, nose and face; eyeball is painful and there is extreme venous congestion)

Caroticocavernous fistula (pulsating exophthalmos).

Unilateral

Retro-orbital tumour (the protrusion measured with the Hertel exophthalmometer is usually >5 mm more than the unaffected eye by the time of presentation, whereas Graves' eyes rarely achieve a difference of 5 mm‡)

Orbital cellulitis.

---

* There are some studies that suggest that radioactive iodine therapy for Graves' disease may worsen exophthalmos though this is a controversial area.

† The ophthalmoplegia is due to infiltration, oedema and subsequent fibrosis of the external ocular muscles. It may occur with oedema of the lids and conjunctivae and precede the exophthalmos. For this reason the term 'congestive

ophthalmopathy' may be preferable to 'malignant exophthalmos'.

‡ Unless the diagnosis is unquestionably Graves' disease, the possibility of a retro-orbital tumour should always be investigated with a computerized tomography (CT) scan, etc., regardless of the Hertel exophthalmometer measurement.

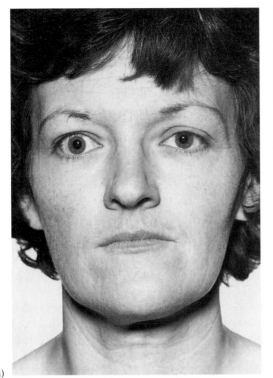

(a)

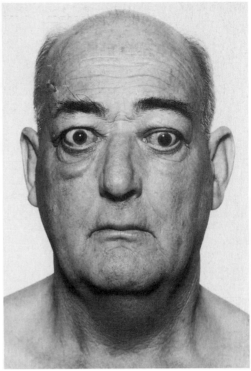

(b1)

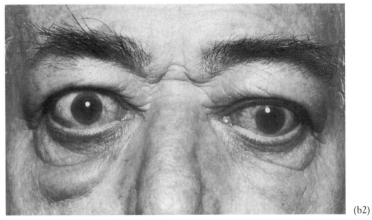

(b2)

Fig. 12.1 (a) Unilateral
exophthalmos. (b1,2) Bilateral
exophthalmos (note proptosis,
ophthalmoplegia, conjunctival
congestion, swelling of the medial
caruncle and periorbital swelling).

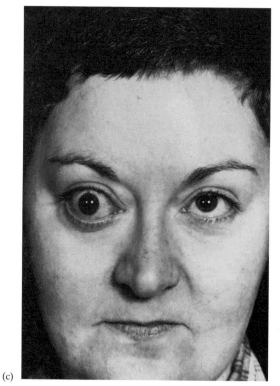
(c)

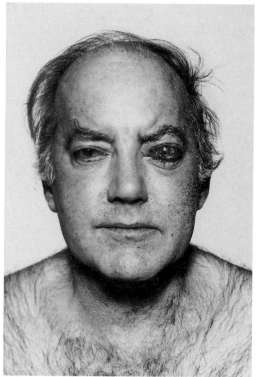
(d)

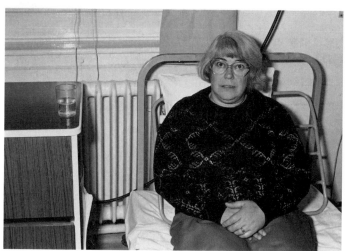
(e)

Fig. 12.1 (*continued*)
(c) Ophthalmoplegia of the right eye.
(d) Severe congestive
ophthalmopathy, chemosis and
corneal ulceration. (e) Tell-tale glass
of water (for examination of the
goitre) in a patient with
exophthalmos.

60 / Ocular palsy

Record 1

The patient has a *convergent strabismus* at rest. There is *impairment* of the *lateral movement* of the R/L eye and *diplopia* is worse on looking to the R/L (the outermost image comes from the affected eye).

The patient has a *VIth nerve palsy*.

Possible causes

1 The causes of **mononeuritis multiplex.***
2 **Multiple sclerosis** (?ipsilateral facial palsy because the VIth and VIIth nuclei are very close in the pons; ?nystagmus, cerebellar signs, pyramidal signs, pale discs, etc. — p. 121).
3 **Raised intracranial pressure** (?papilloedema) causing stretching of the nerve (a false localizing sign) during its long intracranial course.
4 **Neoplasm** (?papilloedema; associated ipsilateral facial palsy if pontine tumour).
5 **Myasthenia gravis** (see below).
6 **Vascular lesions** (probably common as a cause of 'idiopathic' VIth nerve palsy).
7 **Compression by aneurysm** (ectatic basilar artery; uncommon).
8 **Subacute meningitis** (carcinomatous; lymphomatous; fungal (NB acquired immune deficiency syndrome, AIDS); tuberculous; meningovascular syphilis).

Record 2

There is *ptosis.* Lifting the eyelids reveals *divergent strabismus* and a *dilated pupil.* The eye is fixed in a *down and out position* (and there is *angulated diplopia*).

The diagnosis is complete (NB the condition is often partial) *IIIrd nerve palsy.*

Possible causes

1 **Unruptured aneurysm**† of **posterior communicating** (or internal carotid) **artery** (painful).
2 The causes of **mononeuritis multiplex.***

---

* The causes of mononeuritis multiplex include diabetes mellitus, polyarteritis nodosa (gl.) and Churg–Strauss syndrome (gl.), rheumatoid disease, systemic lupus erythematosus (SLE), Wegener's granulomatosis (gl.), sarcoidosis (gl.), carcinoma, amyloidosis (gl.), leprosy (gl.), Sjögren's syndrome (gl.) and Lyme disease (gl.).

† If the ophthalmoplegia is predominant compared to the ptosis/pupil dilatation, the cause is likely to be vascular (intrinsic). If the ophthalmoplegia is minimal compared to the ptosis/pupil dilatation, the cause is more likely to be extrinsic compression by aneurysm, pituitary tumour, meningioma (gl.), etc.

3 Vascular lesion† (if there is a contralateral hemiplegia the diagnosis is Weber's syndrome (gl.)).

4 Midbrain demyelinating lesion‡ (?cerebellar signs, staccato speech, pale discs, etc. —p. 121).

5 Myasthenia gravis (see below).

Other causes of a IIIrd nerve palsy

Subacute meningitis (carcinomatous; lymphomatous; fungal (NB AIDS); tuberculous; meningovascular syphilis—at one time the commonest cause, now very rare)

Ophthalmoplegic migraine (similar to posterior communicating artery aneurysm except that it begins in childhood or adolescence, recovery is more rapid and is always complete; recovery is never complete with an aneurysm)

Parasellar neoplasmata†

Sphenoidal wing meningiomata†

Carcinomatous lesions of the skull base.†

Other causes of ocular palsy

Internuclear ophthalmoplegia (adduction impaired bilaterally but abduction normal or vice versa; ataxic nystagmus is present and distinguishes it from bilateral VIth nerve palsy—see p. 159; ?cerebellar signs)

Exophthalmic ophthalmoplegia (exophthalmos and diplopia—upward and outward gaze most often reduced)

Myasthenia gravis (?ptosis, variable strabismus, facial weakness with a snarling smile, proximal muscle weakness, weak nasal voice, all of which worsen with repetition—p. 162. NB It may superficially resemble IIIrd or VIth nerve palsy)

Cavernous sinus and superior orbital fissure syndromes (total or subtotal ophthalmoplegia which is often painful, together with sensory loss over the first division of the Vth nerve—absent corneal reflex; it is due to a tumour or carotid aneurysm affecting the IIIrd, IVth, Vth and VIth nerves as they travel together through the cavernous sinus into the superior orbital fissure—see Fig. 17.2d, p. 242)

Fourth nerve palsy (adducted eye cannot look downwards—the patient experiences 'one above the other' diplopia when attempting to do this; angulated diplopia occurs when looking down and out; the diplopia is worse when reading and going down stairs)

Ocular myopathy (see footnote, p. 165).

‡ IIIrd nerve palsy is rare in demyelinating disease; internuclear ophthalmoplegia (pp. 121 and 159) is a much commoner result of this condition.

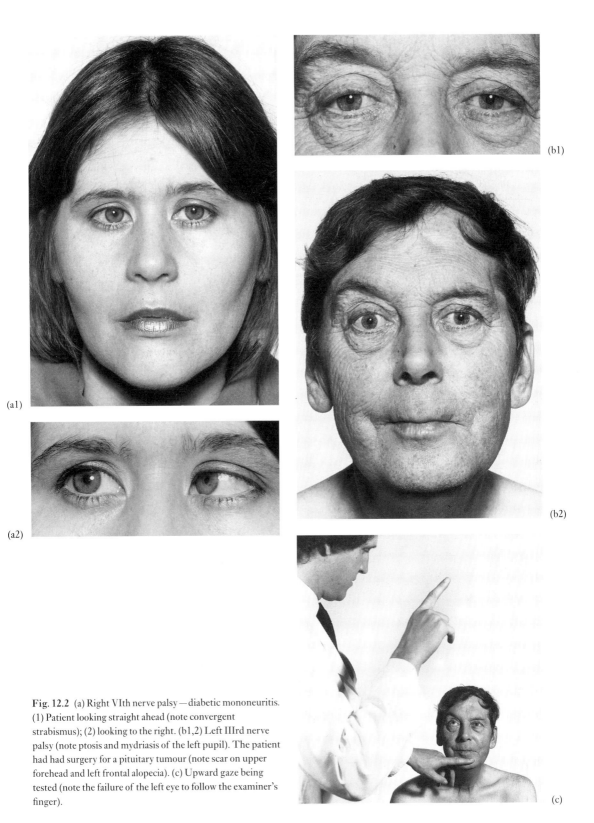

(a1)

(a2)

(b1)

(b2)

(c)

Fig. 12.2 (a) Right VIth nerve palsy — diabetic mononeuritis.
(1) Patient looking straight ahead (note convergent
strabismus); (2) looking to the right. (b1,2) Left IIIrd nerve
palsy (note ptosis and mydriasis of the left pupil). The patient
had had surgery for a pituitary tumour (note scar on upper
forehead and left frontal alopecia). (c) Upward gaze being
tested (note the failure of the left eye to follow the examiner's
finger).

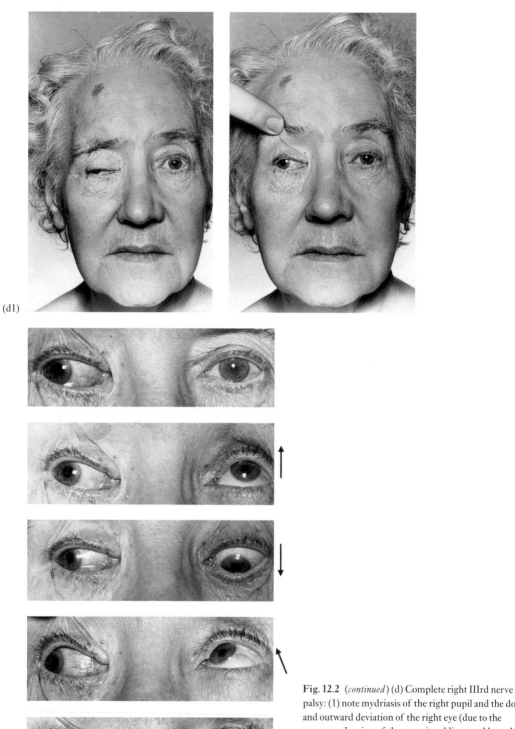

(d1)

(d2)

Fig. 12.2 (*continued*) (d) Complete right IIIrd nerve palsy: (1) note mydriasis of the right pupil and the down and outward deviation of the right eye (due to the unopposed action of the superior oblique and lateral rectus muscles innervated by the IVth and VIth nerves, respectively); (2) testing eye movements (note the failure of the right eye to look straight, upwards, downwards, upwards and laterally, and medially).

61 / Nystagmus

Note: in medical short case examinations nystagmus is most often cerebellar in origin — and usually due to multiple sclerosis.

Record 1

There is nystagmus, greater on the R/L with the fast component to the same side. This suggests:

1 an ipsilateral cerebellar lesion (?cerebellar signs — p. 92),

or

2 a contralateral vestibular lesion (?vertical nystagmus, ?vertigo — see below). (Now, if allowed, *look for cerebellar signs*; occasionally there will be signs of a lesion in the brainstem, e.g. infarction or syringobulbia.*)

Record 2

The nystagmus is *ataxic* in that the *abducting eye has greater nystagmus* than the adducting eye.† With this there is dissociation of conjugate eye movements. There is (may be) a divergent strabismus at rest. On looking to the right, the right eye abducts normally, but there is *impairment of adduction*† of the left eye. On looking to the left, the left eye abducts normally but there is *impairment of adduction*† of the right eye (occasionally the reverse may occur with weakness of abduction on each side but adduction remains normal). When the abducting eye is covered, however, the medial movement of the other eye occurs normally.

The diagnosis is *internuclear ophthalmoplegia*. It suggests multiple sclerosis‡ with a lesion in the medial longitudinal fasciculus. (Now, if allowed, *look for cerebellar signs*, pyramidal signs, pale discs, etc. — pp. 92 and 121.)

Causes and types of nystagmus

A diagramatic representation of conjugate gaze and its various connections is depicted in Fig. 12.3. As can be seen from the multiplicity of these pathways, a disorder within the end-organs (i.e. eye, labyrinth, semicircular canals) or in the medial longitudinal fasciculus anywhere through its long course, or in its nuclear connec-tions (i.e. cerebellar, vestibular nuclei, etc.) can cause nystagmus. Nystagmus can be divided into:

Physiological nystagmus (a few brief jerks can occur in the normal eye at the extreme lateral gaze)

Ocular nystagmus (in patients with a congenital visual defect in one eye, a pendular movement of the eye occurs while gazing straight — fixation nystagmus)

---

* As can be seen from Fig. 12.3, the medial longitudinal bundle extends into the spinal cord so that syringomyelia (gl.) confined to the spinal cord, if extending above C_5, may also cause nystagmus.

† The key sign of the internuclear ophthalmoplegia is the *failure of adduction* — the nystagmus is not essential.

‡ Internuclear ophthalmoplegia is highly characteristic of multiple sclerosis though rarely it may be caused by brainstem gliomata or vascular lesions, or Wernicke's encephalopathy (ocular palsy, nystagmus, loss of pupillary reflexes, ataxia, peripheral neuropathy, Korsakoff's psychosis or other disturbance of mentation; dramatic response to thiamine in the early stages).

Vestibular nystagmus (see below)
Cerebellar nystagmus (*record* 1)
Ataxic nystagmus (*record* 2).

Vestibular nystagmus

This may arise in the periphery (labyrinth or vestibular nerve) or in the central vestibular nuclei and its connections.

Peripheral

The fast component is towards the contralateral side (except with an early irritative lesion when it can be on the side of the lesion) and the nystagmus is fatiguable — it becomes less and less intense on repetition of the test. The patient tends to be unsteady on the ipsilateral side (contralateral to the fast component) as can be revealed whilst assessing Romberg's test (the patient cannot stand on a narrow base even with the eyes open in this situation whereas the patient with sensory ataxia becomes more unsteady when the eyes are closed) and gait (tends to reel on the affected side). Cochlear function is usually affected (diminishes leading to deafness, e.g. Menière's syndrome) and the patient may have vertigo.

Causes of peripheral vestibular nystagmus:

Labyrinthitis (probably viral and self-limiting; nystagmus may be absent and only positional and provoked by movements of the head — often it can be elicited by bending the head backwards about 45° — the nystagmus, as well as the vertigo, may appear but fades with repeated testing)

Menière's syndrome (progressive deafness and tinnitus, with recurrent attacks of vertigo)

Acoustic neuroma (gl.) (progressive tinnitus and nerve deafness; neighbouring nerves — Vth, VIth, VIIth may be involved and there may be cerebellar signs, etc.)

Vestibular neuronitis (acute vertigo without deafness or tinnitus which usually improves within 48 h; full recovery may take weeks or months; may be viral).

Other causes include degenerative middle ear disease, hypertension and head injury.

Central

Lesions affecting vestibular nuclei (cerebrovascular accident, multiple sclerosis, encephalitis, tumours, syringobulbia, alcoholism,§ anticonvulsants, etc.) cause nystagmus which is spontaneous but may be brought on or increased by head movements. It is not adaptable and usually has a vertical component. *Downbeat nystagmus* with the eyes looking straight ahead is characteristic of an Arnold–Chiari malformation. ‖ Downbeat nystagmus on lateral gaze normally indicates a lesion at foramen magnum level (tumour, syringomyelia or cerebellar degeneration).

§Acute alcohol toxicity may cause nystagmus. Nystagmus is also almost always present in Wernicke's encephalopathy. Paradoxically alcohol may reduce congenital nystagmus — a condition which may be gross but symptomless.

‖ An *Arnold–Chiari malformation* may be asymptomatic until adult life when the patient gradually develops cerebellar symptoms and signs. There is cerebellar herniation through the foramen magnum. There may be coexisting syringomyelia of the cervical cord and medulla. Commonly there is radiographic evidence of fusion of the cervical vertebrae, platybasia or basilar impression. Magnetic resonance imaging (MRI) establishes the diagnosis (CT may miss it) when there are no coexisting bony abnormalities. Surgical intervention may benefit selected cases.

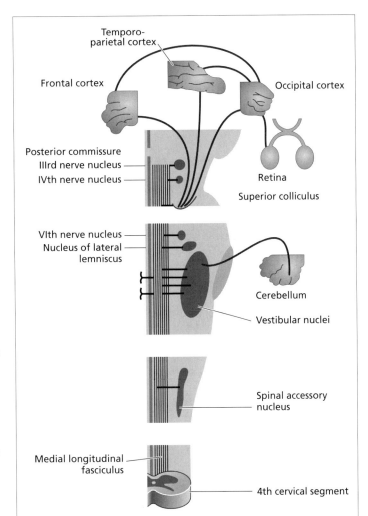

Fig. 12.3 Cortical, brainstem and peripheral control of conjugate gaze. The medial longitudinal bundle starts just below the posterior commissure and ends in the upper cervical spinal cord. During its long course it receives fibres from various nucleii (and the lateral pontine gaze centre) which are concerned with the control of conjugate gaze. Interruption in the cortical or midbrain connections often produces a disorder of conjugate gaze rather than nystagmus. Lesions in the brainstem or below result in nystagmus.

In the figure, the following structures are labelled: Temporo-parietal cortex, Frontal cortex, Occipital cortex, Posterior commissure, IIIrd nerve nucleus, IVth nerve nucleus, Retina, Superior colliculus, VIth nerve nucleus, Nucleus of lateral lemniscus, Cerebellum, Vestibular nuclei, Spinal accessory nucleus, Medial longitudinal fasciculus, 4th cervical segment.

62 / Myasthenia gravis

Record

There is *ptosis* (one or both sides) accentuated by upward gaze, *variable strabismus* (with *diplopia*) and when she tries to screw her eyes up tight, the eyelashes are not buried. The face shows a *lack of expression*, the mouth is slack and there is generalized *facial weakness*. The patient *snarls* when she tries to smile, she cannot whistle, and her *voice* is *weak* and *nasal* (if you ask the patient to count aloud, speech may become progressively less distinct and more nasal). There is *proximal muscle weakness*. Repetitive movements cause an increase in the muscle weakness (myasthenia = abnormal muscular fatiguability).

The diagnosis is myasthenia gravis. A substantial improvement in muscle power in response to a test dose of edrophonium will confirm the diagnosis.

Male to female ratio is 1:2.

Other features of myasthenia gravis

Difficulty with swallowing, chewing and nasal regurgitation

Symptoms worsen as the day progresses

Tendon reflexes are normal or exaggerated (cf. Eaton–Lambert syndrome (gl.))

The *jaw-supporting sign*, if present, is pathognomonic—the patient puts her hand under her chin to support both the weak jaw and neck; this may only become obvious after prolonged conversation

Anti-acetylcholine receptor antibodies are present in 90% of cases

In long-standing cases there may be an element of permanent irreversible myopathic change

Breathlessness is a sinister symptom requiring urgent attention (respiratory deterioration may develop rapidly and should be watched for by monitoring the peak flow rate)

Pathological changes are present in the thymus in 70–80% and some patients are improved by thymectomy; thymomata occur in 10–20% (mostly males) and give a worse prognosis.

Associated immune disorders include thyrotoxicosis (5% of patients), hypothyroidism, rheumatoid arthritis, diabetes mellitus, polymyositis (gl.), SLE, pernicious anaemia, Sjögren's syndrome (gl.), pemphigus and sarcoidosis (gl.).

Crisis

Signs of *cholinergic crisis* are collapse, confusion, abdominal pain and vomiting, sweating, salivation, lachrymation, miosis and pallor. The features which distinguish a *myasthenic crisis* are response to edrophonium and the absence of cholinergic phenomena. Occasionally it is exceptionally difficult to determine whether the collapsed myasthenic has been under- or over-treated. Temporary withdrawal of all drugs and assisted positive pressure respiration is then indicated.

Myasthenic crises may be provoked by:

Infection

Emotional upset

Undue exertion*

Drugs (streptomycin, gentamicin, kanamycin, neomycin, viomycin, polymyxin, colistin, curare, quinine, quinidine, procainamide).

Eaton–Lambert syndrome (myasthenic–myopathic syndrome) is often associated with oat-cell carcinoma of the bronchus. There is proximal muscle wasting, weakness and fatiguability. Often, however, power is initially increased by brief exercise (reversed myasthenic effect). The tendon reflexes are depressed (but increased soon after activity). The electromyographic response to ulnar nerve stimulation shows a characteristic increase in amplitude (it declines in myasthenia gravis). Cholinergic drugs have no effect. Weakness and fatiguability may be greatly improved by guanidine hydrochloride.

---

*Childbirth requires careful management.

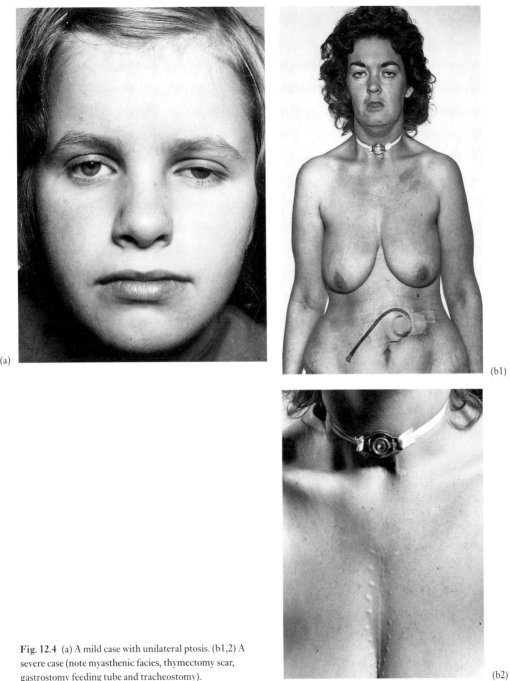

(a)

(b1)

(b2)

Fig. 12.4 (a) A mild case with unilateral ptosis. (b1,2) A severe case (note myasthenic facies, thymectomy scar, gastrostomy feeding tube and tracheostomy).

(c) 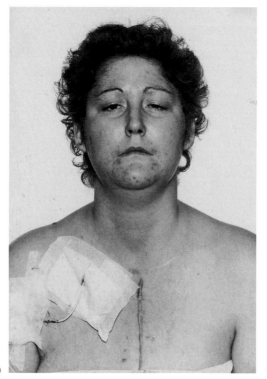 (d)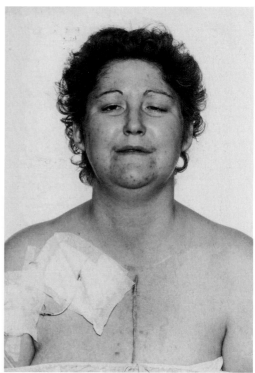

Fig. 12.4 (*continued*) (c) Myasthenic facies (note the
subclavian line which was being used for plasmapherisis).
(d) 'Smile'.

63 / Ptosis

Record 1

There is *unilateral* ptosis.*

Possible causes

1 Third nerve palsy (?dilated ipsilateral pupil, divergent strabismus, etc. — p. 155).
2 Horner's syndrome (?ipsilateral small pupil, etc. — p. 180).
3 Myasthenia gravis (may be the only sign of this condition; ?induced or worsened by upward gaze; variable strabismus, facial and proximal muscle weakness, weak nasal voice, all of which may worsen with repetition, etc. — p. 162).
4 Congenital/idiopathic† (may increase with age; there may be an associated superior rectus palsy).
5 Dystrophia myotonica (usually bilateral).

Record 2

There is *bilateral* ptosis.*

Possible causes

1 Myasthenia gravis.
2 Dystrophia myotonica (?myopathic facies, frontal balding, wasting of facial muscles and sternomastoids, cataracts, myotonia, etc. — p. 209).
3 Tabes dorsalis (gl.) (?Argyll Robertson pupils, etc.).
4 Congenital† (may increase with age).
5 Bilateral Horner's (e.g. syringomyelia (gl.) — ?wasting of small muscles of the hand, dissociated sensory loss, scars, extensor plantars, etc.).
6 Ocular myopathy‡ (?absence of soft tissue in the lids and periorbital region, ophthalmoplegia, mild facial and neck weakness).
7 Oculopharangeal muscular dystrophy (gl.)‡ (similar to ocular myopathy but late onset and dysphagia prominent).

---

* NB Overaction of frontalis with wrinkling of the forehead may be congenital or due to ocular myopathy or syphilis. While testing for ptosis, make sure you hold the head of the patient with one hand, while you ask him to look up at the index finger of the other hand.
† There should be no response to a test dose of edrophonium before this diagnosis is accepted.

‡ Many of the ocular myopathies are associated with characteristic morphological features ('ragged red fibres') and mitochondrial myopathy and are now referred to as chronic progressive external ophthalmoplegia (CPEO). The disorder lies in the cytochromes and the conditions are sometimes termed the mitochondrial cytopathies. Ocular myopathy and oculopharangeal muscular dystrophy may be manifestations of the same condition.

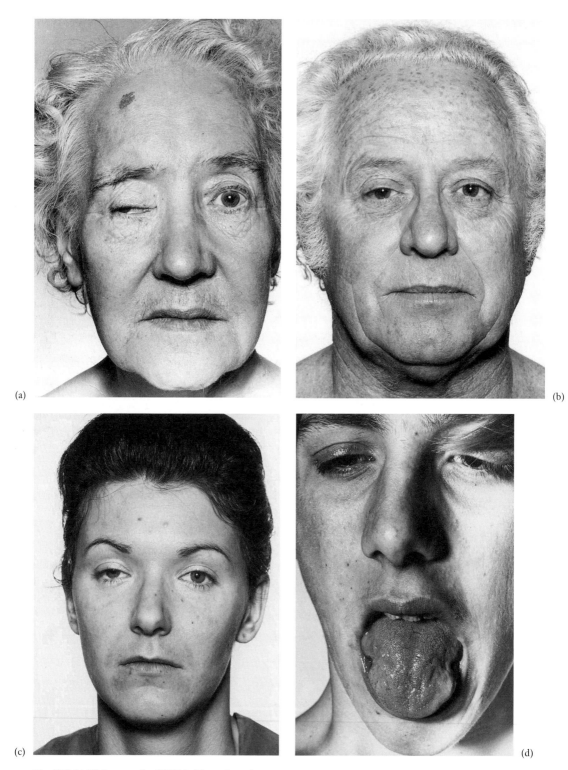

Fig. 12.5 (a) IIIrd nerve palsy. (b) Right Horner's syndrome.
(c) Myasthenia gravis. (d) Dystrophia myotonica.

Other causes of ptosis

Pseudoptosis (following recurrent inflammation or extreme thinning of the lids after repeated angioneurotic oedema)

Voluntary ptosis (to suppress diplopia)

Apraxia of the eyelids (the patient may need to pull down the lower eyelids, tilt back the head or open the mouth to enable the eyes to be opened; there is usually evidence of basal ganglia involvement).

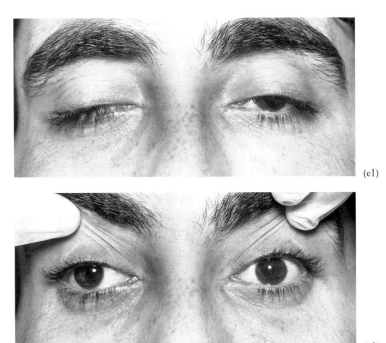

(e1)

(e2)

Fig. 12.5 (*continued*) (e1,2) Ocular myopathy.

64 / Cataracts

Record

There are partial cataracts in both eyes (may be localized to the lens nucleus, or seen as flakes, dots or sector-shaped opacities within the lens periphery).

Commonest causes of cataract

1 Old age (usually nuclear, with a brownish discoloration, or of the cortical spoke variety).

2 Diabetic patients develop senile cataracts at younger ages than non-diabetics and this is the commonest type of cataract in diabetes. Rarely* a 'snowflake' (dot cortical opacities) cataract can develop in a young, poorly controlled diabetic, and progress rapidly to a mature cataract in months or even days (good control may halt and even reverse development).

Other causes of cataract in adults

Trauma

Chronic anterior uveitis

Hypoparathyroidism (gl.) (Chvostek's (gl.) and Trousseau's signs (gl.), tetany, paraesthesiae and cramps, ectodermal changes, moniliasis, mental retardation and psychiatric disturbances, papilloedema, epilepsy, bradykinetic-rigid syndrome)

Radiation (infrared, ultraviolet, X-rays and possibly microwaves)

Dystrophia myotonica (?frontal balding, ptosis, sternomastoid wasting, myopathic facies, myotonia, etc. — p. 209)

Retinitis pigmentosa (including Refsum's disease (gl.) and Laurence–Moon–Biedl syndrome (gl.))

Steroid therapy (10 mg prednisolone daily for more than 1 year)

Chlorpromazine (500 mg daily for 3 years or more)

Chloroquine.

Causes of cataracts in children

These include: perinatal hypoglycaemia, perinatal hypocalcaemia, maternal rubella, galactosaemia (gl.), galactokinase deficiency, genetically inherited, Down's syndrome (gl.) (trisomy 21), Patau's syndrome (trisomy 13), Edward's syndrome (trisomy 18), Alport's syndrome and Lowe's syndrome.

*Rare with modern insulin therapy. A case was seen recently in an insulin-dependent patient who did not take insulin for prolonged periods for personal religious reasons.

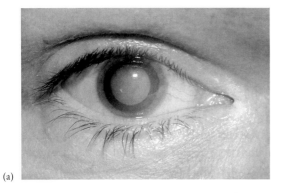 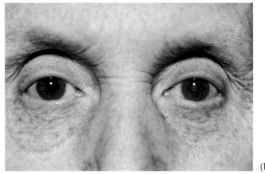

(a)   (b)

Fig. 12.6 (a) Cataract. (b) A cataract is seen in the left eye.

2 scan the face and skull. The abnormality will usually be obvious (see above list) but if you find none then proceed to

3 break down the parts of the face into their constituents and scrutinize each, asking the question to yourself: 'Is it normal?' Thus if you have scanned the eyes and have not been struck by any obvious abnormality (e.g. ptosis or an abnormal pupil), you should look at all the structures such as the *eyelids* (mild degree of ptosis, heliotrope rash on the upper lid in dermatomyositis), *eyelashes* (sparse in alopecia*), *cornea* (arcus senilis, ground-glass appearance in congenital syphilis (gl.)), *sclerae* (icteric, congested in superior vena cava obstruction and polycythaemia), *pupils* (small, large, irregular, dislocated lens in Marfan's syndrome (gl.), cataract in dystrophia myotonica) and *iris* ('muddy iris' in iritis)† on both sides. Look at the *face* for any erythema or infiltrates (lupus pernio, systemic lupus erythematosus (SLE), dermatomyositis, malar flush), around the *mouth* for tight, shiny, adherent skin (systemic sclerosis) or pigmented macules (Peutz–Jeghers) and, if indicated, in the mouth for telangiectases (Osler–Weber–Rendu), cyanosis or pigmentation (Addison's). The whole face can be rapidly covered in this manner. Having spotted the abnormality and, you hope, made the diagnosis you should, if appropriate, try to score extra points by demonstrating

4 additional features in the same way as described under 'What is the diagnosis?' Go through each diagnosis on the list and work out what additional features you would see elsewhere. Thus, if you find a lower motor neurone VIIth nerve lesion, demonstrate the weakness in the upper as well as the lower part of the face (see p. 173), then be seen to examine the ears for evidence of herpes zoster (Ramsay Hunt syndrome (gl.)).

If despite carrying out the above routine there is still no apparent abnormality then examine the facial musculature (see 'Examine this patient's cranial nerves') for evidence of a VIIth nerve lesion which is not obvious.

For *checklist* see p. 277.

---

* May be associated with the organ-specific autoimmune diseases — see p. 214.

† Another uncommon but important sign which may occur in the iris is neovascularization in diabetes (rubeosis iridis). However, it is unlikely that this would occur in the context of 'Examine this patient's face' at an examination.

66 / Lower motor neurone VIIth nerve palsy

Record

On the R/L side there is *paralysis* of the *upper* and lower face*, so that the *eye cannot be closed* (or it can easily be opened by the examiner); the eyeball turns up on attempted closure *(Bell's phenomenon)* and the patient is unable to raise his R/L eyebrow. The corner of the *mouth droops,* the *nasolabial fold is smoothed out*, and the voluntary and involuntary (i.e. including emotional) movements of the mouth are paralysed on the R/L side (the lips may be drawn to the opposite side and the tongue may deviate as well—not necessarily hypoglossal involvement—see footnote, p. 83).

This is a R/L lower motor neurone VIIth nerve lesion (now check the ipsilateral ear for evidence of *herpes zoster*).

Causes of a lower motor neurone VIIth nerve lesion

1 Bell's palsy.†
2 Ramsay Hunt syndrome (gl.) (herpes zoster on the external auditory meatus and the geniculate ganglion—taste to the anterior two-thirds of the tongue is lost; there may be lesions on the fauces and palate).

Other differential diagnoses

Cerebellopontine angle compression (acoustic neuroma (gl.) or meningioma (gl.); Vth, VIth, VIIth, VIIIth nerve palsy, cerebellar signs and loss of taste to the anterior two-thirds of the tongue)

Parotid tumour (?palpable; taste not affected)

Trauma

Pontine lesion (e.g. multiple sclerosis, tumour or vascular lesion)

Middle ear disease (deafness)

The causes of mononeuritis multiplex (diabetes, polyarteritis nodosa (gl.) and Churg–Strauss syndrome (gl.), rheumatoid arthritis, SLE, Wegener's granulomatosis (gl.), sarcoidosis (gl.), carcinoma, amyloidosis (gl.) and leprosy (gl.)).

Causes of bilateral lower motor neurone VIIth nerve paralysis‡

Guillain–Barré syndrome (gl.) (occasionally only VIIth nerves affected)

Sarcoidosis (parotid gland enlargement not always present)

Bilateral Bell's palsy

Myasthenia gravis (?ptosis, variable strabismus, proximal muscle weakness, etc.—p. 162)

Congenital facial diplegia

Some forms of muscular dystrophy (gl.)

Motor neurone disease (rarely)

Lyme disease (gl.) (may be bilateral, alone or with signs of meningoencephalitis or peripheral radiculoneu-

---

* That is, including frontalis ('raise eyebrows'), corrugator superficialis ('frown') and orbicularis oculi ('close your eyes tight'). See also p. 103, especially the footnote.

† In a mild case of Bell's palsy, taste over the anterior two-thirds of the tongue is usually preserved because the lesion is due to swelling of the nerve in the confined lower facial canal.

In cases with more extensive involvement this taste is lost and the patient may also show increased susceptibility to high-pitched or loud sounds (hyperacusis due to stapedius paralysis).

‡ Bilateral lower motor neurone VIIth nerve lesions are easily missed because there is no asymmetry.

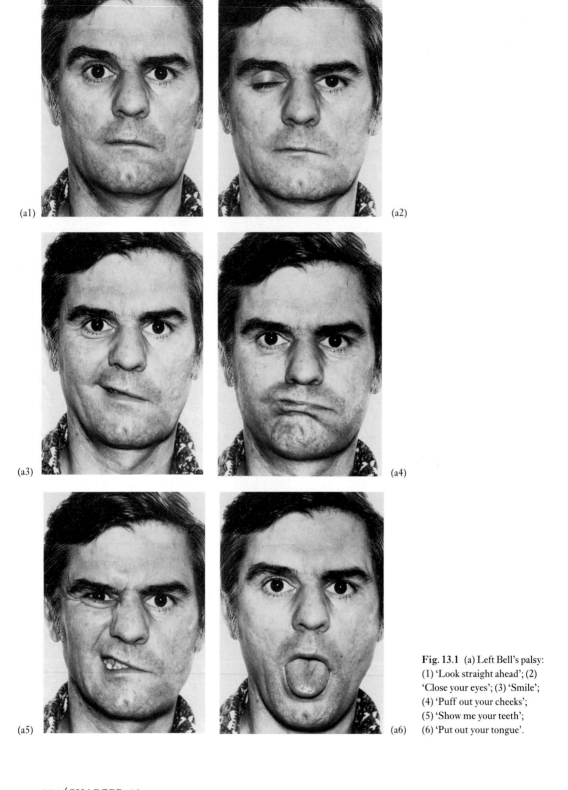

(a1)   (a2)

(a3)   (a4)

(a5)   (a6)

Fig. 13.1 (a) Left Bell's palsy:
(1) 'Look straight ahead'; (2)
'Close your eyes'; (3) 'Smile';
(4) 'Puff out your cheeks';
(5) 'Show me your teeth';
(6) 'Put out your tongue'.

ropathy, knee effusion, Baker's cyst (gl.) rupture, heart block, etc.).

The chorda tympani leaves the facial nerve in the middle ear to supply taste to the anterior two-thirds of the tongue. The superficial petrosal branch to supply the lachrymal glands, and the nerve to the stapedius both leave higher in the facial canal than the chorda tympani. The level of the lesion in the facial canal can sometimes be assessed (very unlikely to be required in an examination) by assessing the relative involvement of these nerves.

Variation of the Ramsay Hunt syndrome
Occasionally facial palsy is associated with trigeminal, occipital or cervical herpes with or without auditory involvement. In some of these cases the geniculate ganglion may be spared—see p. 235.

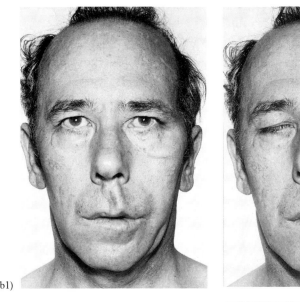
(b1)

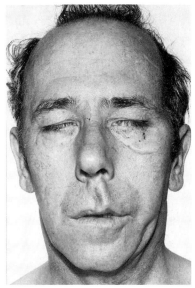
(b2)

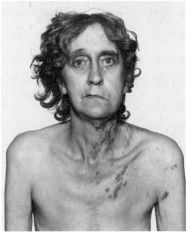
(c)

Fig. 13.1 (*continued*) (b1) Bilateral lower motor neurone VIIth nerve palsy (Guillain–Barré syndrome); (2) 'Close your eyes'. (c) Ramsay Hunt syndrome.

67 / Systemic sclerosis/CRST syndrome

Record

The *skin* over the *fingers and face* (of this middle-aged female) *is smooth, shiny and tight.* There is *sclerodactyly,* the *nails are atrophic* and there is evidence of *Raynaud's phenomenon* (gl.). There is atrophy of the soft tissues at the ends of the fingers. There is *telangiectasia* of the face and pigmentation. There are nodules of *calcinosis** palpable in some of the fingers.

The diagnosis is systemic sclerosis or CRST† syndrome.

Other signs which may be present

Skin ulcers

Vitiligo (p. 214)

Dry eyes and dry mouth (Sjögren's syndrome (gl.))

Dyspnoea or inspiratory crackles (diffuse interstitial fibrosis‡—decreased pulmonary diffusion capacity is the first sign; overspill pneumonitis may also occur).

Other systems which may be involved

Oesophagus (dysphagia or other oesophageal symptoms are present in 45–60%; oesophageal manometry is abnormal and shows diminished peristalsis in 90%)

Kidney (renal failure occurs in 20%—it is late but often fatal; it may be associated with malignant hypertension which tends to be responsive to ACE inhibitors but is otherwise resistant to therapy)

Heart (pericardial effusion is not an uncommon finding if careful echocardiography is performed; cardiomyopathy may occur but is rare)

Musculoskeletal (inflammatory arthritis or myositis—their presence raises the possibility of mixed connective tissue disease§ and therefore an increased likelihood of improvement with steroid therapy)

Intestine (rarely hypomotility with a dilated second part of the duodenum leads to bacterial overgrowth, which in turn leads to steatorrhoea and malabsorption; wide-mouthed colonic diverticuli, and the rare pneumatosis cystoides are other abnormalities which may occur)

Liver (may be associated with primary biliary cirrhosis—p. 70).

---

* If there is diffuse deposition of calcium in subcutaneous tissue in the presence of acrosclerosis this is termed the Thibierge–Weissenbach syndrome.

† CRST or CREST is the association of calcinosis, Raynaud's, oesophageal involvement, sclerodactyly and telangiectasia. It may be a variant of systemic sclerosis associated with a more benign prognosis.

‡ Pulmonary hypertension (gl.) may develop independent of parenchymal changes, suggesting primary pulmonary vessel disease which may respond to steroids. Renal failure has now been replaced by pulmonary complications as the major cause of death in systemic sclerosis. Pleural effusions, pulmonary hypertension, interstitial lung disease, progressive pulmonary fibrosis and obstructive airways disease, all contribute to respiratory failure. Pulmonary hypertension can develop suddenly; all patients should be followed closely for the changes in P_2. The appearance of tricuspid regurgitation is evidence of established pulmonary hypertension. Aggressive vasodilatation therapy should be used to treat pulmonary hypertension.

§ Mixed connective tissue disease is a clinical overlap between systemic sclerosis, SLE and polymyositis (gl.). The serum has a high titre of antiribonuclear protein antibody. The fluorescent antinuclear antibodies are typically distributed in a speckled pattern.

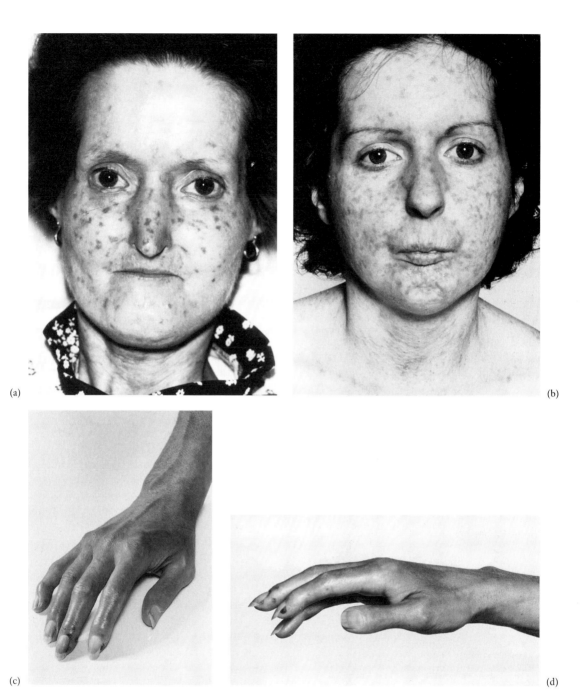

Fig. 13.2 (a) Note the telangiectasia, pinched nose and adherent skin. (b) Perioral tethering with pseudorhagades. (c) Tight, shiny, adherent skin and vasculitis. (d) Atrophy of the finger pulps.

68 / Osler–Weber–Rendu syndrome

Record

There is *telangiectasia* on the face, around the *mouth*, on the lips, on the *tongue* (look under the tongue), the buccal and nasal mucosa and on the fingers, of this (?clinically anaemic) patient (who has none of the features of systemic sclerosis—p. 176).

The diagnosis is Osler–Weber–Rendu syndrome (hereditary haemorrhagic telangiectasia). The lesions may occur elsewhere, especially in the gastrointestinal tract, and may bleed. Patients may present with *epistaxis* (the most common and sometimes the only site of bleeding), *gastrointestinal haemorrhage*, chronic iron deficiency *anaemia* and occasionally with haemorrhage elsewhere (e.g. haemoptysis).

This syndrome is usually considered to be autosomal dominant. In fact it is a family of disorders caused by mutations in various genes.

The telangiectasis consists of a localized collection of non-contractile capillaries and shows a prolonged bleeding time if punctured. In some variants (the pattern in individual families tends to be constant) pulmonary arteriovenous aneurysms are common and increase in frequency (as do the telangiectases) with advancing age. These cases may have *cyanosis* and *clubbing*, and *bruits* over the lung fields. The neurological complications include haemorrhage and the formation of bland or mycotic aneurysms. In the eye there may be bloody tears (conjunctival telangiectasia); retinal haemorrhage or detachment may occur. Cirrhosis (due to telangiectasia or multiple transfusions) and massive intrahepatic shunting may occur.

Treatment

Chronic oral iron therapy may be required. Oestrogens (inducing squamous metaplasia of the nasal mucosa) may be helpful if epistaxis is the main symptom. Also for epistaxis, a low dose of the antifibrinolytic agent, aminocaproic acid, may be successful but should not yet be considered the standard approach. Individual lesions should not be cauterized.

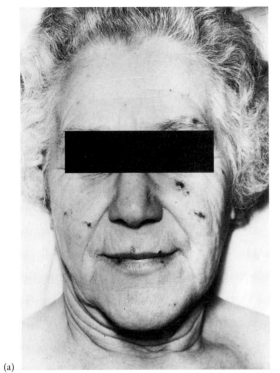

(a)

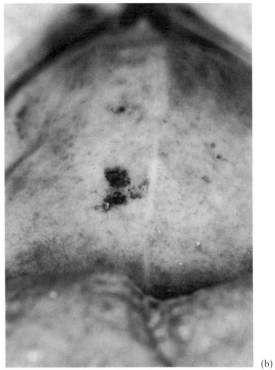

(b)

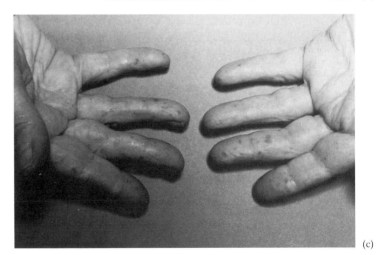

(c)

Fig. 13.3 (a,b) Facial and palatal telangiectasia. (c) Telangiectasiae of the fingers.

69 / Horner's syndrome

Record

There is *miosis,* * *enophthalmos* and slight *ptosis* on the R/L side (the other features are ipsilateral *anhydrosis* and vasodilatation of the head and neck).

This is a R/L-sided Horner's syndrome—now examine the *neck* (scars, nodes, aneurysms), *hands* (wasting of the small muscles) and *chest* (ipsilateral apical signs).

Causes of Horner's syndrome

1 Neck surgery or trauma (?scars).

2 Carotid and aortic aneurysms.

3 Brainstem vascular disease (e.g. Wallenberg's syndrome (gl.)†).

4 Pancoast's syndrome (?wasting of ipsilateral small muscles of the hand, T1 and sometimes C7/C8 sensory loss and pain, clubbing, tracheal deviation, lymph nodes, ipsilateral apical signs).

5 Enlarged cervical lymph nodes especially malignant (?evidence of primary).

6 Idiopathic (common in neurological practice).

7 Syringomyelia (gl.) (?bilateral wasting of the small muscles of the hand, dissociated sensory loss, scarred hands, bulbar palsy, pyramidal signs, nystagmus).

8 Brainstem demyelination (?nystagmus, cerebellar signs, pyramidal signs, pale discs, etc.).

The syndrome can be caused by any other lesion in the sympathetic nervous system as it travels from the sympathetic nucleus, down through the brainstem to the cord, out of the cord at C8, T1 and T2, to the sympathetic chain, stellate ganglion and carotid sympathetic plexus (Fig. 13.4). Some cases of Horner's are idiopathic (usually females).

---

* NB Argyll Robertson pupils in neurosyphilis are usually bilateral, irregular and very small.

† Ipsilateral Vth, IXth, Xth, XIth nerve lesions, cerebellar ataxia and nystagmus. Contralateral pain and temperature loss.

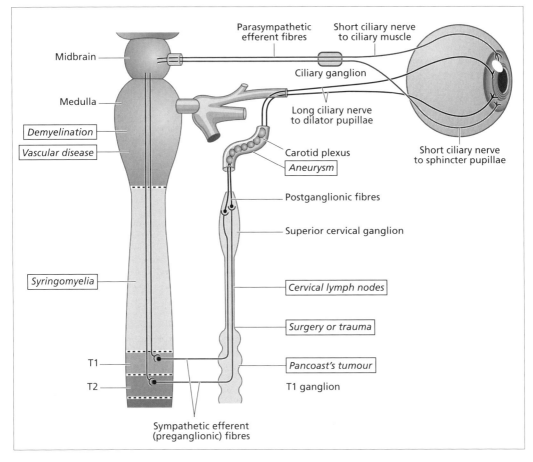

Fig. 13.4 Sympathetic and parasympathetic nerve supply to dilator and sphincter pupillae. The diagram shows the sympathetic pathway and the sites where it may be interrupted to produce Horner's syndrome. (Pathways diagram adapted from *Gray's Anatomy of the Human Body* by kind permission of the publisher, Lea & Febiger.)

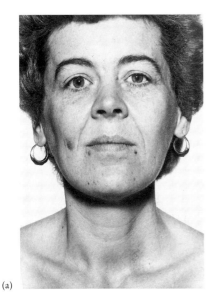

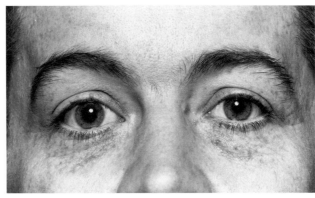

(a)

(b)

Fig. 13.5 (a,b) Left Horner's syndrome (note the scar over the left clavicle).

70 / Systemic lupus erythematosus

Record

There is (in this *young female* patient) a *red, papular butterfly rash* on the face (and elsewhere—especially light-exposed areas) with *scaling, follicular plugging** and *scarring*.

These features suggest lupus erythematosus (chronic discoid lupus erythematosus if only the skin is affected; SLE if there is evidence of multisystem involvement).

Discoid LE—males:females = 1:2.
SLE—males:females = 1:9

Look for other features

Buccal mucosa (sharply defined whitish patches with red borders)
Scalp (scarring alopecia)
Hands and joints (arthritis; deformity may occur but usually mild; Raynaud's (gl.) in 20%)
Skin (vasculitis (gl.)—see below)
Lungs† (pleural effusions, or rarely crepitations from interstitial involvement)
Ankles (oedema—SLE is an important cause of nephrotic syndrome (gl.))
Heart (for pericardial friction rub, rarely pericardial effusion; cardiac enlargement or failure—myocarditis; or murmurs—Libman–Sachs endocarditis)
Proximal muscles (myalgia is common; polymyositis (gl.) may occur)
Eyes (Sjögren's syndrome (gl.); fundal haemorrhages or white exudates called cytoid bodies; papilloedema)

Reticuloendothelial system (lymph nodes; splenomegaly)
Mucous membranes for pallor—anaemia is normochromic normocytic and/or haemolytic (Coombs' test (gl.) is positive or negative); thrombocytopenia often occurs; haematological changes may antedate the other features of the disease by years
Hepatomegaly (chronic passive congestion—usually transient‡)
Urine (proteinuria and haematuria).

NB In SLE vasculitic rashes occur more commonly than the classic butterfly rash. They characteristically affect the elbows, knees, hands and feet. The rash may be a punctate erythematous rash, palmar erythema, periungual erythema or livedo reticularis. Subcutaneous nodules may occur (5%) somewhat resembling those encountered in rheumatoid arthritis.

---

* Very close examination of the butterfly rash reveals that the scales in many areas appear as dots. These dots indicate where the follicle has been plugged by a scale. When the scales are removed (very unlikely to be required in an examination) and the undersurface is inspected, they clearly appear as tiny spicules projecting form the scaly mass. No other scaly condition produces this phenomenon. Healing of the discoid lesions occurs with atrophy, scarring (telangiectasia), hyperpigmentation or hypopigmentation (vitiligo).
† Drug-induced SLE involves the lungs more commonly and kidneys less commonly than classic SLE. The commonest (90%) drugs are hydralazine (slow acetylator), isoniazid, phenytoin and procainamide (rapid acetylators). Other drugs

include hydrochlorothiazide, oral contraceptives, penicillin, practotol, reserpine, streptomycin, sulphonamides, minocycline and tetracycline.
‡ The liver biopsy may be normal or show fatty infiltration and/or fibrosis. These manifestations in SLE should not be confused with the form of chronic active hepatitis, which often has a positive antinuclear factor, called 'lupoid hepatitis'. The liver biopsy in the latter shows an inflammatory infiltrate extending into the liver lobule, causing erosion of the limiting plate and piecemeal necrosis. Fibrous septa isolate rosettes of cells. Cirrhosis is usually present and eventually hepatic failure may develop.

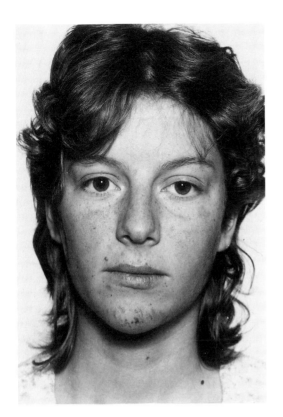

Fig. 13.6 Butterfly rash.

Chapter 14
Examine this patient's hands

Possible short cases include
Rheumatoid hands (p. 189)
Systemic sclerosis/CRST syndrome (p. 176)
Wasting of the small muscles of the hand (p. 192)
Psoriatic arthropathy/psoriasis (p. 195)
Ulnar nerve palsy (p. 198)
Clubbing (p. 200)
Osteoarthrosis (p. 202)
Raynaud's phenomenon (gl.)
Vasculitis (gl.)
Steroid changes (especially purpura)
Acromegaly (p. 257)
Motor neurone disease (p. 110)
Xanthomata (p. 231)
Cyanosis
Chronic liver disease (p. 62)
Thyroid acropachy (gl.)
Carpal tunnel syndrome (p. 204)
Osler–Weber–Rendu syndrome (p. 178)
Tophaceous gout (p. 207)
Dystrophia myotonica (p. 209)

Other diagnoses include: neurofibromatosis (p. 219), systemic lupus erythematosus (SLE) (p. 182), cervical myelopathy (p. 106), dermatomyositis (gl.)
('Examine hands and face'), nail–patella syndrome ('Examine hands and
knees'), Charcot–Marie–Tooth disease (p. 115), superior vena cava obstruction (gl.), facioscapulohumeral muscular dystrophy (gl.), Addison's disease
and Marfan's syndrome (gl.).

Examination *routine*
Experience suggests that when you hear this instruction, rheumatoid arthritis
is likely to be present in about a quarter of the cases, and either scleroderma,
wasting of the small muscles of the hand, psoriasis, ulnar nerve palsy, clubbing
or osteoarthrosis in about a further half. As you approach the patient you
should bear this in mind and look specifically at
1 the **face** for the typical expressionless facies, with adherent shiny skin,
sometimes with telangiectasis (*systemic sclerosis*). It is clear from the list above

that a variety of other conditions may show signs in either the face or in the general appearance, particularly *cushingoid* facies (steroid changes in a patient with rheumatoid arthritis), *acromegalic* facies, *arcus senilis* or *xanthelasma* (xanthomata), *icterus* and *spider naevi* (chronic liver disease) or *exophthalmos* (thyroid acropachy). We leave you to consider the changes you may note as you approach the patient with the other conditions on the list (see individual short cases). Even if the diagnosis is not immediately clear on looking at the face it is likely that in many cases it will become rapidly apparent as you

   2 **inspect the hands**. Run quickly through the six main conditions that make up 75% of cases:

   (a) *rheumatoid arthritis* (proximal joint swelling, spindling of the fingers, ulnar deviation, nodules),
   (b) *systemic sclerosis* (sclerodactyly with tapering of the fingers, sometimes with gangrene of the fingertips, tight, shiny, adherent skin, calcified nodules, etc.),
   (c) generalized *wasting* of the small muscles of the hand, perhaps with dorsal guttering,
   (d) *psoriasis* (pitting of the nails, terminal interphalangeal arthropathy, scaly rash),
   (e) *ulnar nerve palsy* (may be a typical claw hand or may be muscle wasting which spares the thenar eminence; often this diagnosis will only become apparent when you have made a sensory examination), and
   (f) *clubbing*.

The changes that you may see in the other conditions in the list are dealt with under the individual short cases, but if in these first few seconds you have not made a rapid spot diagnosis, study first the dorsal and then the palmar aspects of the hands, looking specifically at

   3 the **joints** for swelling, deformity or Heberden's nodes (gl.) (*osteoarthrosis*);
   4 the **nails** for pitting, onycholysis (gl.), clubbing, nail-fold infarcts (vasculitis — usually rheumatoid) or splinter haemorrhages (unlikely);
   5 the **skin** for *colour* (pigmentation, icterus, palmar erythema), for *consistency* (tight and shiny in scleroderma; papery thin, perhaps with purpuric patches in steroid therapy; thick in acromegaly) and for *lesions* (psoriasis, vasculitis, purpura, xanthomata, spider naevi, telangiectasis in Osler–Weber–Rendu and systemic sclerosis, tophi, neurofibromata, other rashes);
   6 the **muscles** for isolated *wasting* of the thenar eminence (median nerve lesion), for generalized wasting especially of the first dorsal interosseous but sparing the thenar eminence (ulnar nerve lesion), for generalized wasting from a T1 lesion or other cause (p. 192) or for *fasciculation* which usually indicates motor neurone disease, though occasionally it can occur in other conditions such as syringomyelia (gl.), old polio or Charcot–Marie–Tooth disease.

   Before leaving the inspection it is worth looking specifically for *skin crease pigmentation* before moving to

   7 **palpation** of the hands for Dupuytren's contracture (gl.), nodules (may be palpable in the palms in rheumatoid arthritis), calcinosis (scleroderma/ CRST), xanthomata, Heberden's nodes or tophi. In the vast majority of cases

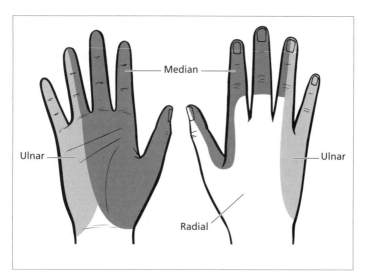

Fig. 14.1 Dermatomes in the hand.

you will have, by now, some findings demanding either specific further action (see below) or a report with a diagnosis. Nonetheless, you should be prepared to continue with a full neurological examination of the hands to confirm a suspected neurological lesion, or if you have still made no diagnosis. If the hands appear normal it may be that there is a sensory defect. In these cases, it is more efficient, therefore, to commence the examination by testing

8 **sensation**. If you feel the examiners will not object, ask the patient if there has been any numbness or tingling in his hands and if so, when (?worse at night — carpal tunnel syndrome) and where. Bearing in mind the classic patterns of sensory defect in ulnar and median nerve lesions (Fig. 14.1) and the dermatomes (see Fig. 7.1, p. 91) seek and define an area of deficit to *pinprick* and *light touch* (dab cotton wool lightly), and check the *vibration* and *joint position* sense. With incomplete sensory loss due to either an ulnar or a median nerve defect, if you stroke the medial border of the little finger and the lateral border of the index finger with your fingers simultaneously, the patient may sense that one side feels different from the other.

9 Check the **tone** of the muscles in the hand by flexing and extending all the joints including the wrist in a 'rolling wave' fashion.

10 The **motor** system of the hands can be tested with the instructions:

(a) 'Open your hands; now close them; now open and close them quickly' (dystrophia myotonica),*

(b) 'Squeeze my fingers' — offer two fingers (C8,T1),†

(c) 'Hold your fingers out straight' (demonstrate); 'stop me bending them' (C7),

(d) 'Spread your fingers apart' (demonstrate); 'stop me pushing them together' (Fig. 14.2) (dorsal‡ interossei — ulnar nerve),

---

* Alternatively, you could miss this step out and go straight to step (b), but then issue the instruction 'Let go' and if there is any suspicion of dystrophia myotonica move to step (a).

† Some neurologists prefer to test the deep finger flexors by trying to extend flexed fingers, whilst steadying the wrist (flexor digitorum profundus C8).

‡ Remember DAB and PAD: DAB = dorsal abduct, PAD = palmar adduct.

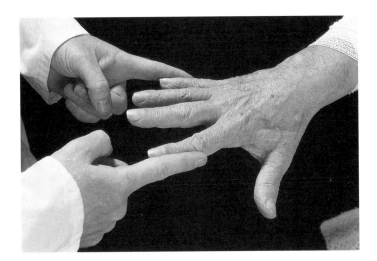

Fig. 14.2 Testing abduction of the fingers — dorsal interossei (ulnar nerve).

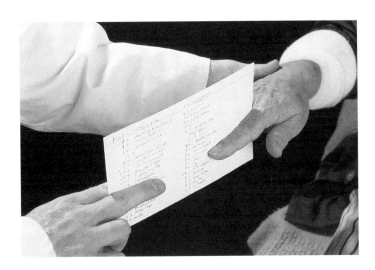

Fig. 14.3 Testing adduction of the fingers — palmar interossei (ulnar nerve).

(e) 'Hold this piece of paper between your fingers; stop me pulling it out' (Fig. 14.3) (palmar‡ interossei — ulnar nerve),

(f) 'Point your thumb at the ceiling; stop me pushing it down' (Fig. 14.4) (abductor pollicis brevis — median nerve),

(g) 'Put your thumb and little finger together; stop me pulling them apart' (Fig. 14.5) (opponens pollicis — median nerve).

Finally, for the sake of completeness, check the

11 radial pulses.

The action you take after finding an abnormality at any stage during the above *routine* will depend on what you find. Most commonly an abnormality found during the inspection will lead to most of the above being skipped in favour of a search for other evidence of the condition you suspect. It is worth emphasizing that there may be clues at

12 the **elbows** in several of the common conditions: rheumatoid arthritis (nodules), psoriatic arthropathy (psoriatic plaques), ulnar nerve palsy (scar,

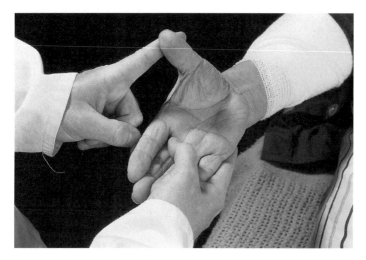

Fig. 14.4 Testing abduction of the thumb—abductor pollicis brevis (median nerve).

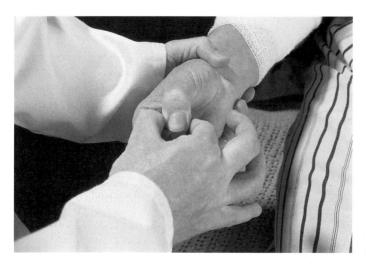

Fig. 14.5 Testing the opponens pollicis (median nerve).

filling of the ulnar groove, restriction of range of movement at the elbow or evidence of fracture) and xanthomata. On the above evidence you will need to examine the elbows in over 40% of cases (do not be put off by rolled-down sleeves). It is worth considering where else you would look, what for and what other tests you would do with the other conditions on the list (see individual short cases), but in particular remember to look for *tophi* on the ears if you suspect gout, and if you have diagnosed acromegaly seek an associated *carpal tunnel syndrome*. If on inspection you suspect a neurological deficit in the hand, you may wish to confirm it by performing only that part of the above *routine* relevant to that lesion, e.g. testing abduction and opposition of the thumb and seeking the classic sensory pattern if you see lone wasting of the thenar eminence and suspect carpal tunnel syndrome.

For *checklist* see p. 277.

71 / Rheumatoid hands

Record

There is a *symmetrical deforming arthropathy*. There is *spindling* of the fingers due to soft tissue swelling at the *proximal interphalangeal* joints and *metacarpophalangeal joints*. There is generalized *wasting* of the *small muscles* of the hand and use is restricted by weakness, deformity and pain. There are *nodules* at the elbow, over the extensor tendons and in the palm. There is *ulnar deviation* of the fingers (consequent upon subluxation and dislocation at the metacarpophalangeal joints). The *terminal interphalangeal joints are spared*. There are arteritic lesions* in the nail folds.

The patient has rheumatoid arthritis.

The ratio of males to females is 1:3.

Other features which may occur

'Swan neck' deformity (*hyperextension of the proximal interphalangeal* joint with fixed flexion of the metacarpophalangeal and terminal interphalangeal joints)

Boutonnière deformity (flexion deformity of the proximal interphalangeal joint with *extension contracture of the terminal interphalangeal* and metacarpophalangeal joints)

Z deformity of the thumb

Triggering of the finger (flexor tendon nodule)

Palmar erythema

Iatrogenic Cushing's (?facies, thin atrophic skin, purpura)

Swollen or deformed knees (p. 117)

Cervical spine disease (upper cervical spine, especially atlantoaxial joint—subluxation can occur with *spinal cord compression*; a lateral X-ray centred on the odontoid peg with the neck in full flexion shows the distance from the odontoid to the anterior arch of the atlas as abnormal at more than 3 mm—general anaesthesia is dangerous and requires extreme care in neck handling)

Anaemia (five causes†)

Chest signs (?pleural effusions; fibrosing alveolitis‡)

Neurological signs (?peripheral neuropathy, mononeuritis multiplex, carpal tunnel syndrome)

Eye signs (episcleritis, painful scleritis, scleromalacia perforans (gl.), cataracts due to chloroquine or steroids)

Sjögren's syndrome (gl.) (?dry eyes, dry mouth)

Felty's syndrome (gl.) (?spleen)

Leg ulceration (vasculitic)*

---

* As well as causing nail-fold infarcts and chronic leg ulceration, the vasculitis (gl.) which is immune complex-induced and may affect small, medium or large vessels, may also lead to digital gangrene. A purpuric rash may occur due to capillaritis. Raynaud's phenomenon (gl.) may occur. Pyoderma gangrenosum (gl.) is a rare cause of ulceration.

† The five causes of anaemia in rheumatoid arthritis are:

1 Anaemia of chronic disease (normochromic normocytic)

2 Gastrointestinal bleeding related to non-steroidal anti-inflammatory agents

3 Bone marrow suppression (gold, phenylbutazone, indomethacin, penicillamine)

4 Megaloblastic anaemia (folic acid deficiency or associated pernicious anaemia; see organ-specific autoimmune disease, p. 214 and footnote)

5 Felty's syndrome.

‡ The lungs may also be affected in other ways. Rheumatoid nodules may occur in the lung fields on chest X-ray and in patients exposed to certain dusts—especially coal miners. The nodules may be accompanied by massive fibrotic reactions (Caplan's syndrome (gl.)). Obliterative bronchiolitis is a severe but rare complication which may be associated with penicillamine therapy.

Cardiac signs (pericarditis is present in up to 40% of patients at autopsy but is rarely apparent clinically; myocarditis, conduction defects and valvular incompetence are rare consequences of granulomatous infiltration)

Secondary amyloidosis (gl.) (?proteinuria, hepatosplenomegaly, etc. — see footnote, p. 61)

Other autoimmune disorders (see pp. 162 and 214).

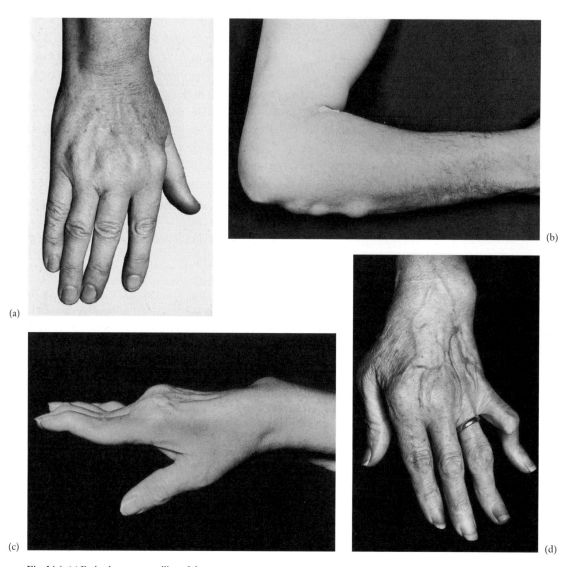

(a)

(b)

(c)

(d)

Fig. 14.6 (a) Early changes — swelling of the metacarpophalangeal joints and slight ulnar deviation. (b) Rheumatoid nodules. (c) 'Swan neck' deformity. (d) Boutonnière deformity.

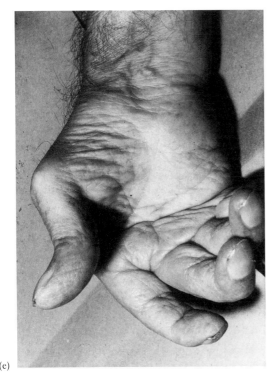

(e)

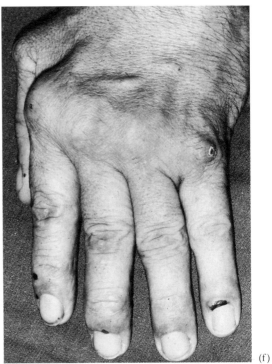

(f)

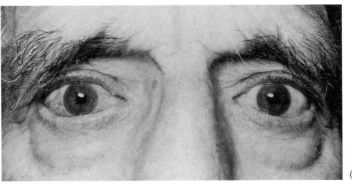

(g)

Fig. 14.6 (*continued*) (e) Z-shaped
thumb. (f) Vasculitis. (g) Episcleritis.

72 / Wasting of the small muscles of the hand

Record
There is *wasting* (and weakness) of the *thenar* and *hypothenar* eminences and of the other small muscles of the hand so that *dorsal guttering* is seen. There is (may be) hyperextension at the metacarpophalangeal joints and flexion at the interphalangeal joints (due to the action of the long extensors of the fingers being unopposed by the lumbricals. In the advanced case a claw hand or *main-en-griffe* is produced).

Generalized wasting of the small muscles of the hand suggests a lesion affecting the lower motor neurones which originate at the level C8,T1 (unless there is arthropathy leading to disuse atrophy).

Causes
A lesion affecting the anterior horn cells at the level C8,T1 such as:

Motor neurone disease (?prominent fasciculation, spastic paraparesis, wasted fibrillating tongue, no sensory signs—p. 110)

Syringomyelia (gl.) (fasciculation not prominent, ?dissociated sensory loss, burn scars, Horner's, nystagmus)

Charcot–Marie–Tooth disease* (?distal wasting of the lower limb, pes cavus, etc.—p. 115)

Other causes are old polio, tumour, meningovascular syphilis and cord compression.

A root lesion at the level C8,T1 such as:

Cervical spondylosis affecting the C8,T1 level (usually affects higher roots—C6,C7—and therefore significant wasting of the small muscles of the hand is uncommon—see p. 106; ?pyramidal signs in the legs, no signs above the level of the lesion, cervical collar)

Tumour at the C8,T1 level (e.g. neurofibroma).

A lesion damaging the brachial plexus (especially the lower trunk and medial cord) such as:

Cervical rib (symptoms provoked by a particular posture or movement, e.g. sleeping on the limb, cleaning windows, etc.; ?supraclavicular bruit though Raynaud's (gl.) and other vascular manifestations are rare in the presence of prominent neurological features)

Pancoast's tumour (?Horner's, clubbing, chest signs, lymph nodes, cachexia, etc.)

Damage caused by violent traction of the arm (e.g. a patient who tried to stop himself falling from a tree by grabbing a passing branch; the same damage in obstetric practice produces Klumpke's paralysis).

Combined ulnar and median nerve lesions (see pp. 198 and 204, respectively).

Arthritis leading to disuse atrophy† (wasting out of proportion to weakness).

Cachexia.

---

* It is not known whether the degenerative process in Charcot–Marie–Tooth disease originates in the distal axons, ventral nerve roots or in the anterior horn cells.
† For example, rheumatoid arthritis. The factors which may contribute to small muscle wasting in the hand in rheumatoid arthritis are disuse atrophy, vasculitis (gl.), peripheral neuropathy, mononeuritis multiplex and entrapment neuropathy (median nerve at the wrist, ulnar nerve at the elbow, and branches—e.g. the deep palmar branch of the ulnar nerve damaged by subluxation of the carpal bones on the radius and ulna).

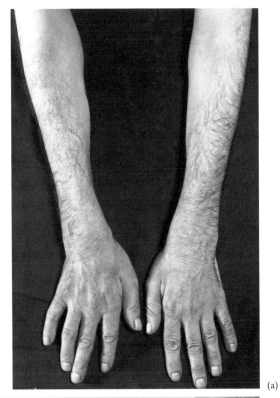

(a)

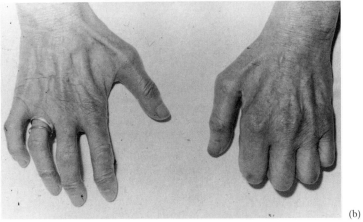

(b)

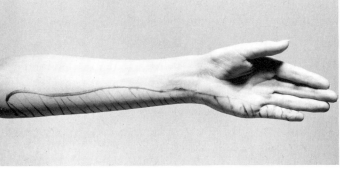

Fig. 14.7 (a) Charcot—Marie—
Tooth disease. (b) Motor neurone
disease. (c) Cervical rib.

(c)

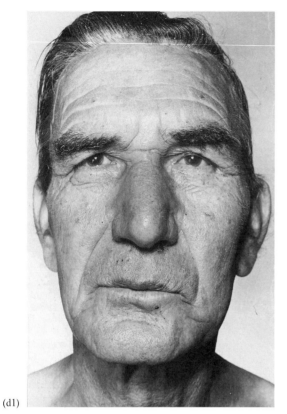

(d1)

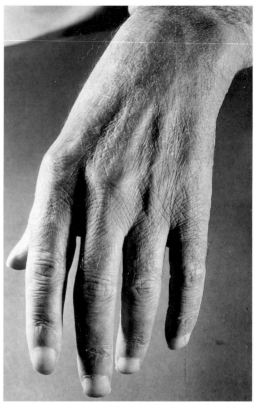

(d2)

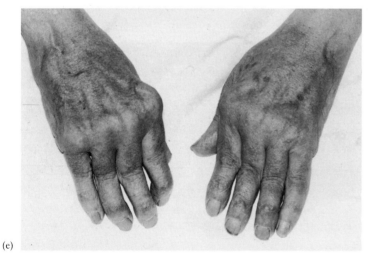

(e)

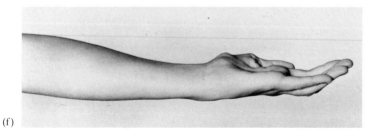

(f)

Fig. 14.7 (*continued*)
(d1,2) Pancoast's tumour (note left
Horner's syndrome and clubbing).
(e) Rheumatoid arthritis. (f) *Main-en-
griffe* (cervical rib).

73 / Psoriatic arthropathy/psoriasis

Note: patients may have arthropathy and/or skin lesions.

Record

There is an *asymmetrical arthropathy* involving mainly the *terminal interphalangeal joints*. There is *pitting* of the fingernails and *onycholysis* (gl.). Some of the nail plates (say which) are thickened and there is a thick scale (*hyperkeratosis*) under them. There are patches of psoriasis at the *elbows*. The plaques are circular with well-defined edges and they are *red* with a *silvery scaly* surface.

The patient has psoriatic arthropathy.

Psoriatic arthropathy (even if severe) can occur with minimal skin involvement.* If there is no obvious psoriasis at the elbows the following areas should particularly be checked for skin lesions:

1 Extensor aspects
2 Scalp
3 Behind the ears
4 In the navel.

Other forms of psoriatic arthropathy

Arthritis mutilans (see Fig. 14.8f)
Arthritis clinically indistinguishable from rheumatoid arthritis but consistently seronegative
Asymmetrical oligo- or monoarthropathy
Ankylosing spondylitis occurring alone or in conjunction with any of the other forms.

Treatment

Treatments of the skin lesions include sunlight, ultraviolet light, coal tar, dithranol, local steroids, calipotriol, PUVA (psoralen and ultraviolet A light). Systemic treatment with acitretin (a retinoid) or antimetabolites (methotrexate, azathioprine, hydroxyurea), because of their side-effects, should be reserved for severe widespread disease unresponsive to topical measures. Analgesic anti-inflammatory agents are used for the pain of the arthropathy. Sulphasalazine and methotrexate are becoming established as effective agents for the treatment of psoriatic arthropathy. Gold and penicillamine may be useful, but few controlled studies have been done. Cyclosporin may also have a place in refractory disease. Choroquine is contraindicated as it may exacerbate the skin lesions (exfoliative dermatitis). Intra-articular steroids are useful for a single inflamed troublesome joint.

Incidence

Found in 1–5% of Caucasians in north-western Europe and the USA, but uncommon among the Japanese, North American Indians and Afro-Americans.

---

* There is no evidence of a link between the activity of the skin lesions and the arthropathy.

74 / Ulnar nerve palsy

Record

The hand shows *generalized muscle wasting** and *weakness* which *spares* the *thenar eminence*. There is sensory loss over the *fifth finger*, the *adjacent half* of the *fourth finger* and the dorsal and palmar aspects of the *medial side* of the *hand*.† (Look for hyperextension at the metacarpophalangeal joints with flexion of the interphalangeal joints in the fourth and fifth fingers—the *ulnar claw hand*.)‡

The patient has an ulnar nerve lesion. (Now examine the elbow for a cause.)

Likely causes

1 Fracture or dislocation at the elbow (?scar or deformity; history of injury).

2 Osteoarthrosis at the elbow with osteophytic encroachment on the ulnar nerve in the cubital tunnel ('filling in' of the ulnar groove due to palpable enlargement of the nerve; limitation of elbow movement is often seen; certain occupations predispose to osteoarthrosis at the elbow—see below).

Other causes

Occupations with constant leaning on elbows (clerks, secretaries on telephone, etc.)

Occupations with constant flexion and extension at the elbow (bricklayer, painter/decorator, carpenter, roofer—shallow ulnar groove will predispose; these occupations may also lead to osteoarthrosis—see above)

Excessive carrying angle at elbow (malunited fracture of the humerus or disturbance of growth leading to cubitus valgus and, over the years, 'tardy ulnar nerve palsy')

Injuries at the wrist or in the palm (different degrees of the syndrome depending on which branches of the nerve are damaged; e.g. occupations using screwdrivers, drills, etc.)

The causes of mononeuritis multiplex (diabetes, polyarteritis nodosa (gl.) and Churg–Strauss syndrome (gl.), rheumatoid arthritis, SLE, Wegener's granulomatosis (gl.), sarcoidosis (gl.), carcinoma, amyloidosis (gl.), leprosy (gl.), Sjögren's syndrome (gl.), Lyme disease (gl.)).

NB Other causes of wasting of the small muscles of the hand (p. 192) may sometimes resemble ulnar nerve palsy. The major features pointing to ulnar nerve palsy as the cause are *sparing of the thenar eminence* and the characteristic sensory loss pattern. The main distin-

---

* (i) The *hypothenar eminence wastes*, though in the manual worker with thickened skin the hand contour may be preserved and the wasting may only be detected on palpation. Loss of the other small muscles is seen from (ii) *loss of the first dorsal interosseous* in the dorsal space between the first and second metacarpals and (iii) *guttering of the dorsum* of the hand— which becomes more prominent as the lesion advances.

† *Record* (continuation): there is *weakness of abduction* and *adduction of the fingers*, and *adduction of the extended thumb* against the palm (inability to grip a piece of paper between the thumb and index finger without flexing the affected thumb— Froment's 'thumb sign'). Flexion of the fourth and fifth

fingers is weak. When the proximal portions of these fingers are held immobilized, flexion of the terminal phalanges is not possible. There is also *wasting of the medial aspect of the forearm* (flexor carpi ulnaris and half of the flexor digitorum profundus). When the hand is flexed to the ulnar side against resistance the tendon of the flexor carpi ulnaris is not palpable.

‡ The ulnar claw hand or partial *main-en-griffe* is due to the unopposed action of the long extensors and is only seen in the fourth and fifth fingers because the radial lumbricals are supplied by the median nerve.

guishing features of the differential diagnoses which may mimic the muscle wasting of ulnar paralysis are:

Syringomyelia (gl.)—dissociated sensory loss extending beyond the ulnar zone; loss of arm reflexes; ?Horner's

C8 lesion (e.g. Pancoast's syndrome)—sensory loss involves radial side of the fourth finger; ?Horner's

Cervical rib—objective sensory disturbances are usually slight or absent and without characteristic ulnar distribution.

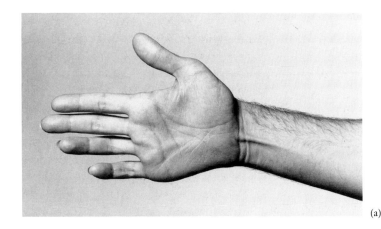

(a)

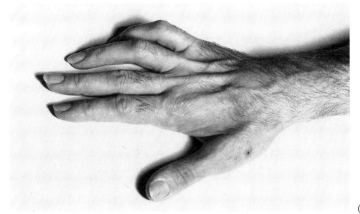

(b)

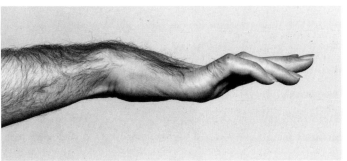

(c)

Fig. 14.9 (a) Loss of the hypothenar eminence. (b) Dorsal guttering. (c) Typical ulnar claw hand.

75 / Clubbing

Record

There is finger clubbing* (*thickening of the nail bed*† with *loss of the obtuse angle* between the nail and the dorsum of the finger—becomes >180°‡; *increased curvature* of the nail bed—both side-to-side and lengthwise; increased *sponginess or fluctuation* of the nail bed; and sometimes, when there is marked swelling of the nail bed, the fingers may have a *drumstick appearance*).

Causes of clubbing

1 Carcinoma of the bronchus (the commonest cause—?nicotine staining, obvious weight loss with temporal dimples, lymph nodes, chest signs, evidence of secondaries, etc.—p. 46).
2 Fibrosing alveolitis (?basal crackles—p. 40).
3 Cyanotic congenital heart disease (gl.) (?cyanosis, thoracotomy scars, Fallot's tetralogy (gl.), Eisenmenger's (gl.)).
4 Bronchiectasis (?productive cough, crepitations, etc.—p. 41).
5 Cirrhosis (?icterus, spider naevi, palmar erythema, Dupuytren's (gl.), xanthelasma—especially in primary biliary cirrhosis, hepatosplenomegaly, etc.—p. 61).

Other causes

Subacute bacterial endocarditis (heart murmur, fever, splenomegaly, petechiae, splinter haemorrhages, Osler's nodes (gl.), Janeway's lesions (gl.), Roth's spots (gl.), etc.)
Empyema
Lung abscess

Crohn's disease
Ulcerative colitis (gl.)
Asbestosis (gl.) (especially with mesothelioma (gl.))
Thyroid acropachy (gl.) (?exophthalmos, pretibial myxoedema, goitre, thyroid status, etc.—p. 247)
Hereditary (rare; dominant).

* Indisputable clubbing is one of the important fundamental clinical signs which, when present, have clear implications. Less clear-cut changes in the finger nails are susceptible to assessment which (even if dogmatic) may be very subjective. Such finger nails are best described as showing 'debatable clubbing' (in that physicians will disagree as to whether there are significant changes or not). Genuine 'debatable clubbing' occurring in an examination may cause trouble if you recognize it as such, but you are not sure what your examiner's opinion is. The safest course in a case of doubt is to use nail bed thickening as your guide and quote the nail angle rule in a way that cannot be argued with. For example:

'The appearance of the nails (e.g. increased curvature) is initially suggestive of clubbing, but the obtuse angle between the nail and the dorsum of the finger is preserved, and therefore by definition (loss of the angle being the "official" first sign) the diagnosis of definite clubbing cannot be accepted in this case.'
† Before palpating always inspect the fingers in profile for a slightly bulbous appearance due to thickening of the nail bed.
‡ *Shamroth's sign*: If you put the fingernails of the same fingers of each of your hands together, against each other, you will see a gap at their base between them. This gap may be lost when the angle is lost in finger clubbing.

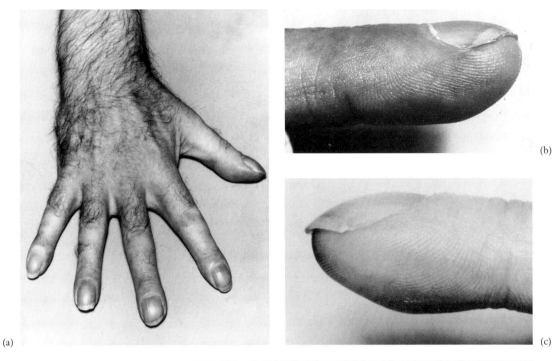

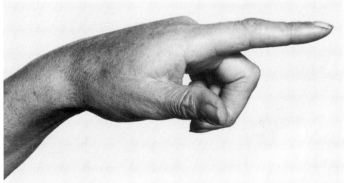

Fig. 14.10 (a) Clubbing (carcinoma of the bronchus). (b) Loss of the angle. (c) Thickening of the nail bed (early drumstick appearance — same patient as in (a)). (d) Clubbing and leuconychia (cirrhosis of the liver).

76 / Osteoarthrosis

Record

There are *Heberden's nodes* (gl.) present at the bases of the distal phalanges (and less commonly Bouchard's nodes at the proximal interphalangeal joints). There is a 'square hand' deformity due to subluxation of the base of the first metacarpal. There is swelling and deformity of the knee joints with development of varus (or valgus) deformity. There is crepitus in these joints. There is wasting and weakness of the quadriceps and glutei, and there is downward tilting of the pelvis when the patient stands on the affected leg (Trendelenberg's sign).

This patients has osteoarthrosis.

Complications

Pain

Deformity

Ankylosis

Entrapment of nerves (e.g. ulnar nerve palsy or carpal tunnel syndrome)

Cervical spondylosis.

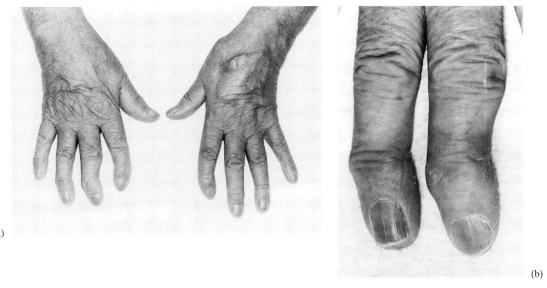

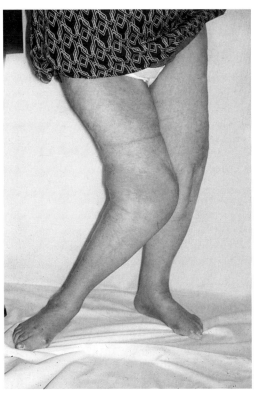

Fig. 14.11 (a,b) Note the square hand deformity, Heberden's nodes and lateral bending of the terminal digits.
(c) Osteoarthrosis of the knee joint with valgus deformity.

(a)

(b)

(c)

77 / Carpal tunnel syndrome

Record

There is (in this ?stout, ?middle-aged lady who complains of pain, numbness or paraesthesiae in the palm and fingers which is particularly bad in the night*) *sensory loss* over the *palmar* aspects of the *first three and a half fingers* and *wasting of the thenar eminence.* There is weakness of *abduction, flexion* and *opposition of the thumb.*

The diagnosis is median nerve palsy. The non-involvement of the flexor muscles of the forearm (i.e. can flex the distal interphalangeal joint of the thumb) suggests that the cause is carpal tunnel syndrome (now check the facies for underlying *acromegaly* or *myxoedema*; underlying *rheumatoid arthritis* should be obvious). *Tinel's sign*† is positive to confirm this.

Though in early cases there may be no abnormal physical signs, usually some impairment of sensation over the affected fingers can be detected. Tenderness on compression of the nerve at the wrist† and thenar atrophy are relatively rare. If the story is characteristic the absence of physical signs should not deter one from advising treatment with intracarpal tunnel steroid injection or carpal tunnel decompression. Investigation with nerve conduction studies may be helpful in cases of doubt.

Causes of carpal tunnel syndrome

Idiopathic (almost entirely females, middle-aged, often obese; or younger women with excessive use of hands; may occur in males after unaccustomed hand use — e.g. house painting)

Pregnancy

Contraceptive pill

Myxoedema (?facies, hoarse croaking voice, pulse, ankle jerks, etc. — p. 251)

Acromegaly (?facies, large spade-shaped hands, bitemporal hemianopia, etc. — p. 257)

Rheumatoid arthritis of the wrists (?spindling of the fingers, ulnar deviation, nodules, etc. — p. 189)

Osteoarthrosis of the carpus (perhaps related to an old fracture)

Tuberculous tenosynovitis

Primary amyloidosis (gl.) (?peripheral neuropathy, thick nerves, autonomic neuropathy; heart, joint and gut (rectal biopsy) involvement may occur — see also footnote, p. 101)

Tophaceous gout (p. 207).

---

* The nocturnal discomfort may be referred to the whole forearm with paraesthesiae extending beyond the cutaneous distribution of the median nerve in the hand. The sensory *signs* however, are confined to the classic median nerve distribution (Fig. 14.1, p. 186).

† *Tinel's sign* is tingling in the distribution of a nerve produced by percussion of that nerve. Percussion over the carpal tunnel sometimes produces a positive Tinel's sign in carpal tunnel syndrome. Other signs are *Phalen's sign* (the patient flexes both wrists for 60 seconds and this produces a prompt exacerbation of paraesthesia which is rapidly relieved when the flexion is discontinued) which is positive in half the patients, and the *tourniquet test* (a sphygmomanometer is pumped above systolic pressure for 2 min and this produces the paraesthesiae). Symptoms may sometimes be induced by *hyperextension* at the wrist.

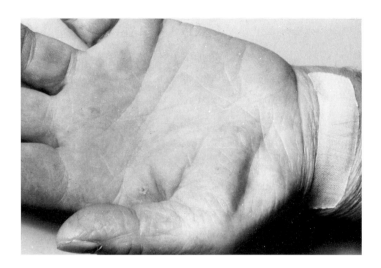

Fig. 14.12 Wasting of the thenar eminence.

78 / Radial nerve palsy

Record

There is *wrist-drop* and sensory loss over the first dorsal interosseous.*
The diagnosis is radial nerve palsy.

The hand hangs limply and the patient is unable to lift it at the wrist or to straighten out the fingers. If the wrist is passively extended he is able to straighten the fingers at the interphalangeal joints (because the interossei and lumbricals still work) but not at the metacarpophalangeal joints where the fingers remain flexed. The patient may feel that his grasp is weak in the affected hand because of the lack of the wrist extension necessary for powerful grip. If the wrist is passively extended the power of grip improves. Abduction and adduction of the fingers may appear weak in radial nerve palsy unless they are tested with the hand resting flat on the table with the fingers extended.

The commonest cause (of this rare condition) is 'Saturday night paralysis' in which the patient, heavily sedated with alcohol, falls asleep with his arm hanging over the back of a chair. The nerve is compressed against the middle third of the humerus, and the brachioradialis (flexion of the arm against resistance — with the arm midway between supination and pronation) and the supinator are also paralysed as well as the forearm extensor muscles. Muscle wasting does not usually occur and complete recovery in a matter of weeks† is usual. If the nerve is injured by a wound in the axilla, paralysis involves the triceps so that extension at the elbow is lost as is the triceps reflex.

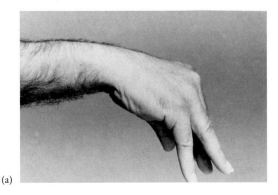
(a)

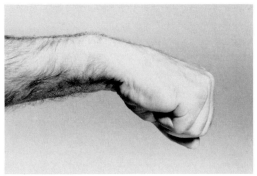
(b)

Fig. 14.13 (a) Wrist-drop. (b) Weak grip due to the missing synergistic effect of an extended wrist.

*Though the cutaneous area supplied by the radial nerve is more extensive than this (Fig. 14.1, p. 186) an overlap in supply by both the median and ulnar nerves usually means that only this small area over the first dorsal interosseous has detectable impaired sensation.

† Usually damage occurs to the myelin sheath only and the Schwann cells will repair the nerve rapidly. If the pressure is prolonged and causes axonal degeneration then the peripheral nerve regeneration rate is about $1 \, mm \, day^{-1}$ (from the undamaged proximal nerve).

79 / Tophaceous gout

Record

There is *asymmetrical swelling* affecting the *small joints* of the *hands* and feet with *tophi* formation (in the periarticular tissues). These joints are (occasionally) severely *deformed*. There are tophi on the *helix* of the *ear* and in some of the tendon sheaths (especially the ulnar surface of the forearm, olecranon bursa, Achilles tendon and other pressure points).

This patient has chronic tophaceous gout.

Chronic tophaceous gout results from recurrent acute attacks. Tophus formation is proportional to the severity and duration of the disease. However, patients with severe tophaceous disease appear to have milder and less frequent acute attacks than non-tophaceous patients. Large tophi may have areas of necrotic skin overlying them and may exude chalky or pasty material containing monosodium urate crystals. Sinuses may form. Tophi may resolve slowly with effective treatment of hyperuricaemia. Effective antihyperuricaemic therapy has reduced the incidence and severity of the tophaceous disease. A major complication is renal disease (urolithiasis, urate nephropathy). Carpal tunnel syndrome may occur.

Associations include obesity, type IV hyperlipidaemia and hypertension. These associations may be the cause of an association which has also been recognized between gout and two other conditions—diabetes mellitus and ischaemic heart disease.

Secondary hyperuricaemia may occur in many situations including:

Drugs—diuretics (especially thiazides), ethambutol, nicotinic acid, cyclosporin

Myeloproliferative and lymphoproliferative disorders (and other conditions with increased turnover of preformed purines)

Chronic renal failure

Alcoholism

Obesity.

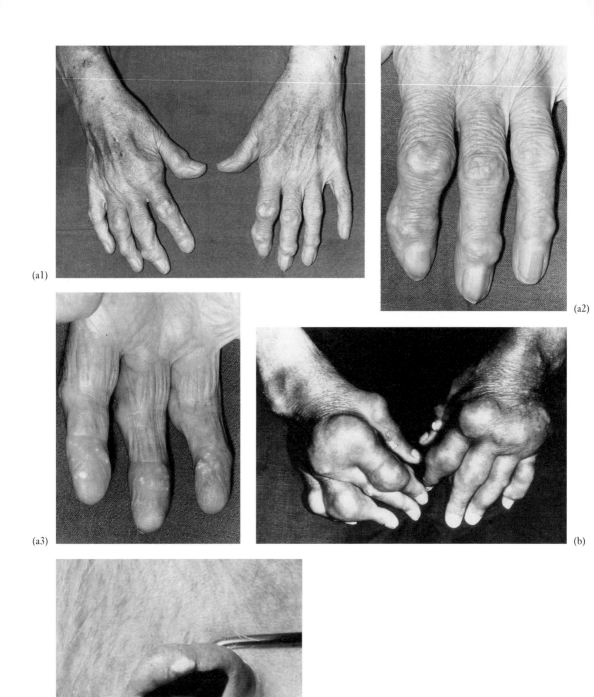

Fig. 14.14 (a1–3) Gouty tophi and arthropathy. (b) An extreme case of tophaceous gout. (c) A tophus on the helix of the ear.

80 / Dystrophia myotonica

Record

The patient has *myopathic facies* (drooping mouth and long, lean, sad, lifeless, somewhat sleepy expression), frontal *balding* (in the male), *ptosis* (may be unilateral) and *wasting* of the *facial muscles*, temporalis, masseter, *sternomastoids*, shoulder girdle and quadriceps. The forearms and legs are involved and the *reflexes* are *lost*. The patient has *cataracts*. After he made a fist he was unable to quickly open it, especially when asked to do this repetitively (this gets worse in the cold and with excitement). He has difficulty opening his eyes after firm closure. When he shook hands there was a delay before he released his grip* (these are all features of *myotonia*). When dimples and depressions are induced in his muscles by percussion, they fill only slowly (*percussion myotonia* —e.g. tongue and thenar eminence).

The diagnosis is dystrophia myotonica.

Males > females.
Autosomal dominant.

Other features

Cardiomyopathy (?small volume pulse, low blood pressure, splitting of the first heart sound in the mitral area; low voltage P wave, prolonged PR interval, notched QRS and prolonged QT_c on the electrocardiogram (ECG); dysrythmias; sudden death may occur)

Intellect and personality deterioration

Slurred speech due to combined tongue and pharyngeal myotonia

Testicular atrophy (small soft testicles but secondary sexual characteristics preserved; usually develops after the patient has had children and thus the disease is perpetuated; evidence regarding ovarian atrophy is indefinite)

Diabetes mellitus (end-organ unresponsiveness to insulin)

Nodular thyroid enlargement, small pituitary fossa but normal pituitary function, dysphagia, abdominal pain, hypoventilation and postanaesthetic respiratory failure may also occur.

The condition may show 'anticipation'— progressively worsening signs and symptoms in succeeding generations; e.g. presenile cataracts may be the sole indication of the disorder in preceding generations.

Myotonia congenita (Thomsen's disease)

There is difficulty in relaxation of a muscle after forceful contraction (myotonia) but none of the other features of dystrophia myotonica (e.g. weakness, cataracts, baldness, gonadal atrophy, etc.). The *reflexes are normal*. Some patients have a 'Herculean' appearance from very developed musculature (?related to repeated involuntary isometric exercise). Myotonia congenita is usually autosomal dominant.

---

* There may be an absence of grip myotonia in advanced disease because of progressive muscle wasting. Though myotonia can be relieved by phenytoin, quinine or procainamide, it is weakness (for which there is no treatment) rather than the myotonia which is the main cause of disability in dystrophia myotonica.

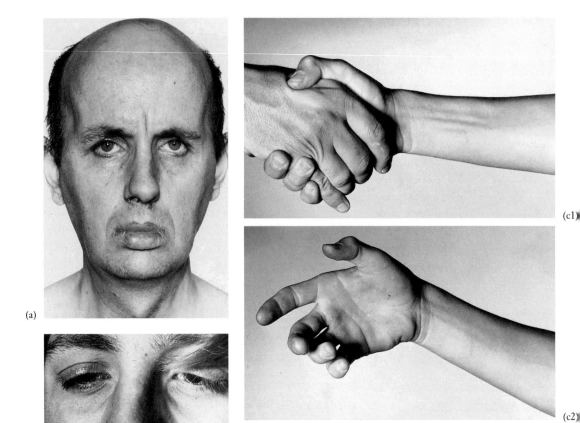

(a)

(b)

(c1)

(c2)

Fig. 14.15 (a–c) Note balding, ptosis and myotonia of the tongue and hands.

Chapter 15
Examine this patient's skin

Possible short cases include
Psoriasis (p. 195)
Vitiligo (p. 214)
Systemic sclerosis/CRST syndrome (p. 176)
Radiation burn on the chest
Purpura (p. 228)
Necrobiosis lipoidica diabeticorum (p. 217)
Granuloma annulare (gl.)
Neurofibromatosis (p. 219)
Pretibial myxoedema (p. 221)
Pemphigus/pemphigoid (p. 223)

Examination *routine*
This instruction is a rather more specific variation of the 'spot diagnosis' *routine*. You should
1 perform a *visual survey* of the patient, from scalp to sole, with regard to the fact that most dermatological lesions have a predilection for certain areas. It is as well to remember some of the regional associations as you *survey* the patient:

Scalp   Psoriasis (look especially at the hairline for redness, scaling, etc.), alopecia,* ringworm (very uncommon)

Face   Systemic sclerosis (tight shiny skin, pseudorhagades, beaked nose, telangiectasis), discoid lupus erythematosus (raised, red, scaly lesions with telangiectasis, scarring and altered pigmentation), xanthelasma, dermatomyositis (gl.) (heliotrope colour to eyelids), Sturge–Weber (gl.), rodent ulcer (usually below the eye or on the side of the nose, raised lesion with central ulcer, the edges being rolled and having telangiectatic blood vessels)

Mouth   Osler–Weber–Rendu, Peutz–Jeghers (gl.), lichen planus (gl.) (white lace-like network on mucosal surface), pemphigus, candidiasis (white exudate inside the mouth usually associated with a disease requiring multiple antimicrobial therapy, or an immunosuppressive disorder, e.g. leukaemia, acquired immune deficiency syndrome (AIDS), etc.), herpes simplex, Behçet's (gl.)

---

*Some causes of alopecia:
1 Diffuse—male-pattern baldness, cytotoxic drugs, hypothyroidism, hyperthyroidism, iron deficiency

2 Patchy—alopecia areata, ringworm; with scarring— discoid lupus erythematosus, lichen planus.

Neck	Pseudoxanthoma elasticum (gl.), tuberculous adenitis with sinus formation (?ethnic origin)
Trunk	Radiotherapy stigmata, morphoea (gl.), neurofibromatosis, dermatitis herpetiformis (gl.) (itching blisters over scapulae, buttocks, elbows, knees), herpes zoster along the intercostal nerves, pityriasis rosea (gl.), Addison's (areolar and scar pigmentation), pemphigus (trunk and limbs)
Axillae	Vitiligo, acanthosis nigricans (gl.) (pigmentation and velvety thickening of axillary skin, perianal, areolar and lateral abdominal skin, 'tripe palms', mucous membranes involved, maybe underlying insulin resistance or malignancy)
Elbows	Psoriasis (extensor), pseudoxanthoma elasticum (flexor), xanthomata (extensor), rheumatoid nodules (extensor), atopic dermatitis (flexor), olecranon bursitis, gouty tophi
Hands	Systemic sclerosis (sclerodactyly, infarcts of finger pulps, prominent capillaries at nail folds), lichen planus (wrists), dermatomyositis (heliotrope lesions — Gottron's papules — on the joints of the dorsum of the fingers/hands, nail-fold capillary dilatation and infarction), Addison's (skin crease pigmentation), granuloma annulare (gl.), erythema multiforme (gl.) (polymorphic eruption, 'target' lesions, mucous membrane involvement, macules, vesicles, bullae, etc.), systemic lupus erythematosus (SLE) (erythematous patches over the dorsal surface of the phalanges), scabies (not in student examinations!)
Nails	Psoriasis (pitting, onycholysis (gl.)), iron deficiency (koilonychia (gl.)), fungal dystrophy, tuberous sclerosis (gl.) (periungal fibromata)
Genitalia	Behçet's (iridocyclitis, uveitis, pyodermata, ulcers, etc.), lichen sclerosus (gl.) (white plaques), candidiasis
Legs	Leg ulcer (diabetic, venous, ischaemic, pyoderma gangrenosum (gl.)), necrobiosis lipoidica diabeticorum, pretibial myxoedema, erythema nodosum, Henoch–Schönlein purpura (gl.), tendon xanthomata in the Achilles, erythema ab igne (gl.), pemphigoid (legs and arms), lipoatrophy
Feet	Pustular psoriasis, eczema, verrucae, keratoderma blenorrhagica (gl.) (?eyes, joints, etc.).

During this *survey* you should consider

2 the **distribution** of the lesions (psoriasis on extensor areas, lichen planus on flexor areas, candidiasis in mucous membranes, tuberous sclerosis on nails and face, necrobiosis lipoidica diabeticorum usually bilateral, gouty tophi in the joints of hands, elbows and on the ears, etc.). Then after the *survey* (which should take a few seconds)

3 examine the **lesions** (see 'Examine this patient's rash') looking in particular for the *characteristic* features, e.g. scaling in psoriasis, shiny purple polygonal papules with Wickham's striae (gl.) in lichen planus, etc. If you have made a diagnosis consider whether you need to look for any

4 associated lesions (arthropathy and nail changes with psoriasis, evidence of associated autoimmune disease with vitiligo, etc.). Go through the skin conditions in the above list and make sure that you would recognize each, would know what else to look for, and what to say in your presentation.

For *checklist* see p. 277.

81 / Vitiligo

Record

There are *areas of depigmentation* around the eyes, mouth, on the knees, and on the dorsum of the feet (the hands, axillae, groins and genitalia are the other commonly affected areas).

The patient has vitiligo.

Sites subject to friction and trauma are often affected and Koebner's phenomenon (a lesion appearing at the site of skin damage) is common. Vitiligo is usually symmetrical but occasionally the depigmentation can be unilateral and follow the pattern of a dermatome. It is inherited as a dominant trait and individuals are usually otherwise healthy. Halo naevi (hypopigmented rings surrounding dark naevi), leucotrichia, premature greying of the hair and alopecia areata as well as vitiligo may all be associated with any of the **organ-specific autoimmune diseases:**

Myxoedema (?pulse, ankle jerks, facies—p. 251)

Hashimoto's disease (gl.) (?goitre—p. 251)

Graves' disease (?exophthalmos, fidgety, goitre, tachycardia, etc.—p. 247)

Pernicious anaemia (?pallor, spleen, subacute combined degeneration of the cord (SACD))

Atrophic gastritis associated with iron deficiency anaemia

Addison's disease (?buccal, skin crease, scar and general pigmentation, hypotension, etc.—p. 263)

Idiopathic hypoparathyroidism (gl.) (Chvostek's (gl.) and Trousseau's signs (gl.), tetany, paraesthesiae and cramps, cataracts, ectodermal changes, moniliasis, mental retardation, psychiatric disturbances, bradykinetic rigid syndrome, epilepsy)

Premature ovarian failure

Diabetes mellitus (?fundi)

Renal tubular acidosis (gl.)

Fibrosing alveolitis (?basal crepitations—p. 40)

Chronic active hepatitis (gl.) (?icterus, etc.)

Primary biliary cirrhosis (?xanthelasma, pigmentation, icterus, scratch marks, etc.—p. 70).

The organ-specific autoimmune diseases tend to occur in association with each other (*polyglandular autoimmune disease*) so that patients with one have an above normal chance of also developing another. Some patients are prone to extensive mucocutaneous candidiasis* (candidiasis–endocrinopathy syndrome) and from this two distinct syndromes emerge. The clinical features of the syndromes are compared in Table 15.1.

Vitiligo, the cutaneous marker of organ-specific autoimmune disease, may occur in the non-organ-specific autoimmune disease systemic sclerosis.† Other disorders associated with vitiligo are morphoea (gl.) and malignant melanoma.

---

* The mucocutaneous candidiasis is associated with hypergammaglobulinaemia, IgA deficiency and anergy to *Candida albicans*.

† Rarely there is an overlap between the organ-specific and non-organ-specific autoimmune diseases. Sjögren's syndrome (gl.) occupies an intermediate position being associated with rheumatoid arthritis on the one hand and autoimmune thyroiditis on the other. Primary biliary cirrhosis is another condition which bridges the gap. It is associated with Sjögren's syndrome, Hashimoto's thyroiditis and renal tubular acidosis on the one hand, and systemic sclerosis, CRST syndrome (given in full on p. 176), rheumatoid arthritis, coeliac disease, dermatomyositis and mixed connective tissue disease, on the other.

Table 15.1 Comparison of the clinical features of the major syndromes characterized by multiple endocrine gland hypofunction (adapted from Cecil's *Textbook of Medicine*, 1992, 19th edn, p. 1389)

	Multiple endocrine deficiency syndrome (Schmidt's syndrome)	Polyglandular deficiency with mucocutaneous candidiasis
Hypoadrenalism	Common	Common
Hypothyroidism	Common	Rare
Diabetes mellitus (type I)	Common	Rare
Gonadal failure	Less common	Less common
Hypoparathyroidism	Rare	Common
Pituitary insufficiency	Rare	Rare
Autoantibodies to endocrine tissues and gastric parietal cells	Often present	Often present
Sex distribution	Strong female predominance	Female preponderance about 4 : 1
Inheritance	Usually 'sporadic', but susceptibility related to HLA haplotype and may be inherited as autosomal dominant	Generally inherited as autosomal recessive; no apparent HLA association; siblings characteristically affected
Time of onset	Usually becomes evident during adult life	Typically becomes evident during childhood preceded by chronic mucocutaneous moniliasis
Other associated 'autoimmune' diseases and characteristics	Pernicious anaemia; hyperthyroidism; coeliac disease; alopecia; vitiligo; myasthenia gravis; isolated red-cell aplasia	Pernicious anaemia; malabsorption; alopecia; vitiligo; IgA deficiency; hypergammaglobulinaemia; chronic active hepatitis; proliferative glomerulonephritis

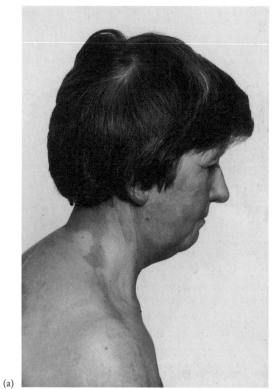
(a)

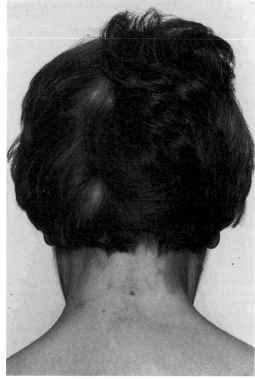
(b)

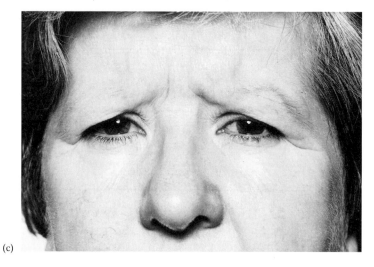
(c)

Fig. 15.1 (a–c) Note the areas of vitiligo and alopecia areata including loss of eyelashes (especially left upper lid) in this patient with diabetes mellitus.

82 / Necrobiosis lipoidica diabeticorum

Record

There are *sharply demarcated*, coalescing *oval plaques* on the *shins* (occasionally arms and elsewhere) of this lady (usually a female aged < 40). The lesions have a *shiny atrophic surface*, with characteristic *waxy yellow centres* and *brownish-red edges*. There is (usually) telangiectasia over the surface.

The diagnosis is necrobiosis lipoidica diabeticorum.

It is rare and usually associated with diabetes, but can occur in the pre-diabetic and on its own. It may have to be differentiated from granuloma annulare (gl.), from nodular vasculitis when small, and from localized scleroderma or sarcoidosis (gl.) when larger.

The lesions may ulcerate. Opinions vary as to whether good diabetic control can improve healing, but this should be tried. Gradual healing, with scarring, occurs over a period of years. Steroids (topical or local injection) administered cautiously (to avoid local atrophy) may help. Severe cases can be treated by excision and skin grafting. The histology varies, some containing large amounts of lipid, some not. There is necrosis of collagen, surrounded by pallisades of granulomatous epithelioid cells, and the aetiology is obscure.

Granuloma annulare

Pale or flesh-coloured papules coalescing in rings of usually 1–3 cm diameter, especially on the backs of the hands and fingers. Blanching by pressure reveals a characteristic beaded ring of white dermal patches. It is sometimes associated with diabetes especially when the lesions are extensive and atypical. The histology is almost identical to necrobiosis lipoidica diabeticorum. The lesions regress spontaneously.

Diabetic dermopathy

Atrophic pigmented patches (start as dull red oval papules; sometimes with a small blister) occurring mostly on the shins of diabetics. It has been suggested that they are precipitated by trauma in association with neuropathy.

Other skin lesions in diabetics

Infective (bacterial—boils, etc.; and fungal—candidiasis)

Foot/leg ulcers (ischaemic and neuropathic)

Vitiligo (?other associated organ-specific autoimmune disease—p. 214)

Fat atrophy (very rare with highly purified insulins)

Fat hypertrophy (recurrent injection of insulin into the same site)

Xanthomata (associated hyperlipidaemia—may disappear with control of diabetes as this causes improvement in the hyperlipidaemia—p. 231)

Insulin allergy (immediate and delayed; though less likely this can even occur in patients on human insulin given subcutaneously)

Sulphonylurea allergy (erythema multiforme (gl.), phototoxic and other eruptions)

Acanthosis nigricans (gl.)

Peripheral anhydrosis (due to autonomic neuropathy)

Chlorpropamide alcohol flush

Pseudoporphyria (diabetic *bullae—bullosis diabeticorum*—resemble burns but are not caused by them. These arise in longstanding diabetics with *neuropathy*. They may be unilateral or bilateral and usually appear on the toes, plantar and dorsal surfaces of the foot, and on the fingers. The blisters are tense, containing serous and sometimes haemorrhagic fluid. The appearances resemble porphyria).

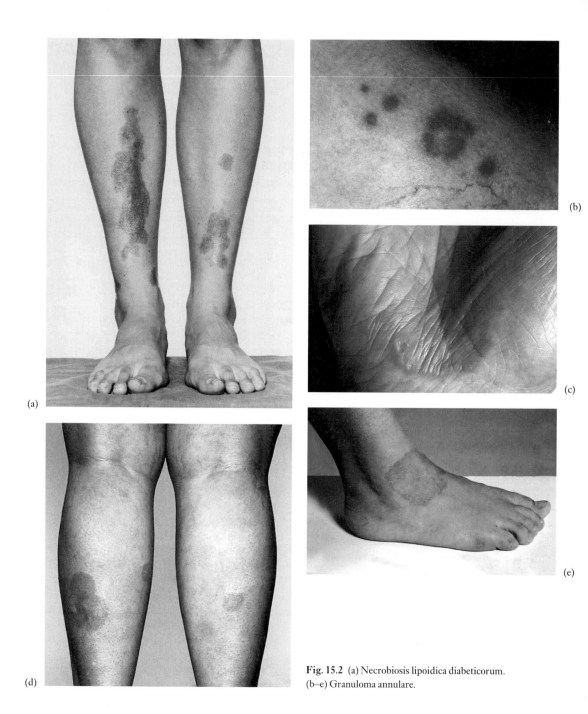

(a)

(b)

(c)

(d)

(e)

Fig. 15.2 (a) Necrobiosis lipoidica diabeticorum.
(b–e) Granuloma annulare.

83 / Neurofibromatosis (von Recklinghausen's disease)

Note: most likely to occur in a short case examination either as a spot diagnosis, with or without a mention of the associated features, or as a case with an associated nerve pressure effect (such as one with an ulnar nerve/T1 lesion).

Record
There are multiple *neurofibromata* and *café-au-lait spots* (normal person allowed up to five of the latter).

The diagnosis is neurofibromatosis.*

Or

There are multiple skin lesions: *sessile* and *pedunculated* cutaneous *fibromata*, as well as neurofibromata which are both *soft* and *firm*, *single* and *lobulated*, and felt both as mobile subcutaneous lumps† and *nodules* along the course of peripheral nerves. There are *café-au-lait* spots (especially in the axillae — axillary freckling).

The diagnosis is neurofibromatosis.*

Autosomal dominant.
The condition is usually asymptomatic.

Complications
Kyphoscoliosis
Pressure effects of the neurofibromata on peripheral nerves and cranial nerves, especially:
(a) acoustic neuroma (gl.) (?Vth, VIth, VIIth, VIIIth nerve lesions, nystagmus and cerebellar signs; may be bilateral)*
(b) Vth nerve neuroma
Spinal nerve root involvement which may cause:
(a) cord compression
(b) muscle wasting
(c) sensory loss (Charcot's joints (gl.) may occur)
Sarcomatous or other malignant change (5–16%)

Lung cysts (honeycomb lung)
Pseudoarthrosis and other orthopaedic abnormalities
Plexiform neuroma.‡

Other intracranial tumours which can occur in this condition are:
Gliomata (optic nerve and chiasma; cerebral)
Meningiomata (gl.)*
Medulloblastomata.

Other features of neurofibromatosis
An association with phaeochromocytoma (gl.) — 5% of cases (?blood pressure)
Nodules of the iris
Hamartomata of the retina
Rib notching.

---

*The phakomatoses or neurocutaneous syndromes are characterized by a disordered growth of the neurocutaneous tissues. More than 20 syndromes have been described, the most important of which are *neurofibromatosis 1 (von Recklinghausen's*—chromosome 17), neurofibromatosis 2 (chromosome 22), tuberous sclerosis (gl.) and Sturge–Weber syndrome (gl.). *Neurofibromatosis 2*, often called *central neurofibromatosis*, is rare and characterized by bilateral acoustic neuromata and often other intracranial tumours such as meningiomata or ependymomata. A few *café-au-lait* spots are present in about 40% of cases. At-risk family members

should be screened regularly with hearing tests, etc.
†Neurofibromatosis should not be confused with lipomatosis with its characteristic soft subcutaneous lumps. In Dercum's disease (usually middle-aged females) subcutaneous lipomata may be painful and associated with marked obesity.
‡An entire nerve trunk and all its branches are involved in diffuse neurofibromatosis with associated overgrowth of overlying tissues leading to gross deformities (temporal and frontal scalp are favourite sites but it may occur anywhere); may grow to lemon or even melon size.

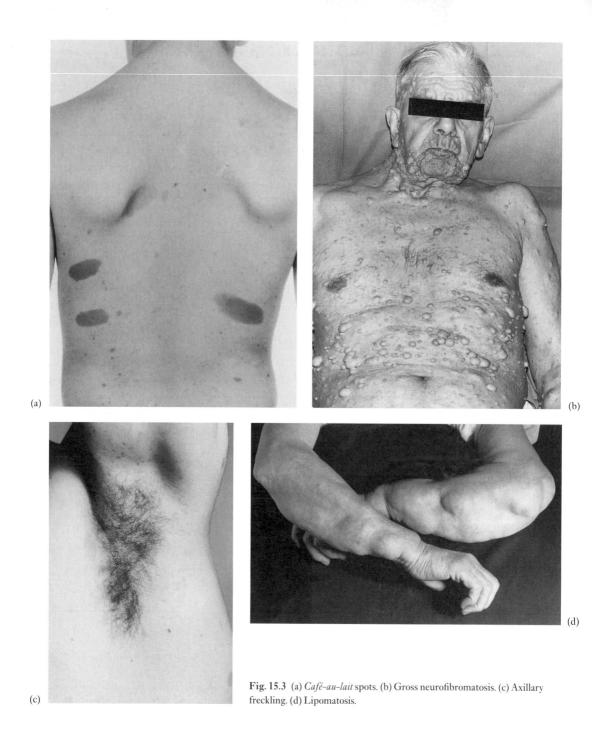

Fig. 15.3 (a) *Café-au-lait* spots. (b) Gross neurofibromatosis. (c) Axillary freckling. (d) Lipomatosis.

84 / Pretibial myxoedema

Record

There are *elevated symmetrical* skin lesions over the anterolateral aspects of the *shins* (may spread onto the feet; may affect other parts of the body, e.g. the face or the dorsa of the hands). The lesions are coarse, *purplish-red* (may be skin colour pink, or rarely brown) in colour and raised with *well-defined* serpiginous *margins*. The skin is *shiny* and has an *orange-peel appearance*. The hairs in the affected areas are coarse and the lesions are *tender* (and itch). The patient has *exophthalmos** (*?thyroid acropachy* (gl.)*) and is likely to have been rendered *euthyroid* (?pulse, etc.) by surgery (*?thyroidectomy scar*) or, more particularly, with *radioactive iodine*.

The diagnosis is pretibial myxoedema (occurs in about 5% of patients with Graves' disease).

The superficial layer of the skin is infiltrated with the mucopolysaccharide, hyaluronic acid. Biopsy scars of the area almost invariably develop keloid.

The latent interval between the treatment for hyperthyroidism and the clinical onset of pretibial myxoedema varies from 4 to 32 months with a mean time of 1 year.

Pretibial myxoedema in its most extreme form clinically resembles lymphoedema. It may be that mucin deposition in the dermis causes compression of the dermal lymphatics which results in dermal oedema and the clinical features of lymphoedema.

* Pretibial myxoedema is almost always accompanied by exophthalmos. Thyroid acropachy (p. 247) is occasionally associated — diffuse thickening of distal extremities, subperiosteal new bone formation simulating clubbing of the digits. Exophthalmos has also been termed *infiltrative ophthalmopathy* and pretibial myxoedema, *infiltrative dermopathy*.

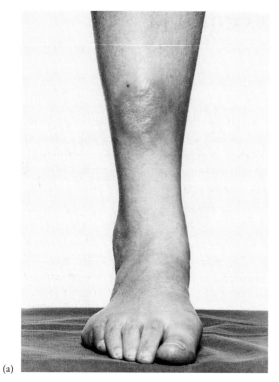
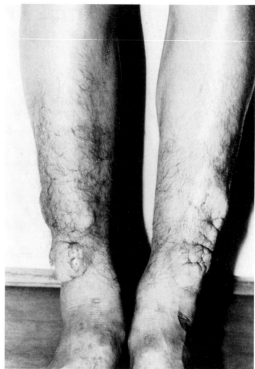

(a)

(b)

Fig. 15.4 (a,b) Pretibial myxoedema.

85 / Pemphigus/pemphigoid

Record 1

This middle-aged (or elderly) patient has flaccid *thin-roofed blisters* (usually over the axillae and trunk), which vary in size (usually 1–2 cm in diameter). Most of the blisters have *burst* leaving *red* and *exuding areas* (which are extremely tender). There are also (not always) red denuded patches in the *mouth* (the first site involved in up to 50%), *pharynx* and *eyes*.

     The patient has pemphigus.

Record 2

This elderly patient has *tense blisters* varying in size from a few millimetres to a few centimetres in diameter involving . . . (describe where—usually it is the limbs but it can be widespread). There are also *reddened* and *urticarial* (sometimes eczematous) *patches* surrounding and separate from the blisters. There are no lesions in the mouth (they do occur but are uncommon).

     The diagnosis is pemphigoid.

Pemphigus vulgaris

This condition occurs most commonly in Jewish people. The site of the blister is in the epidermis. Occasionally lesions may occur without initial blister formation. The mucous membranes never have blisters, only denuded patches. It is a progressive and fatal condition if not treated with corticosteroids in very high doses (initially 100–200 mg daily of prednisolone). Azathioprine may reduce the maintenance dose of steroid. It can be caused by penicillamine, phenylbutazone and rifampicin. There is an increased incidence in patients with thymoma and myasthenia gravis. *Acantholysis* is a characteristic histological feature. Nikolsky's sign* is invariably present. Immunofluorescence of a biopsy shows intercellular immunoglobulins (usually IgG) and/or complement factor C3.

Pemphigoid

The site of the blisters is at the basement membrane between the epidermis and the dermis; therefore the blister is thicker and less likely to rupture than in pemphigus. Mucosal lesions are less common in pemphigoid. Though it is self-limiting (2 years) systemic steroids are usually given (initially 60–80 mg day^{-1}) and azathioprine may reduce the maintenance dose. It does not have a high mortality like pemphigus. It has been alleged that it is sometimes a manifestation of underlying malignancy but this point is not proven. Biopsy shows IgG and complement at the basement membrane zone.

Other bullous disorders

Dermatitis herpetiformis (gl.) (groups of blisters on the elbows, knees and buttocks; associated with coeliac disease)

Epidermolysis bullosa congenita (congenital blistering disorders usually of the hands and feet; genetically determined; range from simple blisters to severe scarring with contractures; teeth and nails abnormal in some forms)

Epidermolysis bullosa acquisita (associated with inflammatory bowel disease, amyloidosis (gl.) and internal malignancy)

Herpes gestationis (pregnancy or early puerperium,

---

* Firm pressure on apparently normal skin causes it to slide off. Nikolsky's sign may also occur in other severe bullous eruptions, such as toxic epidermal necrolysis.

erythematous/urticarial lesions with blistering; no relation to herpes virus; resolves in a few weeks; may require steroids; recurs with increased severity in subsequent pregnancies)

Porphyria cutanea tarda (vesicles, bullae, crusts and scarring in exposed areas such as the backs of the hands and ears. May have areas of hyper- and hypopigmentation and excessive hair growth over the temples and cheeks).

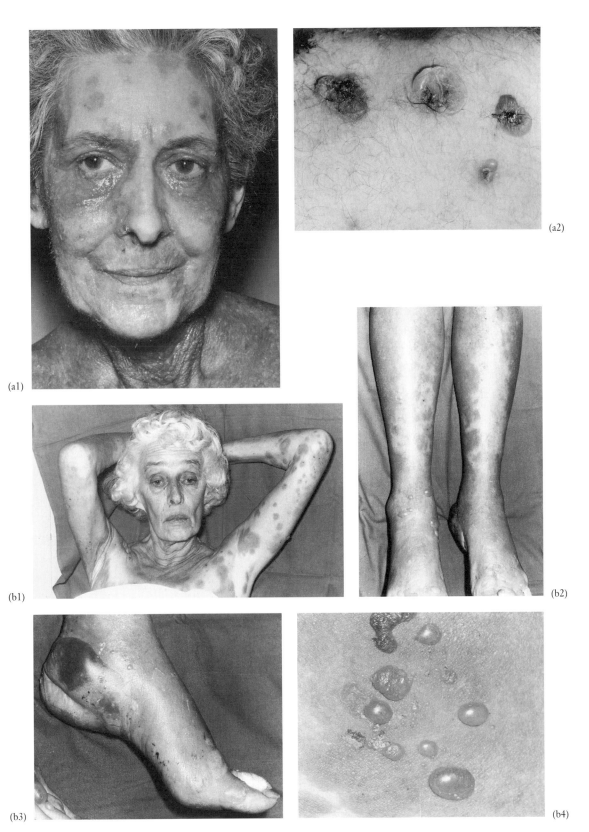

(a1)

(a2)

(b1)

(b2)

(b3)

(b4)

Fig. 15.5 (a1,2) Pemphigus. Note denuded areas and ruptured blisters. (b1–4) Pemphigoid. Note the tense blisters.

Chapter 16
Examine this patient's rash

Possible short cases include
Psoriasis (p. 195)
Purpura (p. 228)
Vasculitis (gl.)
Neurofibromatosis (p. 219)
Juvenile chronic arthritis (Still's disease) (gl.)
Xanthomata (p. 231)
Necrobiosis lipoidica diabeticorum (p. 217)
Granuloma annulare (gl.)
Radiation burn on the chest
Erythema nodosum (p. 233)
Herpes zoster (p. 235)

Examination *routine*
This *routine* is generally the same as that discussed under 'Examine this patients's skin'.
1 You should quickly conduct a *visual survey* as described under 'skin' and note if there are any similar or related lesions elsewhere. Look at the
2 distribution of the lesions, whether confined to a single area (morphoea (gl.), erythema nodosum, rodent ulcer, melanoma, alopecia areata, etc.) or present in other areas such as psoriasis, neurofibromatosis, acanthosis nigricans (gl.), dermatomyositis (gl.), etc. While concentrating on the lesion in question, it is important to look at the
3 surrounding skin for any helpful clues such as *scratch marks* as evidence of itching,* *radiotherapy field markings* on the skin in the vicinity of a radiation burn, or *paper-thin skin* with purpura (corticosteroid therapy), etc. You should now
4 examine the lesion in detail. To determine the *extent* of the lesion you may have to ask the patient to undress, a procedure which will provide you with a little more time to survey other areas. Decide if the rash is *pleomorphic* or *monomorphic* (all the lesions are similar). If so examine one typical lesion carefully in terms of:

---

* Some causes of itching:
1 Dermatological—scabies, dermatitis herpetiformis (gl.), lichen planus (gl.), eczema

2 Medical—cholestasis, chronic renal failure, lymphoma (gl.), polycythaemia rubra vera (gl.).

(a) *colour*, e.g. erythematous or pigmented
(b) *size*
(c) *shape*, e.g. oval, circular, annular, etc.
(d) *surface*, e.g. scaling or eroded
(e) *character*, e.g. macule, papule, vesicle, pustule, ulcer, etc.
(f) *secondary features*, e.g. crusting, lichenification, etc.

It is advisable to be familiar with the correct use of the terms to describe rashes (especially if you do not recognize the lesion!). To say 'skin lesion' or 'skin rash' conveys no diagnostic meaning. In your presentation you should be able to describe the lesion with respect to the above six features, especially if you do not know the diagnosis. The following are some of the useful terms employed in describing skin lesions:

Macules: flat, circumscribed lesions, not raised above the skin—size and shape varies

Papules: raised, circumscribed, firm lesions up to 1 cm in size

Nodules: like papules but larger; usually lie deeper in skin

Tumours: larger than nodules, elevated or very deeply placed in the skin

Weals: circumscribed elevations associated with itching and tingling

Vesicles: small well-defined collections of fluid

Bullae: large vesicles

Pustules: circumscribed elevations containing purulent fluid which may, in some cases, be sterile (e.g. Behçet's (gl.))

Scales: dead tissue from the horny layer which may be dry (e.g. psoriasis) or greasy (e.g. seborrhoeic dermatitis)

Crusts: these consist of dried exudate

Ulcers: excavations in the skin of irregular shape; remember that every ulcer has a shape, an edge, a floor, a base and a secretion, and it forms a scar on healing

Scars: the result of healing of a damaged dermis.

5 Finally, if indicated, look for **additional features** (arthropathy in psoriasis or Still's disease, cushingoid facies if purpura is due to steroids, clubbing with radiation burns on the chest, etc.)

For *checklist* see p. 277.

86 / Purpura

Record

There are numerous reddish-purple macules (which appeared *spontaneously*) which do not fade with pressure.

The appearance is suggestive of purpura.*

Now look at the patient and note:

?*Age* ('senile purpura')

?*Cushingoid features* with thin skin (if present observe for features of underlying steroid-treated disease, e.g. asthma, rheumatoid arthritis, cryptogenic fibrosing alveolitis)

?*Rheumatoid arthritis* (phenylbutazone and gold as well as steroids)

?*Anaemia* (leukaemia, bone marrow aplasia or infiltration)

—as well as the distribution and type of purpura.

Causes of purpura

Thrombocytopenic purpura, such as:

Idiopathic thrombocytopenic purpura (purpuric rash in a young female, ?spleen—may respond to steroids and/or splenectomy)

Marrow replacement by leukaemia (acute and chronic; ?spleen, nodes, liver, anaemia, oral and pharyngeal infection)

Marrow replacement by secondary malignancy (?cachexia, evidence of primary)

Marrow aplasia (idiopathic, secondary to drugs, hepatitis A or B).

Capillary defect (vascular; platelet count normal), such as:

Senile and steroid-induced purpura (purpura over loose skin areas)

Henoch–Schönlein purpura (gl.) (children > adults; purpuric rash (a haemorrhagic vasculitis, sometimes papular) over the extensor surfaces of the limbs particularly at the ankles and on the buttocks; associated with arthritis of medium-sized joints, colicky abdominal pains, occasionally gastrointestinal bleeding and acute nephritis)

Coagulation deficiency, such as: †

Haemophilia (gl.)

Christmas disease (gl.)

Anticoagulant therapy.

---

* Purpura refers to a spontaneous extravasation of blood from the capillaries into the skin; petechiae = pin-head size, ecchymoses = large lesions.

† These conditions may cause ecchymoses rather than purpura.

Other causes of purpura

Other drugs (e.g. sulphonamides, chloramphenicol, thiazides)

Hypersplenism (large spleen)

Von Willebrand's disease (gl.)

Infective endocarditis (?heart murmur, splenomegaly, splinters, clubbing, Osler's nodes (gl.), etc.)

Systemic lupus erythematosus (SLE) (?typical rash)

Polyarteritis nodosa (gl.) (?arteritic lesions)

Osler–Weber–Rendu syndrome (p. 178)

Venous stasis (ankle and lower legs; obesity or varicose veins; accompanied by progressive pigmentation due to deposition of haemosiderin)

Scurvy (gl.) (NB the neglected elderly patient with ecchymoses on the legs)

Paroxysmal nocturnal haemoglobinuria

Amyloidosis (gl.) (periorbital purpura)

Uraemia (pale, brownish-yellow tinge to skin)

Disseminated intravascular coagulation

Thrombotic thrombocytopenic purpura

Haemolytic–uraemic syndrome (gl.)

Paraproteinaemia (gl.)

Meningitis (especially meningococcal)

Septicaemia (especially meningococcal)

Viral haemorrhagic fevers

Kaposi's sarcoma

Factitious purpura

Ehlers–Danlos syndrome (gl.)

Scarlet fever

Measles

Rubella

Glandular fever

Typhoid

Cyanotic congenital heart disease (gl.).

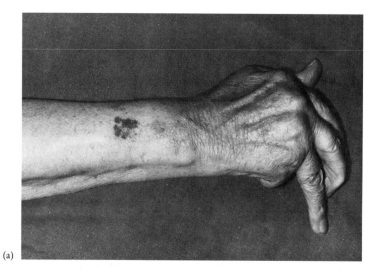

(a)

(b)

Fig. 16.1 (a) Purpura on forearm (note rheumatoid arthritis). (b) Henoch–Schönlein purpura.

87 / Xanthomata

Record 1

There are *tendon xanthomata* (?corneal arcus, xanthelasma) in the *extensor tendons* on the back of the *hand*, and on the *Achilles* and *patella* tendons.

They suggest *familial hypercholesterolaemia*. (In this condition raised and nodular *tuberous xanthomata* may also occur, usually symmetrically, over the *extensor aspects of the joints* and on the *buttocks*. They may be several millimetres to several centimetres in size.)

Record 2

There are (orange or) *yellow papules* (up to 5 mm in diameter) on the *extensor surfaces* particularly over the *joints*, on the *limbs* and on the *buttocks* and *back*. They are (sometimes) surrounded by a rim of erythema (and may be tender).

This is *eruptive xanthomatosis* (?lipaemia retinalis on fundoscopy. There is often abdominal pain and there is a risk of acute pancreatitis. It suggests severe *hypertriglyceridaemia* — plasma triglycerides of the order of 20–25 mmol l^{-1} — 'milky plasma' syndrome).*

Familial hypercholesterolaemia is associated with premature development of vascular disease. Familial hypertriglyceridaemia does not appear to be an important risk factor for atherosclerosis but equivalent hypertriglyceridaemia due to familial combined hyperlipidaemia† is associated with an increased risk.

Order of priorities in treating hyperlipidaemia‡

1 Identify and treat any causes of secondary hyperlipidaemia such as:
  (a) diabetes mellitus (?fundi)
  (b) alcoholism (may be the occult underlying cause of treatment failure)
  (c) nephrotic syndrome (gl.) (?generalized oedema)
  (d) myxoedema (?facies, pulse, ankle jerks)
  (e) cholestasis (?icterus)
  (f) myelomatosis (gl.)
  (g) oral contraceptives
2 Dietary treatment for obesity
3 Dietary treatment for hyperlipidaemia
4 Lipid-lowering drugs.§

Types of hyperlipidaemia simplified

Comparatively common

Type IIa (e.g. familial hypercholesterolaemia) — raised cholesterol only
Type IIb (e.g. familial combined hypercholesterolaemia) — raised cholesterol and triglycerides
Type IV (e.g. familial hypertriglyceridaemia) — raised triglycerides.

---

*This level of hypertriglyceridaemia is usually due to overproduction of triglycerides occurring at the same time as hindrance of removal. For example, the coexistence of familial hypertriglyceridaemia (type IV), diabetes and/or alcohol consumption. Treatment of the secondary cause usually leads to a dramatic reduction in triglyceride levels and greatly reduces the risk of acute pancreatitis which is the main threat of this condition.

† Affected family members show either a combined rise in plasma cholesterol and triglycerides, or hypercholesterolaemia alone, or hypertriglyceridaemia alone.
‡ NB The screening and treatment of families with hypercholesterolaemia.
§ There is increasing evidence that, by lowering cholesterol, statins reduce cardiovascular morbidity and mortality in patients at risk of cardiovascular disease.

Rare

Type I—raised chylomicrons

Type III‖—an inherited defect in apolipoprotein E synthesis resulting in a rise in cholesterol (mostly intermediate density remnants) and triglycerides to an equal extent. It is characteristically associated with palmar xanthomata and is very responsive to fibrates

Type V—raised chylomicrons and triglycerides.

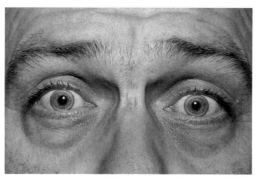

(a)

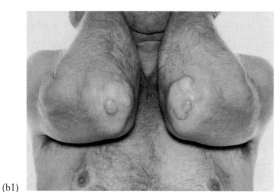

(b1)

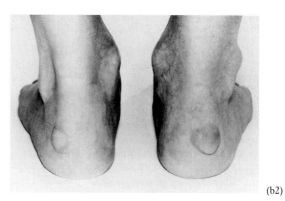

(b2)

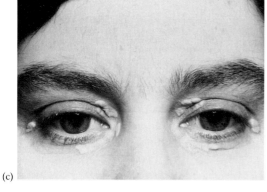

(c)

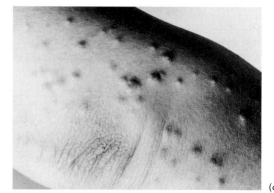

(d)

Fig. 16.2 (a) Arcus senilis. (b1,2) Elbows and Achilles of the same patient. (c) Xanthelasma. (d) Eruptive xanthomata.

‖ Type III is not as rare as types I and V.

88 / Erythema nodosum

Record

There are in this (usually) female patient *raised* (become flat with healing), *red* (pass through the changes of a *bruise* with healing), *tender* lesions 2–6 cm in diameter on the *shins* (and occasionally thighs and upper limbs).

The diagnosis is erythema nodosum (?fever, arthralgia).

Possible causes

1 Acute sarcoidosis (gl.) (bilateral hilar lymphadenopathy; fever, arthralgia, palpable cervical and axillary lymph nodes, mild iridocyclitis).
2 Streptococcal infection (e.g. throat).
3 Rheumatic fever (gl.) (tachycardia, murmur, nodules, etc.).
4 Primary tuberculosis (?ethnic origin, chest signs, etc.).
5 Drugs (sulphonamides, penicillin, oral contraceptives, codeine, salicylates, barbiturates).

Other causes

Pregnancy
Ulcerative colitis (gl.)
Crohn's disease
Yersinia enterocolitis
Malignancies (lymphoma (gl.) and leukaemia)
Syphilis
Leprosy (gl.) (important cause on a worldwide basis)
Tinea and other fungal infections
Coccidiomycosis (gl.)
Toxoplasmosis
Lymphogranuloma venereum (gl.)

Behçet's syndrome (gl.) (orogenital ulceration, iridocyclitis, etc.)
Idiopathic.

Histology

Perivascular mixed cell infiltrate followed by giant cell formation. There is oedema and a variable amount of extravascular blood. The inflammation spreads into the subcutaneous fat.

Or

In a nutshell: subcutaneous inflammatory changes which are vasculitic in origin.

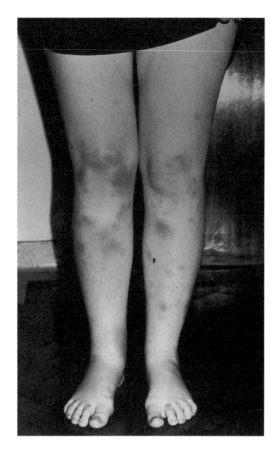

Fig. 16.3 Erythema nodosum.

89 / Herpes zoster

Record

This elderly (or middle-aged) patient has a *vesicular rash* in the *area supplied by the . . . nerve* (say which/where).* The lesions are in *clusters* at different stages of development—the stages each cluster goes through is papule → vesicle → (pustule, sometimes haemorrhagic) → crusting → scar. The regional lymph nodes are enlarged.

The diagnosis is herpes zoster.

Complications

Cranial nerve palsy—especially facial nerve palsy which may occur not only with lesions of the external auditory meatus (Ramsay Hunt syndrome (gl.)), but also with trigeminal zoster and zoster of the head, neck and mouth†

Peripheral motor palsy (lower motor neurone deficit from involvement of motor root—sometimes permanent)

Post-herpetic neuralgia (10%; commoner in the elderly; can be very severe and difficult to treat)

Eye damage (ophthalmic zoster)

Zoster sine herpete (typical pain, etc., but no rash—serological evidence confirms).

Other complications include visceral nerve involvement (pain or dysfunction in an organ), myelitis (transverse or ascending—rare), disseminated encephalitis (rare), cerebellar ataxia (rare) and diffuse polyneuritis (rare).

Generalized herpes zoster is usually associated with an underlying reticulosis (especially Hodgkin's (gl.)), leukaemia or carcinoma (especially bronchogenic).

---

* The commonest is a thoracic dermatome. Cranial nerve involvement is next in frequency. The ophthalmic division of the trigeminal nerve is the commonest cranial nerve. With cranial nerve involvement there are often signs of meningeal irriation and sometimes mucous membranes are affected.

† In true Ramsay Hunt (see p. 173) the zoster is probably of the geniculate ganglion. In other cases there may be multiple cranial ganglia involvement and an associated localized encephalitis and neuronitis. VIIIth nerve involvement (vertigo and deafness) is a particularly common association with facial palsy due to herpes zoster. Acyclovir given as soon as possible after the start of the infection is the treatment of choice.

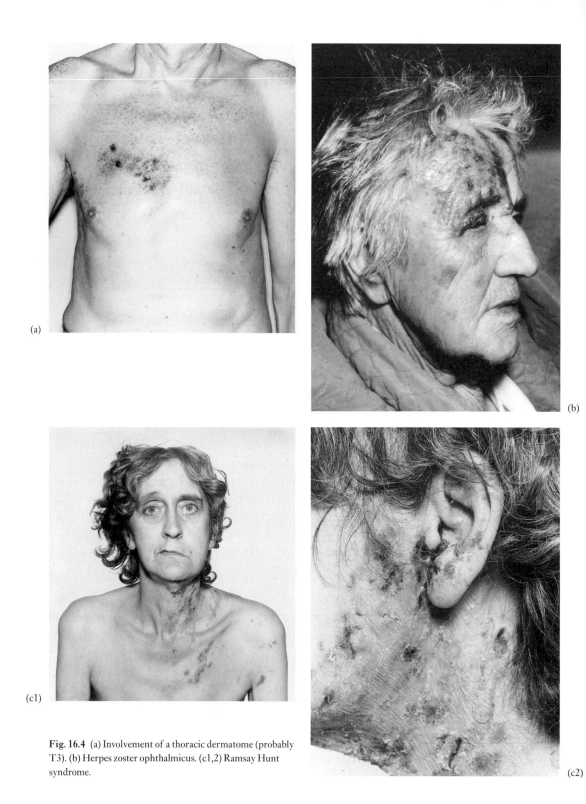

Fig. 16.4 (a) Involvement of a thoracic dermatome (probably T3). (b) Herpes zoster ophthalmicus. (c1,2) Ramsay Hunt syndrome.

Chapter 17
Examine this patient's neck

Possible short cases include

Examination *routine*

As usual the first step is to

1 *survey* the patient quickly from head to foot (exophthalmos, myxoedematous facies, ankle oedema, etc.) and then to

2 **look at the neck.** We believe that the reason for the instruction in half of the cases will be a *goitre.* If another abnormality is visible your further action will be dictated by what you see and we suggest you go through the list and establish a sequence of actions for each abnormality (e.g. if you see giant *v* waves you would wish to examine the heart and liver—see p. 28). If you do see a goitre, offer a drink to the patient:

'Take a sip of water and hold it in your mouth';

look at the neck:

'Now swallow'.

Watch the movement of the goitre, or the *appearance* of a *nodule* not visible before swallowing (behind the sternomastoid—see Fig. 17.2c, p. 242). Next ask the patient's permission to feel the neck, and then approach him from behind. If there has been no evidence of a goitre so far you may wish to palpate the neck for lymph nodes *before* feeling for a goitre. Otherwise

3 **palpate** the thyroid.* With the right index and middle fingers feel below the thyroid cartilage where the isthmus of the thyroid gland lies over the trachea. Then palpate the two lobes of the thyroid gland which extend later-

---

* Some examiners and tutors say that the thyroid gland is best palpated from the side where you can feel it and see its movements.

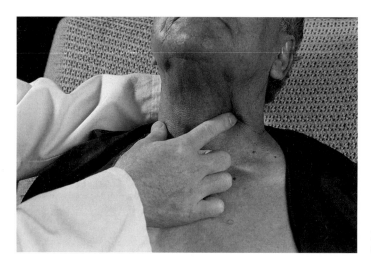

Fig. 17.1 Palpating the left lobe of the thyroid.

ally behind the sternomastoid muscle (Fig. 17.1). Ask the patient to swallow again while you continue to palpate the thyroid, ensuring that the neck is slightly flexed to ease palpation. Remember that if there is a goitre, when you give your presentation you are going to want to comment on its *size*, whether it is *soft* or *firm*, whether it is *nodular* or *diffusely enlarged*, whether it *moves* readily on swallowing, whether there are *lymph nodes* (see below) and whether there is a vascular *murmur* (see below). Extend palpation upwards along the medial edge of the sternomastoid muscle on either side to look for a *pyramidal lobe* which may be present. Apologize for any discomfort you may cause because the deep palpation necessary to feel the thyroid gland causes pain,† particularly in patients with Graves' disease. Next palpate laterally to examine for

4 lymph nodes. If you find lymph node enlargement check not only in the *supraclavicular fossae* and right up the neck but also in the *submandibular, postauricular* and *suboccipital* areas, ensuring that the head is slightly flexed on the side under palpation to allow access and scrutiny of slightly enlarged lymph nodes. Ascertain whether the lymph nodes are *separate* (reactive hyperplasia, infectious mononucleosis, lymphoma (gl.), etc.) or *matted* together (neoplastic, tuberculous), *mobile* or *fixed* to the skin or deep tissues (neoplastic), or whether they are *soft, fleshy, rubbery* (Hodgkin's disease (gl.)) or *hard* (neoplastic). Particularly if you find lymph nodes without a goitre, examine for lymph nodes in the axillae and groins (lymphoma, chronic lymphatic leukaemia (gl.), etc.) and, if allowed, feel for the spleen.

5 Auscultate over the thyroid for evidence of increased vascularity. You may need to occlude venous return to rule out a venous hum, and listen over the

† In viral thyroiditis (rare) the patient may complain of a
painful thyroid and the thyroid may be overtly tender on light
palpation.

aortic area to ensure that the thyroid bruit you hear is not, in fact, an outflow obstruction murmur conducted to the root of the neck.

6 If there is any evidence of thyroid disease begin an assessment of **thyroid status** (see 'Examine this patient's thyroid status') by feeling and counting the pulse (NB do not miss *atrial fibrillation* whether slow or fast). The examiner will soon stop you if he wishes to hear your description of a multinodular goitre in a euthyroid patient.

For *checklist* see p. 278.

90 / Goitre

Record 1

There is a *multinodular* goitre, the R/L lobe being enlarged more than the R/L. There are *no lymph nodes* palpable, there is *no retrosternal* extension, there is *no bruit* and the patient is clinically *euthyroid* (having checked pulse, palms, tremor, lid lag, tendon reflexes).

      The diagnosis (in this middle-aged or elderly patient) is likely to be simple multinodular goitre.

Simple multinodular goitre is due to relative iodine deficiency in a susceptible person. The multinodular nature suggests that it is longstanding. If there has been no recent rapid increase in size and if the gland is not causing symptoms or worrying the patient then no further investigation or treatment is required. The patient should be observed in 6 months or a year to confirm that there is still no change. Fine-needle aspiration should be undertaken if there is any doubt.

Record 2

There is a *firm, diffusely enlarged* goitre without retrosternal extension (check for bruit and if allowed feel the pulse and assess thyroid status).

Possible causes

Simple goitre (euthyroid, no bruit, relative iodine deficiency, especially females, ?puberty, ?pregnancy)

Treated Graves' disease* (?exophthalmos ± bruit, patient is euthyroid—normal pulse, no tremor or sweatiness—or even hypothyroid—slow pulse, facies, ankle jerks)

Hyperthyroid Graves' disease* (?bruit, tachycardia, exophthalmos, tremor, sweatiness, etc.)

Hashimoto's disease (gl.)* (goitre usually but not always, finely micronodular, firm and symmetrical; ?hypothyroid facies, pulse, ankle jerks, etc.)

De Quervain's (gl.) (viral) thyroiditis (gl.) (thyroid tender ± constitutional upset; absent radioactive iodine uptake on scan though the serum thyroxine

may be elevated with thyroid stimulating hormone (TSH) supressed†)

Goitrogens (e.g. lithium, iodide in large doses, phenylbutazone, para-aminosalicylic acid and others are all rare causes)

Dyshormonogenesis (six different types of congenital enzyme defect, all rare).

Record 3

There is a *solitary nodule* in the thyroid (check for lymphadenopathy).

Possible causes

Only one palpable nodule in a multinodular goitre

Thyroid adenoma (scan may show decreased, normal or increased (subclinical toxic nodule) uptake)

Toxic adenoma (hot nodule on scan, tachycardia, sweaty palms, lid lag, etc.)

Thyroid cyst

Thyroid carcinoma (?hard, lymph nodes, recent change, cold on scan).

As well as assessment of thyroid function, fine-needle aspiration to attempt to establish the histological diagnosis should be undertaken in most cases of a solitary thyroid nodule. As an adjunct the nodule may be scanned radioisotopically though this is not usually necessary. If the nodule is hot it is not malignant but if it is cold it may be. In an older patient in whom the nodule has been present without changing for a long

---

*NB The possibility of associated autoimmune disease adds extra interest to the case of goitre, e.g. diabetes mellitus, rheumatoid arthritis, Addison's disease, pernicious anaemia. About 7% of patients with Graves' disease have vitiligo. About 5% of patients with myasthenia gravis have

thyrotoxicosis at some time. (See also pp. 214, 247 and 251.)
† By contrast, when the goitre and raised serum thyroxine is due to Graves' disease there is high radioactive iodine uptake on the scan.

time, observation only (perhaps with full dose thyroxine therapy which will reduce many nodules) may sometimes be justified initially. In any case of doubt, exploration of the neck and biopsy of the nodule are indicated, proceeding to subtotal lobectomy if the nodule is benign.

Types of thyroid carcinoma

Papillary carcinoma is the commonest form. It occurs in children and the middle-aged. It spreads to regional lymph nodes but is often resectable and has a good prognosis. It is often TSH-dependent and may respond to thyroxine

Follicular carcinoma is the next commonest and tends to arise later in life. Blood-borne metastases may occur, but following surgery and suppressive thyroxine treatment, the prognosis is fair. It and its secondaries often take up and respond to radioactive iodine

Anaplastic carcinoma tends to arise in the elderly and is highly malignant

Medullary carcinoma‡ is rare, tends to arise in young adults, secretes calcitonin and sometimes adrenocorticotrophic hormone (ACTH), but usually carries a good prognosis

Lymphoma (gl.) generally arises in a gland affected by Hashimoto's thyroiditis. A rapidly enlarging mass in the thyroid of a patient with Hashimoto's should arouse suspicion.

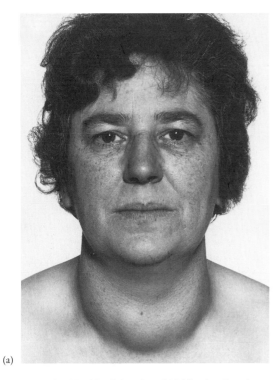
(a)

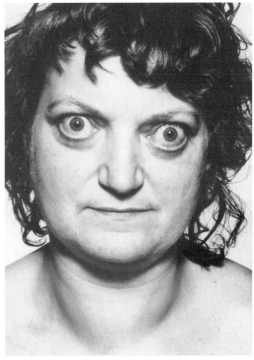
(b)

Fig. 17.2 (a) Multinodular goitre. (b) Diffusely enlarged thyroid (Graves' disease).

‡ MEA (multiple endocrine adenopathy) type IIa (Sipple's syndrome, also known as MEN (multiple endocrine neoplasia) syndrome) describes the association of:
1 Medullary cell carcinoma of the thyroid
2 Phaeochromocytoma (gl.)
3 Parathyroid hyperplasia (50%).
In MEA type IIb, medullary cell carcinoma of the thyroid and sometimes phaeochromocytoma are associated with a variety of neurological abnormalities including mucosal neuromata (lumpy, bumpy lips and eyelids), marfanoid habitus, hyperplastic corneal nerves, skin pigmentation, proximal myopathy and intestinal disorders such as megacolon and ganglioneuromatosis. Parathyroid hyperplasia is less common. In MEA type IIa medullary carcinoma may occasionally secrete other substances such as ACTH, histaminase, vasoactive intestinal peptide (VIP), prostaglandins and serotonin, whereas in MEA type IIb production of hormones other than calcitonin is rare. Both are autosomal dominant. Type IIb is sometimes called type III.

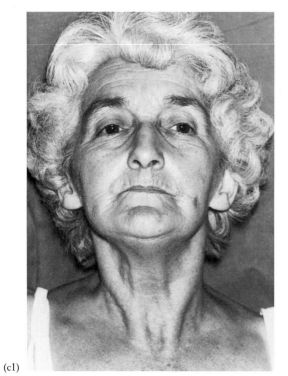

(c1)

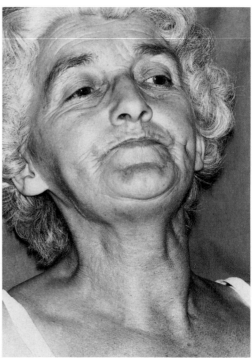

(c2)

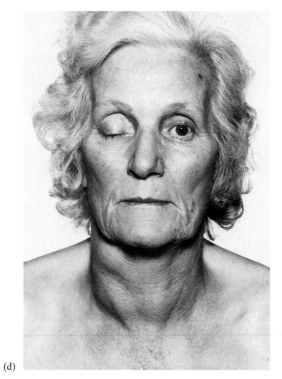

(d)

Fig. 17.2 (*continued*) (c1,2) Solitary nodule only made obvious by swallowing (right). (d) Follicular carcinoma of the thyroid with secondaries in the cavernous sinus (total ophthalmoplegia and absent corneal reflex on the right).

91 / Generalized lymphadenopathy

Record

There is generalized lymphadenopathy with/without . . . cm *splenomegaly* (or hepatosplenomegaly).

The likeliest causes would be a *lymphoreticular disorder* (Hodgkin's (gl.) and non-Hodgkin's lymphoma, etc.) or *chronic lymphatic leukaemia* (gl.).

Other causes

Infectious mononucleosis* (?sore throat)
Sarcoidosis (gl.) (?erythema nodosum or history of)
Tuberculosis (?ethnic origin, lung signs)
Brucellosis (gl.) (?farm worker)
Toxoplasmosis* (glandular fever-like illness)

Cytomegalovirus* (glandular fever-like illness)
Thyrotoxicosis (?exophthalmos, goitre, tachycardia, etc. — p. 247)
Progressive generalized lymphadenopathy in human immunodeficiency virus (HIV) infection.

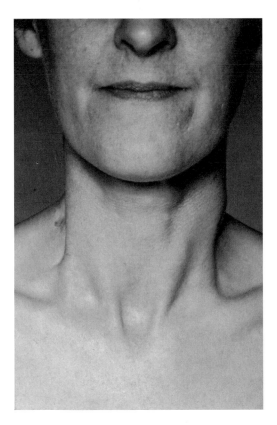

Fig. 17.3 A cervical lymph node seen from the end of the bed.

*Lymph nodes likely to be tender in acute infectious cases.

Chapter 18
Examine this patient's thyroid status

Possible short cases include

Euthyroid **Graves' disease** (p. 247)
Hyperthyroidism
Euthyroid simple **goitre** (p. 240).

Examination *routine*

Although the patient usually has signs of thyroid disease (exophthalmos, goitre), you are not being asked to examine these, but rather to assess whether the patient is clinically hypo-, eu- or hyperthyroid. Perform a speedy

1 *visual survey* looking specifically for *signs of thyroid disease* (exophthalmos, goitre, thyroid acropachy (gl.), pretibial myxoedema—all can occur in association with *any* thyroid status), and ask yourself if the facies are in any way myxoedematous. Observe the patient's

2 **composure**, whether *hyperactive*, *fidgety* and *restless* (hyperthyroid); normal, composed demeanour (euthyroid); or if he is somewhat *immobile* and *uninterested* in the people around him (hypothyroid).

3 Take the **pulse** and *count* it for 15 seconds, noting the presence or absence of *atrial fibrillation* (slow, normal rate or fast). If the pulse is slow (less than 60/min), or if you suspect hypothyroidism, proceed immediately to test

4 for **slow relaxation** of the ankle (Fig. 18.1a),* supinator or other jerks. To test the reflexes you will require the patient's cooperation and the ensuing conversation may provide you with helpful clues (slow hesitant speech, slow movements, etc.). Otherwise

5 feel the **palms**, whether *warm* and *sweaty* or cold and sweaty (anxiety) and then

6 ask the patient to stretch out his hands to full extension of the wrist and elbow. If the **tremor** is not obvious, place your palm against his outstretched fingers to feel for it. Alternatively, you can place a piece of paper on the dorsum of his outstretched hands—it will oscillate if a fine tremor is present.

7 Look at the **eyes**, noting exophthalmos (sclera visible above the lower lid—a

---

* The slow relaxing ankle jerk in hypothyroidism is best demonstrated with the patient kneeling on a chair or bed with the feet hanging over the edge, and the examiner standing behind the patient (Fig. 18.1b). However, this manoeuvre (which is useful for the dressed patient in the out-patient department) is not usually necessary in student clinical examinations.

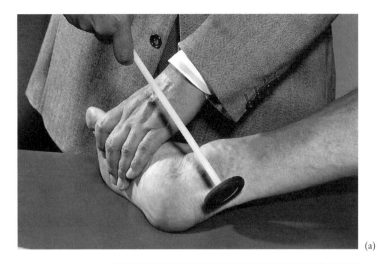

(a)

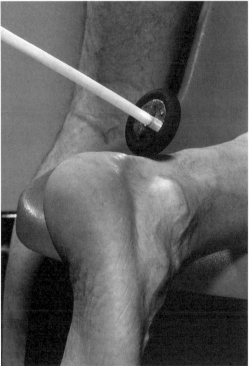

(b)

Fig. 18.1 (a,b) Testing the ankle jerk—watch for the speed of relaxation.

sign not related to thyroid status) but looking specifically for *lid retraction* (sclera visible above the cornea). Test for lid lag (Fig. 18.2) (lid lag and retraction may diminish as the hyperthyroid patient becomes euthyroid).

8 Examine the **thyroid** as described under 'Examine this patient's neck', remembering the steps are: (i) look, (ii) palpate, and (iii) auscultate.*

---

* A thyroid bruit is good evidence of thyroid overactivity; if present it can be heard over the isthmus and lateral lobe of the thyroid; it will not be obliterated by occluding the internal jugular vein (venous hum) or by rotation of the head and it will not be influenced by pressure of the stethoscope (use light pressure to avoid causing non-thyroid bruits).

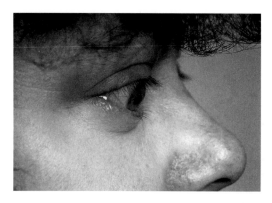

Fig. 18.2 Lid lag. The upper lid lags behind the downward movement of the eyeball (reproduced with permission from A. Mir, *Atlas of Clinical Diagnosis*, 1995, Saunders).

Putting the above findings together it should be possible to provide a definite conclusion about thyroid status; this is considered a very basic skill and it will not be taken lightly if, in your state of nerves, you make fundamental errors. Though the examiner may put you under pressure to test your confidence, keep calm and be particularly wary of being led to diagnose hypo- or hyperthyroidism in the presence of a normal pulse rate.

9 Be prepared with the **standard questions** for assessment of thyroid status (temperature preference, weight change, appetite, bowel habits, palpitations, change of temper, etc. — see pp. 247 and 251) should the examiner wish you to question the patient. Indeed, if there is any doubt about the thyroid status after the above examination, offer to ask the patient these questions.

For *checklist* see p. 278.

92 / Graves' disease

Record 1

The patient (usually female) is *thin*, has *sweaty palms*, a *fine tremor* of the outstretched hands, a *tachycardia** and she is *fidgety* and nervous. There is a small diffuse *goitre* with a *bruit*, and she has *exophthalmos* (p. 152) with *lid lag*.†

This patient is *thyrotoxic* and has Graves' disease.

Record 2

There is *exophthalmos* (?chemosis, ophthalmoplegia, diplopia, lateral tarsorrhaphy), *thyroid acropachy* (gl.),‡ and the lesions on the front of the shins are *pretibial myxoedema* (p. 221). The pulse is regular* and the *pulse rate is normal* (give rate), the palms are *not sweaty*, and there is *no hand tremor* or *lid lag.* There is a *thyroidectomy scar*.

The diagnosis is *euthyroid* Graves' disease,§ the patient having been treated by thyroidectomy in the past.

Male to female ratio is 1:5.

Record 3

This patient with *exophthalmos* (?chemosis, ophthalmoplegia, diplopia, lateral tarsorrhaphy, goitre, thyroidectomy scar, pretibial myxoedema, thyroid acropachy) has *hypothyroid facies*, a *hoarse voice, slow pulse** and *slowly relaxing reflexes.*

The patient has Graves' disease and is clinically *hypothyroid*. It is likely that she had hyperthyroidism treated in the past (?thyroidectomy or radioactive iodine) and is probably now on inadequate thyroxine replacement. (Because of the close links between the autoimmune thyroid diseases—see below—patients with Graves' disease occasionally go on to develop hypothyroidism spontaneously.)

Other signs which may occur

Fever (rarely hyperpyrexia)
Systolic hypertension with wide pulse pressure
Cutaneous vasodilatation
Systolic murmur due to increased blood flow
Proximal muscle weakness (thyrotoxic myopathy)
Hyperactive reflexes

---

* The pulse may be regular or irregular—the patient may have sinus rhythm or atrial fibrillation whatever the thyroid status (hyperthyroid; eu- or hypothyroid due to treatment).
† Graves' disease may be present in the absence of the eye signs and in an elderly male patient. There may be evidence of the humoral autoimmunity, more specifically a circulating antibody to the thyrotrophin (TSH) receptor. The thyroid gland may even have a nodular enlargement but its radioactive iodine uptake is uniformly increased throughout the gland between the nodules in autoimmune disease (Graves' disease). The patient with nodular goitre and thyrotoxicosis due to autonomous hypersecretion of nodule(s) that does not have an autoimmune (thyrotoxicosis) basis, will have some nodules with increased uptake (hot nodules) on the isotope scan. Such patients are more likely to relapse after antithyroid drug therapy than patients with Graves' disease.

‡ Thyroid acropachy may resemble finger clubbing in hypertrophic pulmonary osteoarthropathy (HPOA). However, in thyroid acropachy new bone formation seen on an X-ray has the appearance of soap bubbles on the bone surface with coarse spicules. In HPOA new bone is formed in a linear distribution. Sometimes the new bone formation in acropachy is both visible and palpable along the phalanges.
§ Graves' exophthalmos is due to increased retro-orbital fat and enlarged intraorbital muscles infiltrated with lymphocytes and containing increased water and mucopolysaccharide. It may develop in the absence of hyperthyroidism and remit, persist or develop further despite successful treatment of hyperthyroidism. Pretibial myxoedema tends to develop after the hyperthyroidism has been treated—especially with radioactive iodine.

Choreoathetoid movements (in children)

Fine thin hair (females may show temporal recession of the hairline)

Onycholysis (gl.) (Plummer's nails, typically found bilaterally on the fourth finger)

Palmar erythema

Spider naevi

Splenomegaly (minimal)

Hepatomegaly (minimal)

Palpable lymph nodes (especially axillae)

Thyrotoxic osteoporosis (only rarely causes kyphosis or loss of height).

Important symptoms of hyperthyroidism

(if asked to ask the patient some questions) are heat intolerance, weight loss, increased appetite, diarrhoea, exertional dyspnoea, undue fatiguability, 'can't keep still', irritability and nervousness.

Other organ-specific autoimmune diseases

(see also p. 214) of which autoimmune thyroid disease || is an example include:

Pernicious anaemia

Atrophic gastritis with iron deficiency anaemia

Diabetes mellitus

Addison's disease

Idiopathic hypoparathyroidism (gl.)

Premature ovarian failure

Renal tubular acidosis (gl.)

Fibrosing alveolitis

Chronic active hepatitis (gl.)

Primary biliary cirrhosis.

All of these diseases show a *marked female preponderance*. Premature greying of the hair, alopecia areata and vitiligo (see p. 214) are all associated with this group of diseases. Autoimmune thyroiditis (gl.) is also associated with:

Sjögren's syndrome (gl.)

Myasthenia gravis

Systemic sclerosis

Mixed connective tissue disease

Cranial arteritis (gl.)

Polymyalgia rheumatica (gl.).

|| Graves' disease is one of the three closely related autoimmune thyroid diseases — the others being Hashimoto's thyroiditis and its atrophic variant, myxoedema. Among patients with one of these three it is typical to find relatives with one of the other two. Some patients appear to have a combination which has been termed 'hashitoxicosis'.

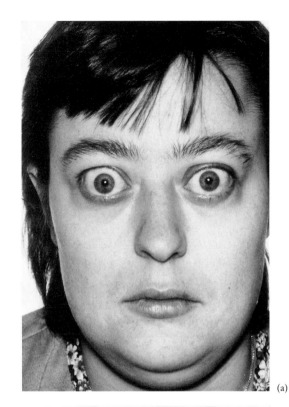

Fig. 18.3 (a) Graves' disease. (b1,2) Hyperthyroidism in a patient who presented with the complaint that she had noticed a staring appearance of her left eye (note thinning of the hair in the temporal region).

(a)

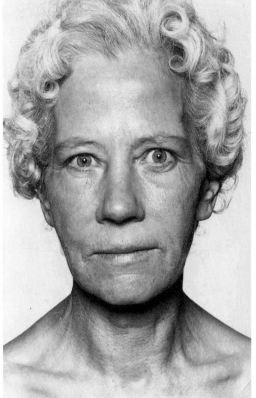

(b1)

(b2)

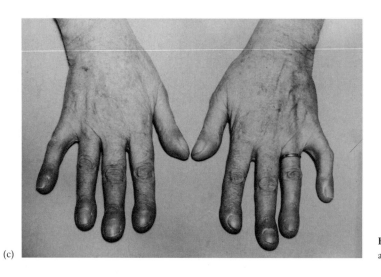

(c)

Fig. 18.3 (*continued*) (c) Thyroid acropachy.

93 / Hypothyroidism

Record 1

The patient is *overweight* with myxoedematous facies (*thickened* and *coarse facial features, periorbital puffiness* and pallor). The *skin* is rough, *dry, cold* and inelastic with a distinct yellowish tint (due to carotenaemia (gl.)), and there is generalized *non-pitting swelling* of the subcutaneous tissues. The patient's voice is *hoarse* and *croaking*, she is somewhat hard of hearing and her movements are *slow*. There is *thinning* of the *hair* which is *dry* and *brittle* and there is (may be) loss of the outer third of the eyebrows (not a reliable sign). The pulse is *slow* (give rate). There is no palpable goitre. The relaxation phase of the *ankle jerks* (and other reflexes) is delayed and *slow*.

This patient has *myxoedema** (?evidence of associated autoimmune disease — see below).

Record 2

As appropriate from the above plus: in view of the symmetrical, firm, finely micronodular (the typical features of a Hashimoto's goitre though there are many exceptions) *goitre* the likely diagnosis is hypothyroidism due to *Hashimoto's thyroiditis* (gl.)* (?associated autoimmune disease — see below).

Record 3

As appropriate from the above plus: in view of the *exophthalmos* it is likely that this patient was treated in the past for *Graves' disease* by radioactive iodine (or thyroidectomy if there is a scar) and is now hypothyroid (occasionally Graves' disease progresses spontaneously to hypothyroidism — see p. 152).

Associated autoimmune diseases†

Pernicious anaemia (?spleen, subacute combined degeneration of the cord (SACD))

Addison's disease (?buccal plus scar pigmentation)

Vitiligo

Rheumatoid arthritis (?hands, nodules)

Sjögren's syndrome (gl.) (?dry eyes and mouth)

Ulcerative colitis (gl.)

Idiopathic (presumed to be autoimmune) chronic active hepatitis (gl.) (?icterus, etc.)

Systemic lupus erythematosus (?rash)

Haemolytic anaemia (gl.)

Diabetes mellitus (?fundi)

Graves' disease

Hypoparathyroidism (gl.)

Premature ovarian failure.

Important symptoms (if asked to ask the patient some questions — NB deafness and hoarse voice):

Cold intolerance

* In hypothyroidism, accumulation of hyaluronic acid in the dermis as well as other tissues alters the composition of the ground substance. This material binds water, producing the mucinous oedema that is responsible for the thickened features and puffy appearance of full-blown hypothyroidism which is termed myxoedema. Hypothyroidism due to autoimmune thyroiditis (gl.) may present as primary thyroid atrophy (*record* 1) or Hashimoto's disease (*record* 2).

† See also p. 214.

Tiredness and depression

Constipation (may occasionally present to the surgeons with faecal impaction)

Angina (treatment may unmask, therefore start with low doses if age >50, or if patient has angina)

Menorrhagia (middle-aged females)

Primary or secondary amenorrhoea (younger patients).

Other features

Anaemia (normochromic, iron deficient—atrophic gastritis, or megaloblastic—frank pernicious anaemia; slight macrocytosis may occur in hypothyroidism without a megaloblastic change in the marrow)

Carpal tunnel syndrome (p. 204)

Peripheral cyanosis (there may be a malar flush)

Raynaud's phenomenon (gl.)

Hypertension

Accident proneness (may present to the casualty department)

Hypothermia (especially the elderly living alone)

Hoffman's syndrome (pain, aching and swelling in muscles after exertion together with signs of myotonia)

Psychosis (myxoedematous madness)

Hypothyroid coma.

A variety of other central nervous system disorders may occur,‡ such as peripheral neuropathy, cerebellar ataxia, pseudodementia, drop attacks and epilepsy.

‡ Always exclude concomitant vitamin B_{12} deficiency as the association with pernicious anaemia is strong. If you find peripheral neuropathy think also of concomitant diabetes mellitus before putting it down to the hypothyroidism.

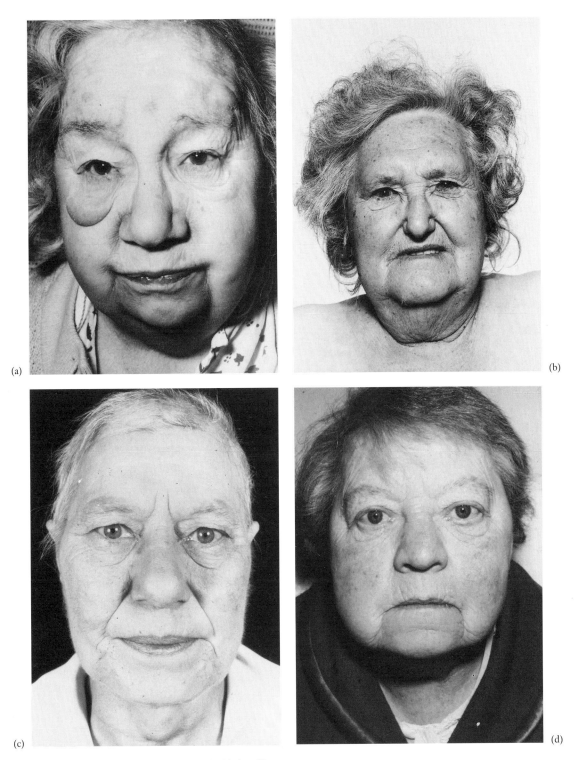

Fig. 18.4 (a–d) Note the thickened skin, periorbital swelling, sparse eyebrows and alopecia. The patient in (d) had a malar flush.

Chapter 19
What is the diagnosis?

Possible short cases include
Acromegaly (p. 257)
Parkinson's disease (p. 260)
Hemiplegia (p. 103)
Goitre (p. 240)
Jaundice
Dystrophia myotonica (p. 209)
Pigmentation
Graves' disease (p. 247)
Exophthalmos (p. 152)
Paget's disease (p. 99)
Ptosis (p. 165)
Choreoathetosis (gl.)
Drug-induced parkinsonism (p. 260)
Breathlessness
Purpura (p. 228)
Hypopituitarism
Addison's disease (p. 263)/Nelson's syndrome (gl.)
Cushing's syndrome (p. 265)
Psoriasis (p. 195)
Hypothyroidism (p. 251)
Systemic sclerosis/CRST syndrome (p. 176)
Sturge–Weber syndrome (gl.)
Spider naevi and ascites (p. 68)
Marfan's syndrome (gl.)
Neurofibromatosis (p. 219)
Cyanotic congenital heart disease (gl.)
Pretibial myxoedema (p. 221)
Uraemia and dialysis scars
Horner's syndrome (p. 180)
Cachexia
Osler–Weber–Rendu syndrome (p. 178)
Ankylosing spondylitis (p. 268)
Ulnar nerve palsy (p. 198)
Turner's syndrome (p. 270)
Down's syndrome (gl.)
Bilateral parotid enlargement/Mikulicz's syndrome (gl.)

Old rickets
Torticollis
Congenital syphilis (gl.)
Syringomyelia (gl.)
Herpes zoster (p. 235)
Pemphigus/pemphigoid (p. 223)
Bell's palsy
Necrobiosis lipoidica diabeticorum (p. 217)
Primary biliary cirrhosis (p. 70)

Examination *routine*

Advice commonly given to students facing a 'spot diagnosis' is to 'keep calm'. When you stand before a patient with a condition from the above list and hear the instruction under consideration you are being asked to do what you should do every day of your medical life. There are two differences, however, between everyday medical life and the examination: (i) the patients in an examination usually have classic, often florid, signs and should be easier to diagnose than most patients seen in the clinic or on the wards; and (ii) in an examination you may be overwhelmed by nerves and as a result make the most fundamental errors. You must indeed try to keep calm and remind yourself that this is likely to be an easy case, and that you will not only make a diagnosis (as you would with ease in the clinic or on the wards), but will also find a way of scoring some extra marks. Unlike some of the instructions requiring long examination *routines*, the 'spot diagnosis' may be solved in seconds leaving time for something extra which you may be able to dictate, rather than leaving it to the examiner to lead. You should start with

1 *a visual survey* of the patient, running your eyes from the head via the neck, trunk, arms and legs to the feet, seeking the areas of abnormality, and thereby the diagnosis. We would suggest that you rehearse presenting the *records* for the various possibilities on the list (see individual short cases). If you are well prepared with the features of these short cases, then in the majority of instances you should be able to make a diagnosis, or likely diagnosis, which you can confirm or highlight by demonstrating additional features (see below). If you have scanned the patient briefly and not found any obvious abnormality, then

2 retrace the same ground scrutinizing each part more thoroughly and asking yourself at each stage, 'Is the head normal?', 'Is the face normal?', etc. If it is not normal describe the abnormality to yourself in your mind trying to match it up with one of the short case *records*. In this way cover the

(a) head (think especially of *Paget's* and *dystrophia myotonica* with frontal balding),

(b) face (think especially of *acromegaly*, *Parkinson's*, the facial asymmetry of *hemiplegia*, the long lean look of dystrophia myotonica, tardive dyskinesia, hypopituitarism, Cushing's, hypothyroidism, systemic sclerosis),

(c) eyes (*jaundice*, *exophthalmos*, ptosis, Horner's, xanthelasma),

(d) neck (*goitre*, Turner's, ankylosing spondylitis, torticollis),

(e) trunk (pigmentation, ascites, purpuric spots, spider naevi, wasting, pemphigus, etc.),

(f) arms (choreoathetosis, psoriasis, Addison's, spider naevi, *syringomyelia*),

(g) hands (acromegaly, *tremor*, clubbing, sclerodactyly, arachnodactyly, claw hand, etc.),

(h) legs (bowing, purpura, pretibial myxoedema, necrobiosis), and

(i) feet (pes cavus).

If you still do not have the diagnosis

3 specifically consider **abnormal colouring** such as *pigmentation*, *icterus* or pallor, and then cover the same ground again but in even more detail

4 **breaking down each part into its constituents**, scrutinizing them, and continually asking yourself the question: 'Is it normal?' This procedure is most profitable on the face (see p. 172).

Once you have the diagnosis, the natural impulse for most people is to give it in one word, and then stand back and wait for the applause. However, it is worth remembering that the majority of students, who have all worked hard and prepared for the examination, are likely to 'spot' the diagnosis. Do not let this opportunity pass you by; try to make more of the case yourself by proceeding to

5 look for **additional** and **associated features**, and then by making your presentation more elaborate. Describe the findings in detail (see individual short cases) and highlight the key features to support your diagnosis (lenticular abnormalities in dystrophia myotonica and Marfan's; thyroid bruit in Graves' disease; webbed neck in Turner's syndrome, and so on). It is worth going through the diagnoses on the list yourself, and considering what additional features you would look for, and how you could really go to town on an easy case. For example, if you diagnose acromegaly you could demonstrate the massive sweaty palms, commenting on the increased skin thickening and on the presence or absence of thenar wasting (carpal tunnel syndrome) and then proceed to test the visual fields. If you suspect Parkinson's disease, take the hands and test for cog-wheel rigidity at the wrist, demonstrate the glabellar tap sign (despite its unreliability) and then ask the patient to walk. If you diagnose hemiplegia, confirm that facial weakness is upper motor neurone (see p. 103), and then check for atrial fibrillation. If you see a goitre, examine it and then assess the thyroid status.

For *checklist* see p. 278.

94 / Acromegaly

Note: you may sometimes be asked questions on areas such as presentation, investigation and complications.

Record

The patient has prominent *supraorbital ridges* and a *large lower jaw*. The facial wrinkles are exaggerated and the lips are full. There is *poor occlusion* of the teeth, the *lower teeth overbiting* in front of the upper (prognathism). The *nose, tongue* and *ears* are enlarged and the patient is *kyphotic*. The *hands* are *large, doughy* and *spade-shaped,** and the *skin* over the back of them is *thickened* (shake hands and examine the dorsum). There is (may be) loss of the thenar eminence bilaterally with impaired sensation in the median nerve distribution (*carpal tunnel syndrome*). The patient is *sweating* excessively and is mildly *hirsute* (one-third of cases). The *voice* is husky and cavernous. There is a *bitemporal peripheral visual field defect*.

The diagnosis is acromegaly.

Other physical signs which may be present

Bowed legs
Rolling gait
Goitre
Gynaecomastia
Galactorrhoea (gl.)
Small gonads
Greasy skin
Acne
Acanthosis nigricans (gl.)
Osteoarthrosis
Prominent superficial veins of the extremities
Proximal muscle weakness
Cardiomegaly (hypertension and cardiomyopathy)
Third nerve palsy.

Other features

Diabetes mellitus (glycosuria, glucose intolerance or frank diabetes may occur; it is usually mild and ketoacidosis is rare; it is somewhat resistant to insulin)
Hypertension (20–50%)
Hypercalciuria (common)
Hypercalcaemia† (occasionally)
Diabetes insipidus (gl.) (normally due to hypothalamic pressure effect; if there is impaired cortisol secretion symptoms may be masked)
Hypopituitarism
Osteoporosis (gl.).

Symptoms before presentation‡

Excessive sweating

---

* Shaking hands with the patient may give the impression of losing one's hands in a mass of dough.

† In some this disappears when the acromegaly is successfully treated. In others it is due to associated hyperparathyroidism as part of *multiple endocrine adenopathy (MEA) type I* (Werner's syndrome) which is two or more of:

1 Pituitary tumour (eosinophil or chromophobe)
2 Islet-cell tumour (gastrin or insulin)
3 Primary hyperparathyroidism (adenoma or hyperplasia)

4 Adrenocortical adenoma (see also p. 265 and footnote). MEA type I should probably be regarded as a complex of separate genetic abnormalities rather than as a consequence of a single primary disease. It should not be confused with MEA type 2 which is usually an autosomal dominant trait with a high degree of penetrance (see footnote, p. 241).

‡ The mean age of onset has been estimated at about 27 years whereas the mean age of presentation is over 40 years, i.e. there is an average pre-presentation lapse of 13–14 years.

Increasing size of shoes, gloves, hats, dentures and rings

Paraesthesiae of the hands and feet

Digital pain and stiffness (of slowly expanding fingers and toes)

Arthralgia

Hypogonadism (amenorrhoea, loss of libido)

Headache (may be severe; may occur without clinically detectable enlargement of the pituitary tumour; the mechanism is not clear)

Visual field or acuity disturbance.

Investigations

Comparative study of old photographs of the patient

Skull X-ray

Computerized tomography (CT) scan or magnetic resonance imaging (MRI) scan of pituitary fossa

X-ray for heel pad thickness (increased) is rarely carried out nowadays

Visual fields

Glucose tolerance test with growth hormone response (lack of suppression; sometimes a paradoxical rise)

Tests of anterior pituitary function (*adrenocorticotroph*: short Synacthen test,§ insulin tolerance test; *thyrotroph*: thyroid-stimulating hormone (TSH) plus total or free T_4; *gonadotroph*: menstrual history plus oestrodiol, luteinizing hormone (LH) and follicle-stimulating hormone (FSH) (female), potency plus testosterone (male); *lactotroph*: prolactin‖).

Treatment

Trans-sphenoidal hypophysectomy

Transfrontal hypophysectomy in some cases with large extensive adenomata

External irradiation (especially if surgery fails; takes 1–10 years to take effect)

Radioactive gold or yttrium implants (very restricted in terms of availability)

Bromocriptine (50% respond but the size of the tumour is not reduced; useful for growth hormone hypersecretion after surgery)

Long-acting somatostatin analogues (require parenteral administration); effective in lowering growth hormone until surgery/radiotherapy; tumour may shrink in some cases.

§ In hypopituitarism, the adrenal cortex does not respond sufficiently in the short Synacthen test. It needs to be primed continually by adrenocorticotrophic hormone (ACTH) from a functioning pituitary in order to be responsive.

‖ The prolactin level may be low in hypopituitarism. However, production may also be elevated because: (i) some growth hormone-secreting pituitary tumours co-secrete prolactin, and (ii) any pituitary macroadenoma which presses on the pituitary stalk will interfere with dopamine suppression of prolactin production and lead to hyperprolactinaemia.

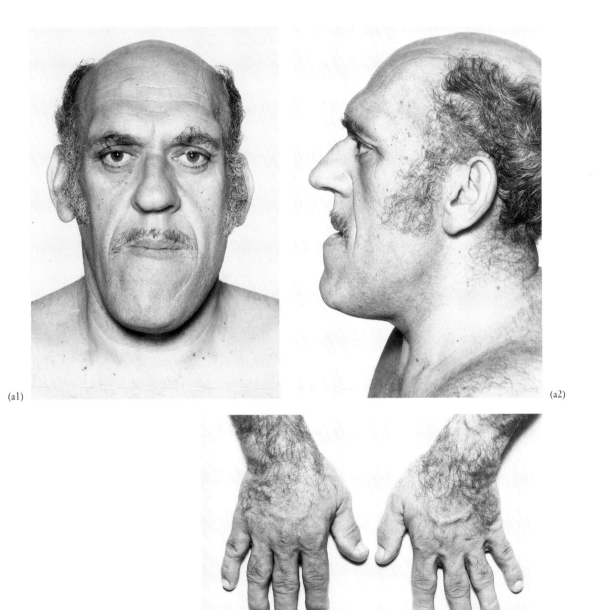

Fig. 19.1 (a1,2) Acromegalic facies.
(b) Large hands with thickened skin.

(a1)

(a2)

(b)

95 / Parkinson's disease

Record 1

This man has an *expressionless, unblinking face* and slurred *low volume monotonous speech*. He is drooling (due to excessive salivation and some dysphagia) and there is *titubation*. He has difficulty starting to walk ('freezing') but once started, progresses with quick shuffling steps as if trying to keep up with his own centre of gravity. As he walks he is *stooped* and he *does not swing his arms* which show a continuous *pill-rolling tremor*. (He has poor balance and tends to fall, being unable to react quickly enough to stop himself.) His arms show a *lead-pipe rigidity* at the elbow but *cog-wheel rigidity* (combination of lead-pipe rigidity and tremor—i.e. worse with anxiety) at the wrist. He has a positive glabellar tap sign (an unreliable sign) and his signs generally are *asymmetrical*— note the greater tremor in the R/L arm. (The tremor is decreased by intention but hand-writing may be small, tremulous and untidy.) There is *blepharoclonus* (tremor of the eyelids when the eyes are gently closed).

    The diagnosis is Parkinson's disease.

Male to female ratio is 3:1.

The features of Parkinson's disease are

1 Tremor
2 Rigidity
3 Bradykinesia.

Bradykinesia (the most disabling) can be demonstrated by asking the patient to touch his thumb successively with each finger. He will be slow in the initiation of the response and there will be a progressive reduction in the amplitude of each movement and a peculiar type of fatiguability. He will also have difficulty in performing two different motor acts simultaneously.

Record 2 (drug-induced extrapyramidal syndrome)

There are (in this ?elderly, chronic schizophrenic) stereotyped tic-like *orofacial dyskinesias* (involuntary movements) including *lip-smacking, chewing, pouting* and *grimacing*. There is (may be) *choreoathetosis* (gl.) of the limbs and trunk.

    The diagnosis is tardive dyskinesia.* (It is likely that the patient has been on sustained phenothiazine treatment for at least 6 months. The condition often persists when the drug is withdrawn, in which case tetrabenazine may help.)

Neuroleptics which may cause abnormal involuntary movements (by inhibiting dopamine function):

Phenothiazines (e.g. chlorpromazine)
Butyrophenones (e.g. haloperidol)
Substituted benzamides (e.g. metoclopramide)
Reserpine
Tetrabenazine.

---

* Called tardive (late) because it does not appear until at least 3 months, or more often a year, after the start or withdrawal of long-term treatment with neuroleptic drugs. This distinguishes tardive dyskinesia from acute dystonias and parkinsonism which develop early. The latter respond to anticholinergic drugs, while tardive dyskinesia responds poorly, or not at all.

Other neuroleptic-induced extrapyramidal adverse reactions (apart

from tardive dyskinesia):

Acute dystonias (soon after starting the drug; e.g. oculogyric crises)

Akathisia (uncontrollable restlessness with an inner feeling of unease)

Parkinson's syndrome (indistinguishable from Parkinson's disease though tremor is less common; tends to respond to anticholinergics rather than L-dopa).

Other causes of parkinsonian syndrome

Postencephalitic (increasingly rare; definite history of encephalitis—encephalitis lethargica pandemic 1916–1928; there may be ophthalmoplegia, pupil abnormalities and dyskinesias; poor response to L-dopa)

Brain damage from anoxia (e.g. cardiac arrest), carbon monoxide or manganese poisoning (dementia and pyramidal signs likely with all)

Neurosyphilis

Cerebral tumours affecting the basal ganglia.

Other conditions which may have some extrapyramidal features

Arteriosclerotic Parkinson's (stepwise progression, broad-based gait, pyramidal signs; may be no more than simply two common conditions occurring in the same patient—cerebral arteriosclerosis and idiopathic parkinsonism)

Normal pressure hydrocephalus (may have a number of causes including head injury, meningitis or subarachnoid haemorrhage, though in many instances the cause cannot be determined; the classic triad is *urinary incontinence*, *gait apraxia* and *dementia*; diagnosed by CT or MRI scan; important to diagnose because it may respond to ventriculosystemic shunting)

Steele–Richardson–Olszewski syndrome (gl.) (supranuclear gaze palsy, axial rigidity, a tendency to fall backwards, pyramidal signs, subtle dementia or frontal lobe syndrome)

Shy–Drager syndrome (gl.) (idiopathic orthostatic hypotension, impotence, urinary incontinence, anhidrosis, cerebellar and pyramidal signs and peripheral neuropathy; L-dopa contraindicated)

Alzheimer's disease (gl.) (severe dementia, mild extrapyramidal signs)

Olivopontocerebellar degeneration (sometimes familial; cerebellar and extrapyramidal signs)

Wilson's disease (gl.) (Kayser–Fleischer rings (gl.), cirrhosis, chorea, psychotic behaviour, dysarthria, dystonic spasms and posturing; leading, if untreated, to dementia, severe dysarthria and dysphagia, contractures and immobility)

Jakob–Creutzfeldt disease (prion protein encephalopathy leading to rapidly progressive dementia with myoclonus and multifocal neurological signs including aphasia, cerebellar ataxia, cortical blindness and spasticity)

Hypoparathyroidism (gl.) (basal ganglia calcification).

NB A condition which is often misdiagnosed as Parkinson's disease in the elderly is *benign essential tremor* (often autosomal dominant, intention tremor worse with stress, no other neurological abnormality; usually improves when alcohol is taken and sometimes with diazepam or propranolol).

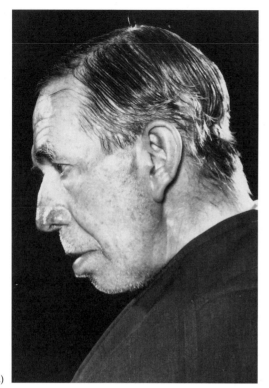
(a)

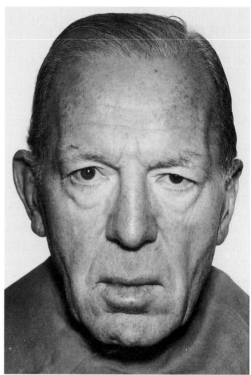
(b)

Fig. 19.2 (a,b) Parkinson's disease.

96 / Addison's disease

Record

There is *generalized pigmentation* (due to the direct action of ACTH causing increased melanin in the skin), which is more marked in the *skin creases* (e.g. palmar), in *scars* (especially more recent ones), in the *buccal mucosa* (look in the mouth), in the *nipples* and at *pressure points*.

This suggests Addison's disease or Nelson's syndrome (gl.) (?temporal field defect, ?abdominal scar of bilateral adrenalectomy).

Patchy, almost symmetrical, areas of skin depigmentation surrounded by areas of increased pigmentation may occur due to vitiligo (15% of patients with idiopathic Addison's) which is one of the associated organ-specific autoimmune diseases. (For the others, which include autoimmune thyroiditis (gl.), diabetes mellitus, pernicious anaemia and hypoparathyroidism (gl.), see p. 214. Premature ovarian failure is particularly associated with Addison's disease.)

Common causes of primary hypoadrenalism

Autoimmune adrenalitis
Tuberculosis (?lung signs).

Other causes of primary hypoadrenalism

Bilateral adrenalectomy (malignant disease, e.g. breast cancer; Cushing's syndrome)
Secondary deposits
Amyloidosis (gl.) (hypoadrenalism preceded by nephrotic syndrome (gl.) — see footnote, p. 61)
Haemochromatosis (gl.)
Granulomatous disease (rarely sarcoidosis (gl.))
Fungal diseases (e.g. histoplasmosis (gl.))
Congenital adrenal hyperplasia*
Meningococcal and pseudomonal septicaemia
Adrenal haemorrhage (newborn especially breech delivery; patients on anticoagulants)
Adrenal vein thrombosis after trauma or adrenal venography.

Skin pigmentation is usually racial (including buccal pigmentation) or due to sun-tanning. Other causes of abnormal generalized pigmentation include:

Endocrine

ACTH therapy (e.g. asthma)
Cushing's disease (?facies, truncal obesity, striae, etc. — p. 265)
Thyrotoxicosis (?exophthalmos, goitre, etc. — p. 247)
Ectopic ACTH (especially oat-cell carcinoma).

Chronic debilitating disorders (also, like Addison's, associated with lassitude and weight loss)

Malignancy (including reticuloses and leukaemias)
Malabsorption syndromes
Chronic infections (especially tuberculosis)
Cirrhosis (?icterus, spider naevi, etc. — pp. 62 and 70)
Uraemia (pale, brownish-yellow tinge to skin).

Pigments other than melanin, such as

Haemochromatosis (gl.) (slate-grey pigmentation, hepatosplenomegaly, etc.)
Argyria (gl.)
Chronic arsenic poisoning.

Drugs

Phenothiazines (blue-grey pigmentation)
Antimalarials (blue-grey pigmentation)
Amiodarone (grey pigmentation)
Cytotoxics
Minocycline (purple-blue pigmentation; may get blue oral discoloration due to blue-black discoloration of alveolar bone and hard palate — 'black-bone disease').

---

* Series of inherited defects in adrenocortical steroidogenesis (e.g. 21-hydroxylase deficiency). Homozygotes present neonatally with salt wasting, hypotension and ambiguous genitalia in females.

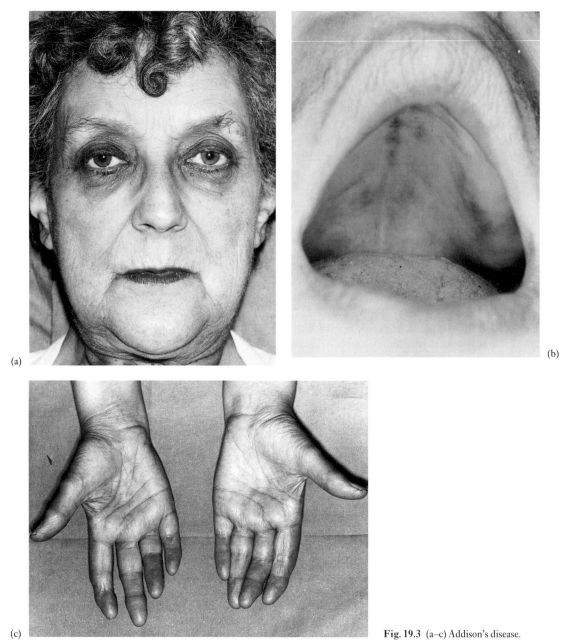

(a)

(b)

(c)

Fig. 19.3 (a–c) Addison's disease.

97 / Cushing's syndrome

Note: sometimes there may be a patient with Cushing's disease* or an adrenal tumour* but usually almost all cases are secondary to therapeutic steroids—especially for asthma and rheumatoid arthritis, but also for cryptogenic fibrosing alveolitis and chronic active hepatitis (gl.), amongst others.

Record

The patient has a *moon face* with *acne* and *truncal obesity* with a *buffalo hump*. The skin is thin (demonstrate by raising a skinfold at the back of the patient's hand) and shows excessive bruising (*purpuric patches*—often at venesection sites), and there are purple *striae* on the abdomen (must be differentiated from the pale pink striae of obese adolescents and the stretch marks of pregnancy and simple obesity). She is *hirsute* with a *deep voice*. There is *proximal muscle weakness* (few patients with Cushing's syndrome can rise normally from the squatting position).

The diagnosis is Cushing's syndrome (?evidence of underlying steroid-responsive inflammatory or immunological disorder).

Other features of Cushing's syndrome
Hypertension and peripheral oedema (salt retention)

Irregular menstruation

Impotence

Back pain (osteoporosis (gl.) and vertebral collapse leading to kyphosis and loss of height)

Diabetes mellitus

Pigmentation (especially ectopic or exogenous ACTH)

Psychiatric disorder (commonly depressive illness).

Causes of Cushing's syndrome*
Therapeutic corticosteroids

Therapeutic ACTH

Cushing's disease*—pituitary (basophilic or chromo-phobe pituitary adenoma) or hypothalamic lesion leading to excessive ACTH

Adrenocortical adenoma* (occasionally part of *MEA type I* with one or more of: primary hyperparathyroidism, islet-cell tumour, pituitary tumour—see also p. 257†)

Adrenocortical carcinoma*

Ectopic ACTH-secreting non-endocrine tumours*:

1 Oat-cell carcinoma of bronchus (weight loss, pigmentation, hypokalaemic alkalosis and oedema)

2 Bronchial adenoma

3 Carcinoid tumour (gl.) (usually bronchial)

4 Carcinoma of the pancreas

5 Non-teratomatous ovarian tumour.

---

* When the syndrome is not iatrogenic, then in about 80% of affected adults the cause is Cushing's disease; whereas adrenal adenoma, carcinoma and ectopic ACTH syndrome contribute equally to the remaining 20%.

† The islet-cell tumour may secrete gastrin (Zollinger–Ellison syndrome) or insulin (insulinoma). The pituitary tumour may be eosinophilic (acromegaly) or a chromophobe adenoma which is non-secreting (bitemporal hemianopia, headaches, blindness, hypopituitarism and other pressure symptoms—the tumour may become very large). Pituitary tumours may also secrete prolactin (impotence, amenorrhoea, galactorrhoea (gl.)) or ACTH (Cushing's disease).

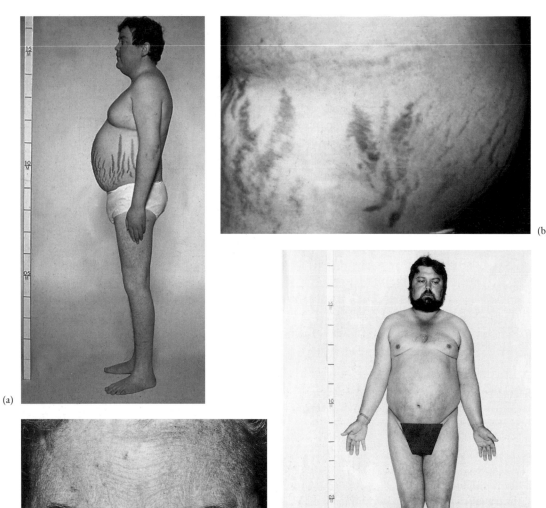

(a)

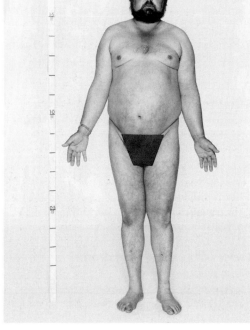

(b)

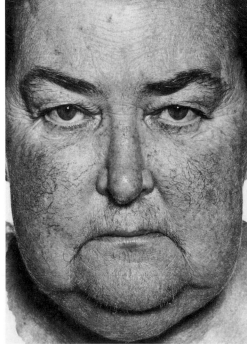

(c)

(d)

Fig. 19.4 (a) Cushing's syndrome. (b) Abdominal striae.
(c) Cushingoid facies (steroid therapy for cerebral lupus
erythematosus). (d) Truncal obesity (Cushing's disease).

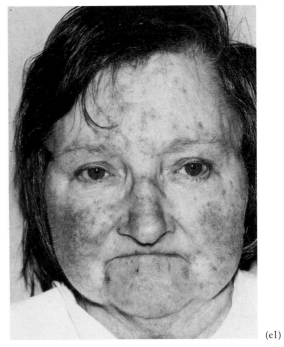

(e1)

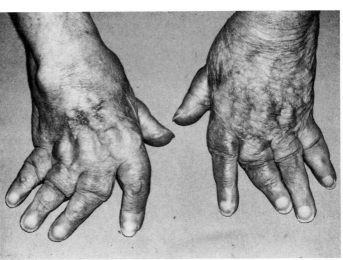

(e2)

Fig. 19.4 (*continued*) (e1,2) Corticosteroid therapy in a patient with rheumatoid arthritis.

98 / Ankylosing spondylitis

Note: you may be asked to examine either the chest, the back, the neck, to watch the patient walk, or to watch the patient 'look at the ceiling'. The diagnosis may not be apparent with the patient lying down.

Record

There is (in this male patient) *loss of lumbar lordosis* and *fixed kyphosis* which is compensated for by extension of the cervical spine (to attempt to keep the visual axis horizontal) producing a *stooped*, 'question mark' posture. When I ask the patient to turn his head to look to the side his whole body turns as a block (the spine being rigid with little movement). *Chest expansion is reduced*; the patient breathes by increased diaphragmatic excursion which is the cause of the *prominent abdomen*.

The diagnosis is ankylosing spondylitis. (If allowed, look at the *eyes*—iritis; listen to the *heart*—aortic incompetence; and examine the *chest*—apical fibrosis).

Ratio of males to females is 8 : 1.

Complications and extra-articular manifestations

Iritis—30% (acute, deep aching pain, redness, photophobia, miosis, sluggish pupillary reflex, circumcorneal conjunctival injection; may result in synechiae or cataracts)

Aortitis—4% (?collapsing pulse and early diastolic murmur of aortic incompetence; ascending aortic aneurysm)

Apical fibrosis—rare (?apical inspiratory crackles; probably secondary to diminished apical ventilation; there may be calcification and cavitation; may get secondary *Aspergillus* infection)

Cardiac conduction defects—10% (usually atrioventricular block; other cardiac abnormalities may occur—pericarditis and cardiomyopathy)

Neurological (atlantoaxial dislocation or traumatic fracture of a rigid spine may injure the spinal cord—tetra/paraplegia; involvement of the sacral nerves at the sacroiliac joints may cause sciatica; rarely cauda equina involvement can cause urinary or rectal sphincter incompetence)

Secondary amyloidosis (gl.) (kidneys, adrenals, liver—?hepatomegaly).

Other features

There is a strong (87%) association with HLA-B27.

There is a familial tendency; 50% of relatives are HLA-B27 and 9% have sacroiliitis which may be symptomless.* Ankylosing spondylitis usually starts before the age of 45.† It may present as an asymmetrical peripheral arthritis usually of large, weight-bearing joints; the small joints of the hands and feet are only rarely involved. It commonly presents with low back pain:

Ankylosing spondylitis—pain worse on waking, eases with exercise,

Compared with

Mechanical back pain—no pain on waking; pain brought on by exercise.

In the '*heels, hips, occiput*' test the patient is asked to demonstrate that he can put all three against a wall at once. *Schober's test* refers to the normal 10 cm excursion of two points 5 cm apart when the patient bends forward.

---

* The disease is more severe in sporadic cases (about 80%) than in the familial form (20%). Sibling pairs concordant for the disease tend to have disease of comparable severity.

† In the early stages, loss of lateral flexion of the lumbar spine is usually the first sign of spinal involvement, followed by loss of lumbar lordosis.

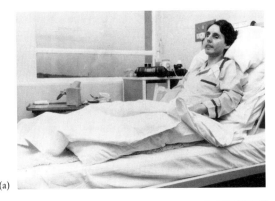

(a)

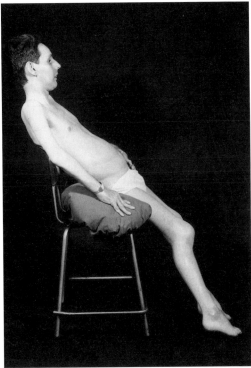

(b)

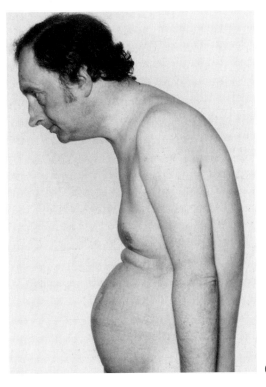

(c)

Fig. 19.5 (a) The ankylosing spondylitis is less obvious when reclining in bed. (b) In the same patient as (a), a rigid and immobile spine was revealed by his attempt at sitting up (note the generalized involvement of the joints in this severe case). (c) Patient attempting to look straight ahead (note the kyphosis, loss of lumbar lordosis and protuberant abdomen).

99 / Turner's syndrome

Record

The patient (who probably presented with primary amenorrhoea) is *short* (usually less than 1.5 m) with a *short webbed neck** (only found in 54%) and shows *cubitus valgus* deformity. She has a *shield-like chest* (and may have widely separated nipples). The *nails are hypoplastic* and she has *short fourth metacarpals* (other metacarpals may also be short). The *hairline is low*, she has a *high-arched palate* and there are *numerous naevi*. The secondary sexual characteristics are underdeveloped (unless the patient has been treated with oestrogens).

The diagnosis is Turner's syndrome. (If allowed: examine the cardiovascular system—abnormal in 20%; especially coarctation of the aorta (p. 31) but also atrial septal defect (gl.), ventricular septal defect (p. 30) and aortic stenosis (p. 22).)

The patient with Turner's syndrome is likely to have streak gonads and a chromosome constitution which is mostly 45,XO,† though mosaicism (XO,XX) does occur. Red–green colour blindness (an X-linked recessive character) occurs as frequently in Turner's as it does in normal males, and other X-linked conditions may occur.

Other features which sometimes occur

Lymphoedema
Genitourinary abnormality (e.g. horseshoe kidney)
Hypertelorism (gl.)
Epicanthal fold
Mental retardation (rare)
Strabismus
Ptosis
Intestinal telangiectasia
Premature osteoporosis (gl.)
Premature ageing in appearance
Higher incidence of diabetes mellitus and Hashimoto's thyroiditis (gl.).

Noonan's syndrome

This may affect both sexes. Females have a Turner's phenotype but normal 46,XX, normal ovarian function and normal fertility. Patients with Noonan's (gl.) are more likely to have right-sided cardiac lesions (especially pulmonary stenosis) whereas patients with Turner's are more likely to have left-sided lesions. Mental retardation is frequent.

---

* A feature especially associated with cardiovascular abnormalities in this condition.

† Most 45,XO pregnancies end in spontaneous abortion.

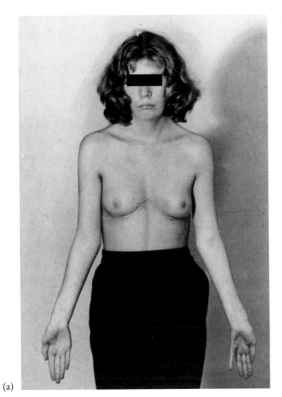

(a)

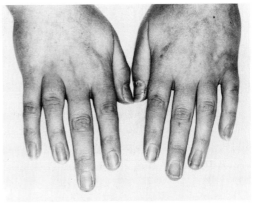

(b)

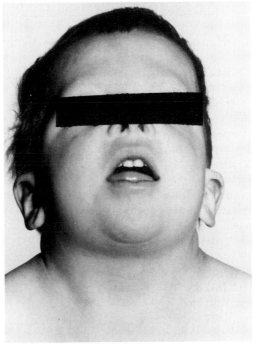

(c)

Fig. 19.6 (a) XO,XX mosaic. Note the webbed neck, increased carrying angle and scar under the breasts (special incision for atrial septal defect repair). (b) The hands of another patient showing a short fourth metacarpal. (c) Noonan's syndrome.

Record

There is gynaecomastia (may be unilateral). This is confirmed on palpation by the presence of *increased glandular tissue*. Now look for signs of *cirrhosis, heart failure* (spironolactone), *atrial fibrillation* (digoxin), *clubbing and cachexia* (carcinoma of the lung), *absence of body hair* (hypogonadism, oestrogen therapy) or evidence of an *endocrine disorder*—see below.

There may be feminization of the nipples and tenderness of the breasts. Gynaecomastia must be differentiated from tumours of the breast and simple adiposity.

Causes of gynaecomastia

Pubertal (very common*—due to transient dominance of circulating oestradiol over testosterone)

Senile (normal rise in oestrogens and fall in androgens with age)

Cirrhosis of the liver (?stigmata—p. 62)

Thyrotoxicosis (?exophthalmos, goitre, etc.—p. 247)

Carcinoma of the lung (5% of patients; sometimes with hypertrophic pulmonary osteoarthropathy; human chorionic gonadotrophin (hCG) secreted by the tumour)

Carcinoma of the liver (hCG secreting)

Klinefelter's syndrome (gl.) (47,XXY, small testes, mental deficiency, incomplete virilization, raised LH and FSH)

Pituitary disease,† i.e. acromegaly, hypopituitarism (?visual field defect)

Isolated gonadotrophin deficiency (e.g. Kallman's syndrome (gl.)—hypogonadotrophic hypogonadism and anosmia, often with harelip or cleft palate)

Testicular tumours (due to hCG secretion, oestrogen secretion or excess aromatase activity in the tumour tissue)

Addison's disease (?pigmentation—buccal and scar; p. 263)

Adrenal carcinoma

Testicular feminization (androgen insensitivity)

Drug-induced:‡
(a) oestrogen therapy (carcinoma of the prostate)
(b) digoxin
(c) griseofulvin
(d) alkylating agents (cause testicular damage)
(e) antiandrogens (including cyproterone acetate, spironolactone, ketoconazole, metronidazole and cimetidine)

Other drugs include phenothiazines, reserpine, tricyclics, methyldopa, isoniazid, amphetamines, aromatizable androgens, anabolic steroids, penicillamine, captopril, calcium channel blockers, diazepam, marijuana and heroin.

---

*Thirty-nine per cent of 1855 adolescent boys of different ages at one boy scout camp, though other surveys have found it less common.

†NB Prolactin excess in the absence of oestrogens produces galactorrhoea (gl.) rather than gynaecomastia.

‡The letters of the word MADRAS form a useful mnemonic: methyldopa, aldactone, digoxin, reserpine, alkylating agents, stilboestrol.

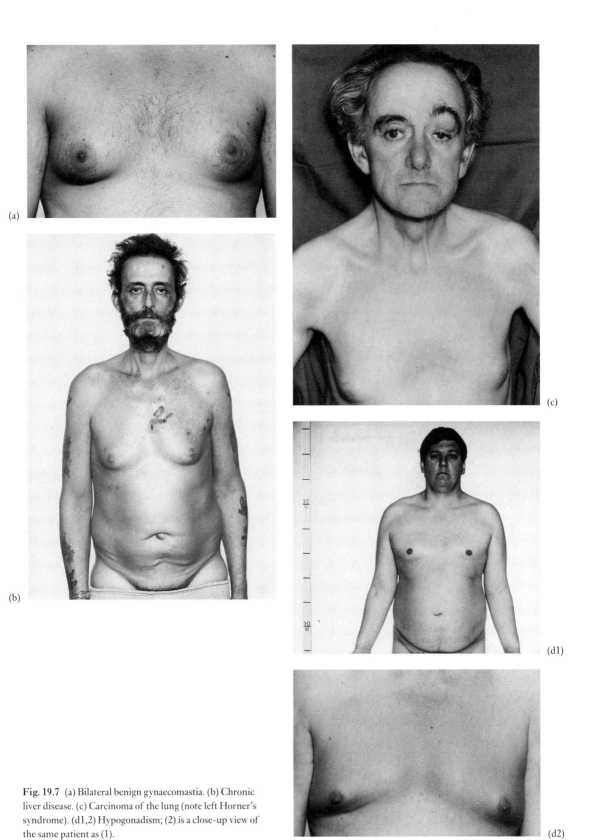

(a)

(b)

(c)

(d1)

(d2)

Fig. 19.7 (a) Bilateral benign gynaecomastia. (b) Chronic liver disease. (c) Carcinoma of the lung (note left Horner's syndrome). (d1,2) Hypogonadism; (2) is a close-up view of the same patient as (1).

Appendices

1 / Checklists

1 / Pulse (p. 1)

Observe

1 Face (malar flush, thyroid facies).
2 Neck (Corrigan's pulse, raised JVP, thyroidectomy scar, goitre) and chest (thoracotomy scar).

Palpate and assess

3 Pulse.
4 Rate.
5 Rhythm (?slow atrial fibrillation).
6 Character (normal, collapsing, slow rising, jerky).
7 Carotid.
8 Opposite radial.
9 Radiofemoral delay.
10 All the other pulses.
11 Additional diagnostic features.

2 / Heart (p. 9)

1 *Visual survey*:
   (a) breathlessness
   (b) *cyanosis*
   (c) pallor
   (d) *malar flush*
   (e) carotids
   (f) jugulars
   (g) *valvotomy scar*, midline scar
   (h) ankle oedema
   (i) clubbing; splinter haemorrhages.
2 Pulse (rate and rhythm).
3 Lift up the arm (?collapsing).
4 Radiofemoral delay.
5 Brachials and carotids (?slow rising).
6 Venous pressure.
7 Apex beat.
8 Tapping impulse.
9 Right ventricular lift.
10 Other pulsations, thrills, palpable sounds.
11 Auscultation (time heart sounds, etc.; turn patient onto left side; lean patient forwards).
12 Sacral oedema (?ankle oedema).
13 Lung bases.
14 Liver.
15 Blood pressure.

3 / Chest (p. 32)

1 *Visual survey*—general appearance (cachexia, superior vena cava obstruction, systemic sclerosis, lupus pernio, kyphoscoliosis, *ankylosing spondylitis*).
2 Dyspnoea.
3 Lip pursing.
4 Cyanosis.
5 Accessory muscles.
6 Indrawing (intercostal muscles, supraclavicular fossae, lower ribs).
7 Chest wall (upward movement, asymmetry, scars, radiotherapy stigmata).
8 Clubbing (tobacco staining, coal dust tattoos, rheumatoid deformity, systemic sclerosis).
9 Pulse (flapping tremor).
10 Venous pressure.
11 Trachea (deviation, tug, notch–cricoid distance).
12 Lymphadenopathy.
13 Apex beat.
14 Asymmetry.
15 Expansion.
16 Percussion (do not forget clavicles, axillae).
17 Tactile vocal fremitus.
18 Breath sounds.
19 Vocal resonance.
20 Repeat 14–19 on back of chest (feel for lymph nodes in the neck).

4 / Abdomen (p. 51)

1 *Visual survey* (pallor, jaundice, spider naevi, etc.).
2 Pigmentation.
3 Hands (Dupuytren's contracture, clubbing, leuconychia, palmar erythema, flapping tremor).
4 Eyes (anaemia, icterus, xanthelasma).
5 Mouth (cyanosis, etc.).
6 Cervical lymph nodes.
7 Gynaecomastia.
8 Spider naevi.
9 Scratch marks.
10 Body hair.
11 Look at the abdomen (pulsation, distension, swelling, distended abdominal veins).
12 Palpation (light palpation, internal organs, inguinal lymph nodes).
13 Percussion.
14 Shifting dullness.

15 Auscultation.
16 Genitalia.
17 Rectal.

5 / **Visual fields** (p. 74)
Observe
1 *Visual survey* (acromegaly, hemiparesis, cerebellar signs).
Test
2 Peripheral visual fields by confrontation.
3 Central scotoma with a red-headed hat pin.
4 Additional features.

6 / **Cranial nerves** (p. 79)
1 Look.
2 Smell and taste (I, VII, IX).
3 Visual acuity (II).
4 Visual fields (II).
5 Eye movements (III, IV, VI).
6 Nystagmus (VIII, cerebellum and its connections).
7 Ptosis (III, sympathetic).
8 Pupils (light, accommodation—III).
9 Discs (II).
10 Facial movements (VII, V).
11 Palatal movement (IX, X).
12 Gag reflex (IX, X).
13 Tongue (XII).
14 Accessory nerve (XI).
15 Hearing (Weber, Rinné—VIII).
16 Facial sensation (including corneal reflex—V).

7 / **Arms** (p. 88)
Observe
1 Face (hemiplegia, nystagmus, wasting, Parkinson's, Horner's).
2 Neck (pseudoxanthoma elasticum, lymph nodes).
3 Elbows (psoriasis, rheumatoid nodules, scars, deformity).
4 Tremor.
5 Hands (joints, nails, skin).
6 Muscle bulk.
7 Fasciculation.
Test
8 Tone.
9 Arms out in front (winging, myelopathy hand sign, sensory wandering).
10 Power:
   (a) arms out to the side (C5)
   (b) bend your elbows (C5,6)
   (c) push out straight (C7)
   (d) squeeze fingers (C8,T1)
   (e) hold the fingers out straight (radial nerve, C7)

(f) spread fingers apart (ulnar nerve)
(g) piece of paper between fingers (ulnar nerve)
(h) thumb at ceiling (median nerve)
(i) opposition (median nerve).
11 Coordination (rapid alternate motion, finger–nose).
12 Reflexes.
13 Sensation (light touch, pinprick, vibration, joint position).

8 / **Legs** (p. 94)
Observe
1 *Visual survey* (*Paget's disease*, hemiparesis, exophthalmos, nystagmus, thyroid acropachy, rheumatoid hands, nicotine-stained fingers, wasted hands, muscle fasciculation).
2 Obvious lesion (see group 1 diagnoses).
3 Bowing of the tibia.
4 Pes cavus.
5 One leg smaller than the other.
6 Muscle bulk.
7 Fasciculation.
Test
8 Tone.
9 Power:
   (a) lift your leg up (L1,2)
   (b) bend your knee (L5,S1,2)
   (c) straighten your leg (L3,4)
   (d) bend your foot down (S1)
   (e) cock up your foot (L4,5).
10 Coordination (heel–shin).
11 Tendon reflexes (clonus).
12 Plantar response.
13 Sensation (light touch, pinprick, vibration, joint position).
14 Gait (ordinary walk, heel-to-toe, on toes, on heels).
15 Rombergism.

9 / **Gait** (p. 123)
1 *Visual survey* (cerebellar signs, Parkinson's, Charcot–Marie–Tooth, ankylosing spondylitis).
2 Check patient can walk.
3 Observe ordinary walk (ataxia, spastic, steppage, parkinsonian).
4 Arm swing (Parkinson's).
5 Turning (ataxia, Parkinson's).
6 Heel-to-toe (ataxia).
7 On toes (S1).
8 On heels (L5).
9 Romberg's test (sensory ataxia).
10 Gait with eyes closed.
11 Additional features.

10 / **Ask questions** (p. 129)

1 *Visual survey* (from top to toe, ?obvious diagnosis).
2 Specific questions (Raynaud's, systemic sclerosis/CRST, hypo- or hyperthyroidism, Crohn's, nephrotic syndrome).
3 General questions (name, address).
4 Questions with long answers (last meal).
5 Articulation ('British Constitution', 'West Register Street', 'biblical criticism').
6 Repetition.
7 Additional signs.
8 Comprehension ('put out your tongue', 'shut your eyes', 'touch your nose').
9 Nominal dysphasia (keys).
10 Orofacial dyspraxia.
11 Higher mental functions.

11 / **Fundi** (p. 136)
Observe
1 *Visual survey* (medic-alert bracelet, etc.).
Ophthalmoscopy
2 Lens.
3 Vitreous (opacities, haemorrhages, fibrous tissue, new vessels).
4 Disc (optic atrophy, papillitis, papilloedema, myelinated nerve fibres, new vessels).
5 Arterioles and venules (AV nipping, silver wiring).
6 Each quadrant and macula (haemorrhages, microaneurysms, exudates, new vessels, photocoagulation scars, choroidoretinitis, retinitis pigmentosa, drusen).
7 Do not stop until you have finished and are ready.

12 / **Eyes** (p. 150)
Observe
1 Face (e.g. myasthenic, tabetic, hemiparesis).
2 Eyes (exophthalmos, strabismus, ptosis, xanthelasma, arcus senilis).
3 Pupils (Argyll Robertson, Horner's, Holmes–Adie, IIIrd nerve).
Test
4 Visual acuity.
5 Visual fields.
6 Eye movements (ocular palsy, diplopia, nystagmus, lid lag).
7 Light reflex (direct, consensual).
8 Accommodation reflex.
9 Fundi.

13 / **Face** (p. 171)
1 *Visual survey* of the patient.
2 Scan the head and face.

3 Break down and scrutinize the parts of the face:
   (a) eyelids (ptosis, rash)
       eyelashes (scanty)
       cornea (arcus, interstitial keratitis)
       sclerae (icteric, congested)
       pupils (small, large, irregular, dislocated lens, cataracts)
       iris (iritis)
   (b) face (erythema, infiltrates)
       mouth (tight, shiny, adherent skin; pigmented patches, telangiectasia, cyanosis).
4 Additional features.

14 / **Hands** (p. 184)
Observe
1 Face (*systemic sclerosis*, Cushing's, acromegaly, arcus senilis, icterus and spider naevi, exophthalmos).
2 Inspect the hands (rheumatoid, sclerodactyly, wasting, psoriasis, claw hand, clubbing).
3 Joints (swelling, deformity, Heberden's nodes).
4 Nails (pitting, onycholysis, clubbing, nail-fold infarcts).
5 Skin (colour, consistency, lesions).
6 Muscles (wasting, fasciculation).
Palpate and test
7 Hands (Dupuytren's contracture, nodules, calcinosis, xanthomata, Heberden's nodes, tophi).
8 Sensation (light touch, pinprick, vibration, joint position).
9 Tone.
10 Power.
11 Pulses.
12 Elbows.

15 / **Skin** (p. 211)
1 *Visual survey* (regional associations; scalp, face, mouth, neck, trunk, axillae, elbows, hands, nails, legs, feet).
2 Distribution (psoriasis on extensor areas, lichen planus on flexural areas, etc.).
3 Lesions: look for characteristic features (scaling, Wickham's striae, etc.).
4 Associated lesions (arthropathy, etc.).

16 / **Rash** (p. 226)
1 *Visual survey* (scalp to sole).
2 Distribution.
3 Surrounding skin (?scratch marks).
4 Examine the lesion (colour, size, shape, surface, character).
5 Additional features.

17 / Neck (p. 237)

1 *Survey* the patient (eyes, face, legs).
2 Look at the neck (swallow).
3 Palpate the thyroid (swallow; size, consistency, etc.; pyramidal lobes).
4 Lymph nodes (supraclavicular, submandibular, postauricular, suboccipital, axillae, groins, spleen).
5 Auscultate the thyroid (distinguish from venous hum and conducted murmurs).
6 Assess thyroid status.

18 / Thyroid status (p. 244)

1 *Visual survey* (exophthalmos, myxoedematous facies, goitre, thyroid acropachy, pretibial myxoedema).
2 Composure (fidgety, normal, immobile).
3 Pulse.
4 Ankle jerks.
5 Palms.
6 Tremor.
7 Eyes (lid retraction, lid lag).
8 Thyroid (look, palpate, auscultate).
9 Questions.

19 / 'Spot' diagnosis (p. 254)

1 *Visual survey*.
2 Retrace the same ground more thoroughly:
   (a) head (*Paget's, dystrophia myotonica*)
   (b) face (*acromegaly, Parkinson's, hemiplegia*, dystrophia myotonica, tardive dyskinesia, hypopituitarism, Cushing's, hypothyroidism, systemic sclerosis)
   (c) eyes (*jaundice, exophthalmos*, ptosis, Horner's, xanthelasma)
   (d) neck (*goitre*, Turner's, spondylitis, torticollis)
   (e) trunk (pigmentation, ascites, purpuric spots, spider naevi, wasting, pemphigus)
   (f) arms (choreoathetosis, psoriasis, Addison's, spider naevi, *syringomyelia*)
   (g) hands (acromegaly, *tremor*, clubbing, sclerodactyly, arachnodactyly, claw hand, etc.)
   (h) legs (bowing, purpura, pretibial myxoedema, necrobiosis)
   (i) feet (pes cavus).
3 Abnormal colouring (*pigmentation, icterus*, pallor).
4 Break down and scrutinize (especially face).
5 Additional features.

2 / Short cases in the final MB in UK medical schools in 1996/97

The following is a list of the short cases given in the final exams as ascertained in a survey undertaken in 1996/97 across 29 medical schools in the UK (house physician survey results).

Acromegaly
Ankylosing spondylitis
Aortic incompetence
Aortic stenosis
Ascites (± drain) spot diagnosis and questions
Cataracts
Cerebrovascular accident
Clubbing
COAD
Consolidation (pneumonia)
Cranial nerves
Diabetic retinopathy
Facial nerve palsy
Foot ulcer — neuropathic
Glass eye
Graves' eyes
Hepatomegaly
Hypersplenism
Incisional hernia
Jaundice
Lymphoedema
Lymphoma

Mitral regurgitation
Murmur
Ophthalmoplegia
Optic neuritis
Peripheral neurophathy
Pituitary hyperplasia
Pleural effusion
Pneumothorax
Polycystic kidney
Prosthetic heart valves
Psoriasis
Ptosis
Pulmonary fibrosis
Retinitis pigmentosa
Rheumatoid arthritis
Spinal cord compression
Splenomegaly
Still's disease
Thyrotoxicosis
Transplanted kidney
Ulnar nerve lesion

3 / Glossary

ACANTHOSIS NIGRICANS: localized, soft, velvety, brown hyperpigmentation of the body folds especially those of the neck, axillae and groins. There can be a roughness to the skin of the soles and palms. In younger patients (under 40 years) it can be associated with obesity, insulin resistance (high insulin levels in the blood; there may be glucose intolerance or frank diabetes) and some endocrine disorders. Less commonly it is associated with underlying malignancy (usually adenocarcinoma of the stomach, gastrointestinal tract, and less commonly of the ovary, uterus, breast and lung) and there should be suspicion of this possibility in a patient aged over 40 years.

ACNE ROSACEA (ROSACEA): chronic condition of the nose and central part of the face clinically characterized by flushing and a papular rash (follicular). In severe cases there is overgrowth of the skin and subcutaneous tissues leading to a rhinophyma of the nose. Treat with long-term low-dose tetracycline.

ACOUSTIC NEUROMA: a neurofibroma of the VIIIth cranial nerve sheath which grows in the cerebellopontine angle and which causes progressive perceptive deafness, vertigo, ipsilateral facial numbness and weakness, and eventually cerebellar ataxia.

ALPHA 1 ANTITRYPSIN DEFICIENCY: approximately 2% of patients with emphysema have an inherited deficiency of α_1-antitrypsin which is produced in the liver and is circulated to the lungs where it prevents the action of neutrophil elastase—a substance that destroys the connective tissue of alveolar walls. Patients usually present before the age of 40 years with respiratory infections and X-ray evidence of basal emphysema. They are invariably smokers.

ALZHEIMER'S DISEASE (ALZHEIMER'S DEMENTIA, ALZHEIMER'S SYNDROME): a form of presenile dementia, characterized by short-term memory loss, disturbance in emotional behaviour, and focal psychological deficits such as spatial orientation or initiating motor skills. After 2–3 years the dementia becomes well established and more profound symptoms such as aphasia, apraxia and agnosia occur.

AMYLOIDOSIS: primary amyloidosis is a rare condition due to the deposition of amyloid in the tissues such as muscle, bone and cartilage. Restrictive car-diomyopathy with congestive cardiac failure is a characteristic cardiac presentation. Secondary amyloidosis is more common and is often secondary to chronic suppurative or inflammatory conditions such as rheumatoid arthritis, ulcerative colitis or myeloma.

ANDROGEN–INSENSITIVITY SYNDROME: see testicular feminization syndrome.

AORTIC SCLEROSIS: thickening of the aortic valve due to atheromatous changes and ageing of the aortic ring. There is an ejection systolic murmur in the aortic area but no significant gradient across the valve (less than 30mmHg) and no abnormality in the pulse, blood pressure or ECG.

ARGYRIA: slate-grey or bluish discoloration of the skin due to silver deposition after long-term medicinal administration of a soluble silver salt (used to be a common treatment for nasal and sinus conditions).

ASBESTOSIS: can occur in workers in environments exposed to asbestos (used to be seen commonly in shipbuilding yards and power stations). Blue asbestos is more harmful than white. It is a progressive disorder characterized by breathlessness, finger clubbing and bilateral basal inspiratory crackles. Pleural plaques and fibrosis can be seen on chest X-ray. Can cause mesothelioma—a malignancy of the pleura. There is an important relationship between asbestosis and cigarette smoking as there is an almost inevitable progression to adenocarcinoma of the bronchus.

ASPERGILLOSIS: a condition due to the inhalation of the fungus *Aspergillus* which is found on decaying leaves and trees. Causes bronchopulmonary allergic aspergillosis (clinically similar to asthma), aspergilloma (pulmonary mycetoma; *Aspergillus* colonization of a pre-existing cavity) presenting with haemoptysis, and a fulminant variety occurring in immunosuppressed patients and requiring urgent management with intravenous amphotericin.

ASTEROID HYALOSIS: with the opthalmoscope focused in front of the retina, the vitreous is seen to be filled with a myriad of tiny white, discrete, shiny opacities, like a galaxy of stars. A benign finding in a small number of patients which does not disturb vision.

ATRIAL SEPTAL DEFECT: a defect in the septum separating the two atria is a common congenital lesion seen in adults, mostly in females. In the commoner variety, the defect is in the region of the fossa ovalis (ostium secundum defect). The symptoms are usually mild and the condition is often discovered either on a routine chest X-ray (dilatation of the pulmonary segment, increased pulmonary vasculature and enlarged right ventricle), or in elderly patients with the onset of atrial fibrillation which heralds left heart failure. Clinically, there is a systolic murmur over the pulmonary area and a fixed split second heart sound. The sinus venosus defect is high in the septum near the entry of the superior vena cava, and is frequently associated with anomalous connection of the pulmonary vein from the right lung to the junction of the superior vena cava and the right atrium. The ostium primum defect lies immediately adjacent to the atrioventricular valves, either of which may be involved, usually the mitral valve which is incompetent. The ECG shows left axis deviation in contrast to the secondum defect in which there is right bundle branch block and right axis deviation.

AUTOIMMUNE THYROIDITIS: see Hashimoto's disease.

BAKER'S CYST: a collection of synovial fluid which has escaped from the knee joint or a bursa and which has formed a new synovial-lined sac in the semimembranous bursa in the popliteal space. Occasionally it may rupture and dissect into the calf mimicking acute phlebothrombosis.

BEHÇET'S SYNDROME: a rare condition clinically characterized by oral and genital ulceration, iritis, polyarthritis, erythema nodosum, neurological and gastrointestinal symptoms. Treat with steroids but the response is not uniformly successful.

BLALOCK SHUNT: this is a palliative surgical procedure for Fallot's tetralogy in young infants before total correction is performed later on. It is the anastomosis between a subclavian artery and a pulmonary artery. It results in an increased blood flow to the lungs.

BOTULISM: a severe neuroparalytic disease caused by food poisoning due to the preformed toxins of *Clostridium botulinum* in inadequately prepared food. Symptoms include vomiting, ocular palsies and pharyngeal paralysis. It can be fatal (respiratory or bulbar paralysis).

BRUCELLOSIS (UNDULANT FEVER): infectious disease caused by the *Brucella* organisms found in cows and goats. It affects people who are in contact with infected animals and those who drink infected, unpasteurized milk. The majority of patients experience recurrent bouts of fever, malaise, night sweats, chills and excessive fatigue.

BUDD–CHIARI SYNDROME: due to thrombosis of the hepatic vein or the inferior vena cava causing portal hypertension with hepatomegaly and ascites. It may follow abdominal trauma or be in association with a hypercoagulable state (e.g. contraceptive pill, polycythaemia rubra vera, paroxysmal nocturnal haemoglobinuria).

CAPLAN'S SYNDROME: patients with rheumatoid arthritis who have been exposed to various industrial dusts, especially coal dust, can develop a nodular pulmonary fibrosis with characteristic changes of nodules accompanied by massive fibrotic reaction on a chest X-ray.

CARCINOID: a tumour derived from the argentaffin cells of the intestine, appendix, stomach and bronchus. It can metastasize slowly to the liver producing the *carcinoid syndrome* which is characterized by facial flushing, cyanosis, palpitations, pulmonary valve disease and diarrhoea caused by the overproduction and decreased clearance of serotonin, histamine, bradykinin and prostaglandins.

CAROTENAEMIA: increased quantities of carotene in the blood (usually from ingestion of excessive carrots) causing a pale, yellow-red pigmentation of the skin. Carotene is found in many plants and animals, but mainly in carrots.

CEREBELLOPONTINE ANGLE SYNDROME: due to a lesion at the cerebellopontine angle (often an acoustic neuroma) and causing cerebellar signs and nystagmus together with a palsy of one or more of the V, VI, VII and VIII cranial nerves.

CHARCOT'S JOINTS: originally described by Charcot in tabes dorsalis. These are painless, grossly deformed, unstable and abnormally mobile joints damaged by trauma and associated with sensory loss (e.g. peripheral neuropathy in diabetes mellitus and dissociated sensory loss in syringomyelia). X-rays show marked joint disorganization and bony distortion. The joints commonly affected are: knees and ankles in tabes dorsalis, shoulders and elbows in syringomyelia, ankles in diabetes mellitus, and any joint in leprosy.

CHOREOATHETOSIS: abnormal movements of the body of combined choreiform (irregular, brief and involuntary contractions) and athetoid (continual, slow, writhing movements mostly involving the limbs) pattern. The symptoms are associated with a vascular or infiltrative lesion of the pallidum.

CHRISTMAS DISEASE: deficiency of factor IX. Also X-linked recessive and similar clinically to haemophilia. Incidence is approximately 1 in 30 000 men. Treat with factor IX concentrate.

CHRONIC ACTIVE HEPATITIS: a serious disorder that has a potential to cause liver failure and cirrhosis. Histologically recognized by the expansion of portal areas with infiltration of lymphocytes and plasma cells, piecemeal necrosis of the liver cells at the interface of the connective tissue and the parenchyma. Causes include hepatitis B (about 20% of cases), hepatitis C and D, alcohol, ulcerative colitis, hereditary (α_1-antitrypsin deficiency) and drugs (methyldopa, isoniazid, nitrofurantoin and ketoconazole). Liver function tests will be abnormal with positive autoantibodies. The clinical course is highly variable.

CHRONIC LYMPHATIC LEUKAEMIA: usually occurs in older people (rare before age 30 and almost never in children) and is often asymptomatic but with a raised white cell count (mostly lymphocytes). Symptoms include those of anaemia, recurrent infections and painless lymphadenopathy. The liver and/or spleen may be enlarged. The disease may remain stable for 8–12 years. Since treatment (chlorambucil) does not cure the disease, it is withheld until there is a clinical indication of anaemia, infection, bleeding or a disfiguring lymphadenopathy.

CHRONIC MYELOID LEUKAEMIA: about 90% of cases have a very specific and characteristic cytogenetic abnormality, the Philadelphia chromosome rearrangement (Ph). Presents with anaemia, night sweats, fever, weight loss and abdominal discomfort from gross splenomegaly, which may be discovered incidentally in the absence of any symptoms.

CHURG–STRAUSS SYNDROME: the pathology is dominated by an eosinophilic infiltration and occurs in patients with a history of asthma. It is characterized by a high eosinophil count, vasculitis and extravascular granulomata of many organs causing rhinorrhoea, sinusitis, cough, arthralgia and neurological symptoms. Perinuclear antineutrophil cytoplasmic antibodies (pANCA) may be positive. Antineutrophil cytoplasmic antibodies (ANCA) are detected on fixed human neutrophils. There are two major ANCA patterns; one a cytoplasmic or cANCA which is now called proteinase 3 (PR3-ANCA) and the other a pANCA which has now been renamed myeloperoxidase (MPO-ANCA).

PR3-ANCA is present in about 90% of serum from patients with Wegener's granulomatosis, and MPO-ANCA is found in about 60% of patients with other vasculitides (e.g. Churg–Strauss syndrome).

CHVOSTEK'S SIGN: important sign in hypocalcaemia. Gentle tapping over the facial nerve, as it emerges from the parotid gland, produces involuntary twitching of the facial muscles. The patient may also have Trousseau's sign (see p. 293).

COCCIDIOMYCOSIS: caused by the organism *Coccitioides immitis*, a soil saprophyte found mainly in the USA, Central and South America. It is usually asymptomatic but can affect the lungs causing fever, malaise, cough and sputum. It is a cause of erythema nodosum and erythema multiforme. Pulmonary cavitation and meningitis can occur in extreme cases. Mild cases are self-limiting but otherwise treat with amphotericin.

COELIAC DISEASE: due to a congenital or acquired sensitivity to gluten (found in wheat or rye flour). It causes villous atrophy in the duodenum and jejunum and leads to malabsorption. It is treated with a gluten-free diet.

CONGENITAL SYPHILIS: contagious venereal disease with infection acquired *in utero*. Characterized by a saddle-nose, underdeveloped upper jaw making the mandible appear prominent (bull-dog jaw), frontal bossing, rhagades at the corners of the mouth, Hutchinson's teeth, Moon's molars and sabre-shaped tibiae.

COOMBS' TEST (DIRECT ANTIGLOBULIN TEST): an agglutination test used in haematology to diagnose autoimmune haemolytic anaemia.

CORRIGAN'S SIGN: visible distension and collapse of the arterial pulse seen in the neck in conditions with a run-off of ejected blood from the arterial circulation (e.g. aortic incompetence, patent ductus arteriosus, large arteriovenous fistula).

COURVOISIER'S SIGN: palpable gall bladder in association with jaundice indicating long-standing common bile duct obstruction by cancer. Courvoisier's law states that the gall bladder is not palpable if the jaundice is caused by a stone, since cholelithiasis would cause fibrosis and contraction of the bladder.

CRANIAL ARTERITIS: see temporal arteritis.

CRANIOPHARYNGIOMA: a suprasellar congenital tumour, usually benign, which occurs in children and young adults. Commonly presents with impaired gonadal function. A quarter of patients present with visual disturbances.

CREUTZFELD–JAKOB DISEASE: a slowly progressive

dementia pathologically characterized by spongiform encephalopathy. It is an example of a 'prion' disease and is very similar to bovine spongiform encephalitis (BSE) in cattle. Can be transmitted through corneal grafts and human growth hormone treatment before therapeutic human growth hormone was made by genetic engineering. Incubation period is long but once symptoms occur death is usually within 2 years.

CYANOTIC CONGENITAL HEART DISEASE: central cyanosis occurs either with a right-to-left shunt (see Eisenmenger's syndrome) or because of an admixture of pulmonary and systemic blood in perfusion/ventilation mismatch (bronchial asthma, pulmonary embolism, chronic bronchitis, etc.). Fallot's tetralogy (commonest cause in those who survive the neonatal period) is a good example of central cyanosis in early childhood. Right-to-left shunts occur when, for example, in a septal defect pulmonary resistance gradually increases and eventually the pressure on the right side becomes greater than on the left. At this stage the flow then reverses to become a right-to-left shunt (Eisenmenger's syndrome). It is then too late to perform any surgical correction.

CYSTIC FIBROSIS (MUCOVISCIDOSIS): an autosomal recessive disorder in which all exocrine glands produce thick, viscous secretions. Presents in infants and can cause meconium ileus, recurrent bronchopulmonary infections and later pancreatic deficiency. Diagnosis is by positive sweat testing (NaCl >60 mmoll^{-1}) in infancy and later by pancreatic function tests. It is a cause of failure to thrive in infancy.

DE QUERVAIN'S THYROIDITIS: an acute thyroiditis of viral origin giving a transient hyperthyroidism and then often a transient hypothyroidism. Can be associated with fever, malaise, pain in the neck, tachycardia and local tenderness over the gland. The erythrocyte sedimentation rate is usually elevated with an early suppression of uptake on thyroid scanning in the early stages (hyperthyroidism with a 'cold' thyroid isotope scan is found in de Quervain's thyroiditis; hyperthyroidism with a 'hot' thyroid isotope scan in Graves' disease). Treat with aspirin and short-term steroids in severe cases.

DERMATITIS HERPETIFORMIS: presents with groups of intensely itching vesicles and papules occurring on the scalp, buttocks, knees, elbows and shoulders, and occasionally mucous membranes. May be associated with gluten intolerance (coeliac disease) which is often asymptomatic.

DERMATOMYOSITIS: maybe associated with adenocarcinoma in about 10% (usually bronchus, stomach and breast) and is characterized by polymyositis and a violaceous rash (heliotrope) usually around the eyes and across the knuckles (Gottron's papules).

DIABETES INSIPIDUS: a deficiency of vasopressin leads to polyuria (can pass up to 10–15 litres of urine per day), nocturia and polydipsia. Causes include congenital, idiopathic, infections (tuberculous meningitis), infiltration (sarcoid, histiocytosis X), trauma, vascular, tumours (craniopharyngioma, pituitary, metastases, lymphoma). Biochemically there is a raised plasma osmolality with low urinary osmolality, a high plasma sodium and no urinary concentration with fluid deprivation. Treatment with vasopressin restores urinary concentration.

DIPHTHERIA: worldwide infection, mainly of children, caused by *Corynebacterium diphtheriae*. Active immunization has seen a virtual eradication of the disease in developed countries. It is an infection of the upper respiratory tract and associated with toxin production. Neurological manifestations can occur either early or late and may include cranial nerve palsies, peripheral neuropathy and occasionally encephalitis. Treatment is with antitoxin given early together with penicillin.

DIRECT ANTIGLOBULIN TEST: see Coombs' test.

DOWN'S SYNDROME (MONGOLISM, TRISOMY DEFECT OF CHROMOSOME 21): usually seen in the offspring of more elderly mothers. Many characteristics including congenital heart disease, short stature, mental retardation and a typical facial appearance.

DRESSLER'S SYNDROME (POSTMYOCARDIAL INFARCTION SYNDROME): occurs weeks or months after a myocardial infarction (usually a second or subsequent one) and is clinically characterized by pericarditis, fever and pericardial effusion. Due to an immune response to the damaged cardiac muscle. Treat with anti-inflammatory drugs and occasionally steroids.

DUPUYTREN'S CONTRACTURE: thickening of the palmar fascia causing a gradual flexion deformity of the fingers. Usually only affects the ring and little fingers. Sometimes associated with alcoholic liver disease.

EATON–LAMBERT SYNDROME: progressive muscle weakness (usually proximal) in patients with carcinoma (usually bronchial) in the absence of dermatomyositis. It is often referred to as the reversed myasthenic syndrome as the weakness improves on exercise (e.g. tendon reflexes become brisker after exercise).

EBSTEIN'S ANOMALY: rare congenital abnormality of the tricuspid valve which is displaced into the right ventricle. May be associated with an interseptal defect.

EHLERS–DANLOS SYNDROME (CUTIS HYPERELASTICA): a heterogeneous group of diseases with nine different varieties. The condition is characterized by hyperextensible skin which is very thin and elastic, associated with poor wound healing and thin, tissue-paper scars. There can be bruising, bleeding and aortic dissection (due to fragility of the blood vessels), recurrent dislocations of the joints (due to hypermobility of the joints) and mitral valve prolapse.

EISENMENGER'S COMPLEX: Eisenmenger's syndrome due to a ventricular septal defect.

EISENMENGER'S SYNDROME: right-to-left cardiac shunt due to pulmonary hypertension which develops as a result of a congenital defect of the heart in which there is a communication between the two sides of the heart (e.g. ventricular or atrial septal defect, patent ductus arteriosus).

ERYTHEMA AB IGNE: a reticular, erythematous, pigmented rash usually on the lower leg secondary to exposure to heat (e.g. sitting close to a gas fire, using a very hot water bottle for relief of pain). Commonly seen in women and may be associated with hypothyroidism.

ERYTHEMA MULTIFORME: an acute, self-limiting but often recurrent condition affecting the skin and mucous membranes. It is often mediated by circulating immune complexes that evolve in response to infection (herpes simplex 1, *Mycoplasma* pneumonia, streptococcal infections, tuberculosis, histoplasmosis), drugs (sulphonamides, chlorpropamide, barbiturates) and connective tissue diseases. As the name implies the cutaneous rash is pleomorphic with papules, erythematous plaques, blisters and target lesions on the hands, forearms, face and feet. The target lesions are diagnostic and are recognized by a central, dark area or a blister surrounded by a pale, red zone, which in turn is surrounded by a rim of erythema. When the mucous membranes of the mouth and eyes are also involved the condition is referred to as the Stevens–Johnson syndrome.

FACIOSCAPULOHUMERAL MUSCULAR DYSTROPHY (LANDOUZY–DÉJÉRINE MUSCULAR DYSTROPHY): autosomal dominant condition affecting the face, shoulder and pelvic girdles. Starts between the ages of 10 and 40 years. It is slowly progressive with a normal life expectancy.

FALLOT'S TETRALOGY: congenital heart disease consisting of a tetrad of a ventricular septal defect (VSD), an over-riding aorta, pulmonary stenosis with outflow obstruction and right ventricular hypertrophy. There is right-to-left shunting through the VSD and so central cyanosis is a feature.

FELTY'S SYNDROME: this is the association of splenomegaly and lymphadenopathy with rheumatoid arthritis. The large spleen causes hypersplenism leading to neutropenia, anaemia and thrombocytopenia.

FOSTER–KENNEDY SYNDROME: ipsilateral optic atrophy, often with a central scotoma, and contralateral papilloedema, due to a tumour compressing the ipsilateral optic nerve, at the same time raising intracranial pressure to cause papilloedema in the other eye. It usually occurs with a meningioma of the sphenoid ridge.

FRIEDREICH'S ATAXIA: see hereditary ataxias.

GALACTORRHOEA: milk production from the breasts. The patient with galactorrhoea may not complain about it, but on direct questioning she may have noticed crusting over the nipple. Galactorrhoea with hyperprolactinaemia is often due to a prolactinoma.

GALACTOSAEMIA: an inborn error of galactose (a constituent of disaccharide lactose found in milk) metabolism with galactose intolerance which causes galactose to accumulate in the blood. Characterized by failure to thrive, cataracts, irritability, anorexia and eventually mental retardation. Treatment is a lactose-free diet.

GASTRINOMA: see Zollinger–Ellison syndrome.

GAUCHER'S DISEASE: a familial (autosomal recessive) disorder of lipid metabolism affecting the spleen (massive splenomegaly), bone marrow and other organs with an infiltration of Gaucher cells containing lipid.

GENERAL PARESIS OF THE INSANE: a form of neurosyphilis in which there is progressive dementia, brisk reflexes, extensor plantars and tremor. Argyll Robertson pupils are usually seen. There may be fits and patients usually die within 3–4 years. Parenteral penicillin given for 2–3 weeks can halt but not reverse the neurological damage.

GLAUCOMA: this is a term signifying raised intraocular pressure and of which there are many varieties.

GRAHAM STEELL MURMUR: an early diastolic murmur due to pulmonary regurgitation. Often seen in patients with mitral stenosis with secondary pulmonary hypertension.

GRANULOMA ANNULARE: a chronic eruption of papules which grow to form nodules and then coalesce to produce annular lesions and which may finally disappear spontaneously. In its generalized form it is associated with diabetes mellitus.

GUILLAIN–BARRÉ SYNDROME: acute infective polyneuritis occurring after a flu-like illness and causing demyelination in the spinal roots and peripheral nerves. Leads to ascending weakness and paralysis and sometimes respiratory paralysis.

HAEMOCHROMATOSIS: an autosomal recessive condition due to iron deposition in the liver causing cirrhosis. There is a bronzed pigmentation of the skin and diabetes mellitus and cardiac failure can occur because of iron deposition in the pancreas and the heart.

HAEMOLYTIC ANAEMIA: anaemia due to excessive red-cell destruction caused by a haemolytic process in, for example, sickle cell disease, thalassaemia and lymphomata.

HAEMOLYTIC–URAEMIC SYNDROME: disorder of infants and children characterized by intravascular haemolysis and fragmentation of the red blood cells (microangiopathic haemolysis), thrombocytopenia and acute renal failure. It can occur after a febrile illness and the clustering of cases supports an infective association. Treatment is with heparin and fresh frozen plasma but most cases recover spontaneously.

HAEMOPHILIA: due to a deficiency of factor VIII. It is an X-linked recessive condition affecting 1 in 5000 to 1 in 10 000 of the male population. Clinically, there is a haemorrhagic tendency following trivial trauma, especially into the joints (haemarthrosis) and muscles. Factor VIII levels of less than 5% cause severe haemorrhage. Treat with intravenous factor VIII concentrate.

HASHIMOTO'S DISEASE (AUTOIMMUNE THYROIDITIS): presents usually in middle-aged females with a rubbery and firm goitre. Thyroid microsomal antibodies are usually present. Patients can be either hypo- or euthyroid, though there can on rare occasions be an initial hyperactivity of the gland which is often referred to as 'hashitoxicosis'. Treatment with thyroxine can cause the goitre to shrink even when the hypothyroidism is subclinical.

HEBERDEN'S NODES: osteoarthritic bony swellings of the distal interphalangeal joints of the fingers. These are knobbly and painless lesions, though in the acute stages the swellings may be soft, red and warm. They run in families and mostly occur in females in late middle age.

HENOCH–SCHÖNLEIN SYNDROME: this is an allergic, systemic necrotizing vasculitis with purpuric papules mainly on the lower limbs and buttocks. Usually occurs in children as a type III hypersensitivity reaction often following an upper respiratory infection. Associated with abdominal pain, haematuria, nephritis and arthritis. Usually self-limiting and recovery should be spontaneous though a few develop renal impairment.

HEREDITARY ATAXIAS: the most well known is Friedreich's ataxia. This is a familial condition with progressive degeneration of the spinocerebellar and corticospinal tracts presenting in childhood with ataxia, nystagmus, dysarthria, absent joint position and vibration sense in the lower limbs, absent lower limb reflexes and extensor plantar responses, optic atrophy and pes cavus.

HISTIOCYTOSIS X: three varieties all characterized by the presence of granulomata containing histiocytes, eosinophilic granulocytes, giant cells and lymphocytes. Letterer–Siwe disease is a widespread disorder usually seen in infants less than 3 years old and is invariably fatal. There are skin lesions, lymphadenopathy and hepatosplenomegaly. Eosinophilic granuloma is the commonest variety occurring in adults and clinically presents with increasing shortness of breath and cough. The chest X-ray shows diffuse bilateral mottling and there is often recurrent pneumothorax. Hand–Schüller–Christian disease usually starts before the age of 5; there is exophthalmos, diabetes insipidus and bony lesions. The chest X-ray usually shows hilar lymphadenopathy similar to sarcoidosis. It may spontaneously improve. The latter two varieties have a relatively good survival rate (at least 20 years). Treat with steroids and/or cyclophosphamide.

HISTOPLASMOSIS: caused by the fungus *Histoplasma capsulatum*. It occurs worldwide (mainly in the USA—Ohio and the Mississippi basin) with the spores surviving in moist soil for several years. Clinically presents with: (i) primary pulmonary histoplasmosis—usually asymptomatic, can have mild flu-like illness with fever, chills, myalgia and cough; secondary bacterial pneumonia, pleural effusion and erythema nodosum can occur; (ii) chronic pulmonary histoplasmosis clinically very similar to tuberculosis with pulmonary cavities, infiltrates and fibrous streaking from the periphery to the hilum; and (iii) disseminated histoplasmosis resembling disseminated tuberculosis with fever, lymphadenopathy, hepatosplenomegaly, weight loss, leucopaenia and thrombocytopaenia. Diagnose by the histoplasmin skin test and complement fixation tests. Treat with amphotericin, ketoconazole or fluconazole.

HODGKIN'S DISEASE: a potentially curable malignancy of the lymph nodes. Presents usually in the young to middle age groups with painless lymphadenopathy (usually cervical). Prognosis and treatment depends on the staging (I–IV) which is according to the extent of lymph node involvement (single site, multiple sites on one side of the diaphragm, lymph nodes on both sides of the diaphragm, liver and spleen involved) and the association with, or lack of, systemic symptoms such as night sweats, pruritus, fatigue, loss of weight and pain in the affected areas induced by alcohol. Treatment is with radiotherapy for a single node and quadruple chemotherapy (CHOP) if more extensive.

HOLMES–ADIE PUPIL (MYOTONIC PUPIL): it is due to denervation of the ciliary ganglion and is of no clinical significance, except that it comes in the differential diagnosis of unequal pupils. Usually seen in young women and is often associated with reduced or absent tendon reflexes. The pupil is dilated on the affected side, there is no reaction (or sometimes slow reaction) to bright light and incomplete constriction to convergence.

HUNTINGTON'S CHOREA: progressive autosomal dominant disorder beginning in young to middle age characterized by choreoathetosis and dementia.

HURLER'S SYNDROME: an autosomal recessive disorder otherwise known as gargoylism. It is one of the mucopolysaccharidoses and can affect the bones, liver, spleen and brain and can cause aortic incompetence.

HYDATID DISEASE: due to infection with a cestode, *Echinococcus granulosus*. Commonly occurs in sheep-rearing areas (Australia and Wales) and causes calcified cysts in the liver and lungs. Humans are infected at the larval or hydatid cyst stage through intimate contact with infected dogs or sheep.

HYPERTELORISM: a greater than normal distance between two paired organs, and the term is usually applied to the eyes in some conditions such as Turner's syndrome. In this case it results from underdevelopment of the greater wings and overgrowth of the lesser wings of the sphenoid, and should be distinguished from other abnormalities, e.g. underlying meningioma or in the median cleft syndrome.

HYPERTROPHIC OBSTRUCTIVE CARDIOMYOPATHY (HOCM)

(ASYMMETRIC HYPERTROPHY OF THE SEPTUM, IDIOPATHIC SUBAORTIC STENOSIS, HYPERTROPHIC CARDIOMYOPATHY): characterized by marked hypertrophy of the left and/or right ventricle especially the interventricular septum in the absence of any cardiac or systemic cause. It results in vigorous left ventricular (LV) contraction closing in the subaortic area causing obstruction of the outflow tract, and abnormal systolic mitral valve movement with mitral incompetence. 50% of cases are familial. In some families there is a high incidence of sudden death. Patients present with syncope (usually exertional), angina, cardiac arrhythmias or sudden death. Dyspnoea may occur due to left ventricular failure. Classic clinical features include a double apical pulsation producing a palpable fourth heart sound, a jerky carotid pulse due to fast ejection and sudden obstruction to LV outflow during systole, an ejection systolic murmur due to LV outflow obstruction and a pansystolic murmur due to mitral regurgitation. The electrocardiogram shows LV hypertrophy and on echocardiography asymmetric hypertrophy of the septum is diagnostic.

HYPOPARATHYROIDISM: this can be due either to hypofunction of the parathyroid glands or due to their surgical removal. It leads to hypocalcaemia.

JANEWAY'S LESIONS: small (1–4 mm), purplish macules on the palms, soles and ankles seen in acute and subacute bacterial endocarditis and due to infected emboli. Similar to Osler's nodes but non-tender.

JUVENILE CHRONIC ARTHRITIS: see Still's disease.

KALA-AZAR: visceral leishmaniasis caused by *Leishmania donovani* and transmitted by sandfly vectors. Small nodules containing parasites occur near the site of inoculation. The later stages are characterized by fever, lymphadenopathy and gross hepatosplenomegaly.

KALLMAN'S SYNDROME: hypogonadotrophic hypogonadism (due to a deficiency of gonadotrophin-releasing hormone (GnRH)) associated with anosmia or hyposmia (impaired sense of smell) and occasionally associated with colour blindness, cleft palate and renal abnormalities. Often familial (X-linked). Patients can be fertile.

KAYSER–FLEISCHER RING: a brown ring at the outer edge of the cornea due to the deposition of a copper-containing pigment and seen only in Wilson's disease.

KERATODERMA BLENNORRHAGICA: a cutaneous feature of, and seen in 10% of patients with, Reiter's syndrome. Clinically characterized by scaling and brownish-red macules (early), but in fully developed cases resembles pustular psoriasis with vesiculopustular lesions, crusts and limpet-like masses of yellowish-brown scales.

KLINEFELTER'S SYNDROME: another example of hypogonadism. It is a chromosomal disorder (47,XXY) which can affect 1 in 1000 males. They clinically present with small, pea-sized, firm testes which may be undescended, sexual underdevelopment, occasionally mental retardation (20%), gynaecomastia and infertility. The diagnosis is made by chromosomal analysis. Often associated with increased maternal age. Treatment can be with androgens but the infertility is irreversible.

KOILONYCHIA: thin, spoon-shaped nails present congenitally or acquired in severe iron deficiency anaemia. Can also occur with trauma.

LAURENCE–MOON–BIEDL SYNDROME: this is characterized by the combination of obesity, sexual underdevelopment, retinitis pigmentosa, mental retardation and polydactyly or syndactyly.

LEBER'S OPTIC ATROPHY: a hereditary form of optic atrophy thought to involve mitochondrial inheritance and to be exclusively matrilineal, affecting young males. The onset is usually subacute and visual loss is not progressive.

LEPROSY: a chronic granulomatous infection due to Mycobacterium leprae. It affects mainly the skin and peripheral nerves. There are several types, mainly lepromatous and tuberculoid. Transmission occurs through prolonged close contact.

LICHEN PLANUS: itchy, papular rash usually seen on the anterior aspect of the wrists. Unknown aetiology. A white, lacy, linear appearance on the buccal mucosa and pterygium (proximal nail-fold invagination of the nail) are characteristic lesions.

LICHEN SCLEROSUS: an irregular, polygonal flat-topped, ivory-white papular eruption with comedo-like plugs on the surface (black heads). Cause is unknown. May be pruritic.

LITTLE'S DISEASE: spastic diplegia in which the legs are more affected than the arms. The causes include low birth weight, perinatal asphyxia and cerebral infections such as encephalitis and meningitis. Sometimes it is hard to distinguish cerebral paraplegia from tetraplegia, and the distinction may even be academic in cases where, for example, meningitis may have affected both the cerebrum as well as the spinal cord.

LUPUS PERNIO (CUTANEOUS SARCOID): a chilblain-like lesion often affecting the nose and cheeks and seen in about 10% of cases of sarcoidosis.

LYME DISEASE: caused by Borrelia burgdorferi and transmitted by ticks on deer and sheep. Originally described in Lyme, Connecticut, but now known to occur in Europe particularly in forests and woodland (e.g. the New Forest). Prompt removal of the tick from the skin prevents the infection. Clinically characterized by erythema chronicum migrans, headache, fever, malaise, arthralgia and lymphadenopathy in the early stages. Later there are neurological (meningoencephalitis, cranial nerve palsies) and cardiac problems (myocarditis). Arthritis develops in the last stage. Diagnose by finding the organism in blood or cerebrospinal fluid. Also IgM and IgG antibodies can be raised. Treat with penicillin or tetracycline.

LYMPHOGRANULOMA VENEREUM: a sexually transmitted infection caused by Chlamydia trachomatis which is endemic in the tropics. The primary lesion is usually an ulcer on the genitalia with regional lymphadenopathy (painful and fixed) which may rupture. The nodes may be involved both above and below the inguinal ligament, and fibrosis may result, producing the 'groove sign' (linear depression parallel to the inguinal ligament). Can also present with proctitis and perirectal abscesses which appear similar to Crohn's disease. Treat with 2 weeks of tetracycline. Chronic infection may persist with fistula and sinus formation.

LYMPHOMA: abnormal malignant proliferation of the lymphoid system presenting either as Hodgkin's or non-Hodgkin's disease, depending on the histological appearances. Characterized by lymphadenopathy affecting either a single group or multiple sites on the same or both sides of the diaphragm, splenomegaly and, in advanced cases, by systemic features of night sweats, malaise, weight loss and fever.

MACLEOD'S (SWYER–JAMES) SYNDROME: unilateral lobar emphysema usually due to an obliterating bronchiolitis caused by an adenovirus infection in childhood. There is increased translucency in one hemithorax due to diminished vascular markings in the lung on that side.

MALADIE DE ROGER: pure, uncomplicated and mild (usually very small) ventricular septal defect. There is a loud, long systolic murmur in an otherwise asymptomatic patient. The defect usually closes spontaneously in most cases.

MALARIA: infectious disease characterized by recurrent paroxysms of fever, shivering and sweating. Caused by one of the four species of Plasmodium. Of these P. falciparum is the most dangerous, causing black water fever and cerebral malaria. It can be a cause of a pyrexia of unknown origin in a patient returning from travel in an affected country.

MARFAN'S SYNDROME: autosomal dominant condition characterized by long extremities, arachnodactyly, hypotonic muscles, hyperextensible joints, lens dislocation and cardiac lesions, e.g. aortic incompetence, aortic dissection and mitral valve prolapse.

MEIG'S SYNDROME: fibromyoma of the ovary associated with pleural effusion and ascites.

MENINGIOMA: benign primary tumour of the arachnoid membrane. Commonly arises along the dorsal surface of the brain, the base of the skull, the falx cerebri, the sphenoid ridge or within the lateral ventricles. Although benign, meningiomata can cause damage because of their large size. They grow over several years and can erode adjacent bone. They can also be found along the intracranial venous sinuses which they can invade.

MESOTHELIOMA: a tumour of the mesothelium of the pleura, pericardium or peritoneum associated with asbestos exposure. Spreads locally and causes exudative effusions. Treatment is unsatisfactory.

MIKULICZ'S SYNDROME: bilateral parotid gland enlargement combined with lacrimal gland enlargement and dry eyes and mouth. Occurs in sarcoidosis and lymphoma.

MITRAL VALVE PROLAPSE: discovered by hearing a midsystolic click, due to the sudden prolapse of the posterior cusp of the mitral valve into the left atrium, followed by a murmur during systole. The valve is usually congenitally deformed (may have large leaflets) or have undergone myxomatous change. The chordae are usually abnormally long. The prolapsing (billowing) mitral valve syndrome is also known as Barlow's syndrome. Common, especially in young women. Can occur with Marfan's syndrome, thyrotoxicosis, rheumatic or ischaemic heart disease, atrial septal defect or hypertrophic obstructive cardiomyopathy. Atypical sharp chest pain in the submammary region is a common complaint. Confirm diagnosis on echocardiography. If necessary treat with β-blockers and antiarrhythmics; occasionally repair of the valve is needed. Antibiotic prophylaxis is important as for any other valvular heart problem.

MORPHOEA: localized 'scleroderma' (thickening) of the skin with no systemic features. It is more common in women (3:1) and affects mainly the limbs and trunk. There are plaques of thickened blue-red skin occasionally with central pallor. The skin may become waxy. Plaques resolve eventually but usually leave some degree of hyperpigmentation. Steroids may be given if lesions are severe with much swelling.

MUCOVISCIDOSIS: see cystic fibrosis.

MUSCULAR DYSTROPHY: inherited, progressive weakness of skeletal muscle with destruction and regeneration of the muscle fibres and their eventual replacement by fibrous and fatty tissue. There are several types of which Duchenne muscular dystrophy is the most common and the most severe. This is an inherited X-linked recessive disorder occurring in 1 in 3000 male infants. Symptoms occur by the age of 4 years and include difficulty in running and getting up to a standing position. Gower's sign is when the child has to 'climb up his legs with his hands'. A proximal limb weakness is associated with pseudohypertrophy of the calves. There is no cure and death occurs usually by the age of 20. Limb-girdle and facioscapulohumeral dystrophies are much milder.

MYCOSIS FUNGOIDES: cutaneous manifestation of a T-cell lymphoma. Commonly presents as erythematous, well-circumscribed, scaly, indurated, itchy plaques which may remain confined to the buttocks, thighs or trunk. Tumours may eventually occur. There can be visceral spread and ultimately death. It is a disease of middle to old age. Treatment with cytotoxics is not very helpful.

MYELOFIBROSIS: fibrosis of the bone marrow occurring in the later stages of some of the myeloproliferative conditions such as polycythaemia rubra vera. Haemopoiesis is taken up by the liver and the spleen which become grossly enlarged.

MYELOMATOSIS: multiple myeloma. A malignant tumour that infiltrates the bone marrow with plasma cells. Presents with anaemia and lytic bone lesions. Bence Jones protein (monoclonal light chain in the urine) is often present in the urine—when the urine is heated it precipitates at 40–60°C then dissolves at 100°C, but then re-precipitates with cooling. In lower concentration in the urine it is not shown on the Albustix but is readily demonstrated by salicylsulphonic acid.

NELSON'S SYNDROME: hyperpigmentation due to excess adrenocorticotrophic hormone secretion after adrenalectomy has been performed for the treatment of Cushing's syndrome of pituitary origin (Cushing's disease).

NEPHROTIC SYNDROME: the principal features of this condition seen in patients with glomerular disease are generalized oedema, massive albuminuria, hypoalbuminaemia and hyperlipidaemia. The primary abnormality is an increased capillary wall permeability resulting in the excretion of large amounts of protein (greater than 3.5 g day^{-1}) in the urine.

NOONAN'S SYNDROME: an autosomal recessive disorder, occurs in karyotypically normal males and females, and is characterized by many of the features of the female Turner's syndrome. Sometimes referred to as 'male Turner's syndrome' though it can occur in both sexes. The commonest cardiovascular complications are pulmonary stenosis, left ventricular hypertrophy and cardiomyopathy. Webbing of the neck is common and there may be marked mental retardation. The facial appearance (hypertelorism, ptosis, low-set ears, micrognathia, etc.) and short stature are similar to Turner's and males have undescended, hypoplastic testes.

OCULOPHARYNGEAL MUSCULAR DYSTROPHY: a milder form of ocular myopathy (starts with ptosis and progresses to ophthalmoplegia) associated with dysphagia which can be quite troublesome. Starts late in life; there is often French-Canadian ancestry. Some patients with this syndrome have spinal muscular atrophy.

ONYCHOLYSIS: loosening and dystrophy of the nails, usually incomplete and beginning at the free border. It can cause the free edge to appear white. Causes include trauma (commonest), psoriasis, fungal infections, thyrotoxicosis and porphyria (rare).

OSLER'S NODES: small, elevated and tender red lesions found on the finger pads in subacute bacterial endocarditis.

OSTEOGENESIS IMPERFECTA: a congenital abnormality of the bones making them very brittle and resulting in multiple fractures. Associated with blue sclerae (the bluish choroid shows through the very thin sclerae) and with joint and muscle laxity.

OSTEOPOROSIS: thin bones due to a reduction in bone mass. It is a common problem affecting nearly 50% of all elderly women. 40% of all Caucasian women will have an osteoporosis-induced fracture at some time. Type 1 is the typical postmenopausal variety and type 2 is the now recognized osteoporosis occurring in women over the age of 70. This is due to a lack of contact with sunshine, or related to low calcium intake and less vitamin D-containing foods. Fractures (vertebral, Colles', femoral neck) are common after falls. Serum calcium and alkaline phosphatase are normal. Diagnosis is confirmed with bone densitometry (DEXA scanning). Pre-vention includes hormone replacement therapy, increased intake of dietary or supplemental calcium and treatment with diphosphonates.

PARAPROTEINAEMIAS: these include multiple myeloma and Waldenström's macroglobulinaemia. Both are diseases of older people. Myeloma is part of a spectrum of disorders characterized by the presence of a paraprotein in the serum which can be seen on electrophoresis. This paraprotein is produced by abnormal proliferating plasma cells. There may also be excretion of light chains in the urine (Bence Jones protein). Clinical features reflect bone marrow infiltration (anaemia, infections, bleeding), bone destruction (fractures and symptoms of hypercalcaemia) and renal impairment which can be multifactorial (amyloid deposition, hypercalcaemia, hyperuricaemia and dehydration). Treatment is with chemotherapy, radiotherapy for bone pain and more recently with bone marrow transplantation. Waldenström's macroglobulinaemia (proliferation of lymphocytes and plasma cells secreting IgM) is usually seen in older people with features similar to lymphoma (lymphadenopathy, splenomegaly, bone marrow infiltration) and disorders related to hyperviscosity (headaches, visual and neurological impairment, bleeding) caused by the circulating macroglobulin. Diagnosis is from bone marrow aspiration and electrophoresis of the serum. Treat with alkylating agents and plasmapheresis for hyperviscosity.

PATENT DUCTUS ARTERIOSUS: persistence of the foetal ductus arteriosus beyond the first few weeks of life. Associated with a flow of blood from the aorta to the left pulmonary artery which causes a continuous 'machinery' murmur heard widely over the precordium and a collapsing peripheral pulse. It may be complicated by infective endocarditis and a reversed (right-to-left) shunt (Eisenmenger's syndrome).

PEUTZ–JEGHERS SYNDROME: rare autosomal dominant condition of childhood characterized by multiple brownish-black macules (lentigines) in the circumoral skin together with intestinal (jejunum) polyposis which can present as intussusception.

PHAEOCHROMOCYTOMA: rare tumour of the sympathetic nervous system (<1 in 1000 cases of hypertension). 90% come from the adrenal gland with 10% arising elsewhere in the sympathetic chain. 25% are multiple and 10% malignant. They usually release noradrenaline and adrenaline. Clinical features are due to catecholamine excess and include paroxysms of palpitations, sweating, headache, pallor, tremor, chest pain and increments in blood pressure. Diagnosis is by measuring urinary metanephrines (screening test) and plasma catecholamines. Computerized tomography scanning can localize the tumour which should be removed if possible.

PITYRIASIS ROSEA: a self-limiting condition with a scaling maculopapular eruption seen mainly in children. It is less common in the summer and may have a viral aetiology but it is not contagious. It usually starts with a large herald patch on the trunk followed by smaller round or oval, pink or salmon-coloured scaling papules and plaques over the trunk and upper limbs. Clears spontaneously with no treatment in 6–8 weeks.

POLYARTERITIS NODOSA: a condition characterized pathologically by inflammation and fibrinoid necrosis of the walls of medium-sized and small arteries. More common in males. Causes hypertension, renal failure, skin rash, migratory arthralgia and peripheral neuropathy.

POLYCYTHAEMIA RUBRA VERA: primary polycythaemia presenting with raised haemoglobin, white cell count and platelets often in association with thrombotic events due to the high haemoglobin level and hyperviscosity. There is often splenomcgaly and diminished iron stores due to the unchecked formation of red blood cells. It belongs to the group of myeloproliferative disorders and can eventually lead to acute myeloid leukaemia.

POLYMYALGIA RHEUMATICA: polymyalgia rheumatica and temporal arteritis are two conditions at each end of a spectrum with giant cell arteritis as the underlying pathological lesion. The cause is unknown. It usually presents suddenly with pain and severe early morning stiffness (proximal muscles of pelvic and shoulder girdle) to the extent that getting out of bed is difficult. It is a condition of older age (rare under 50 years). The ratio of women to men is 3 : 1. Systemic symptoms include malaise, anorexia, weight loss and low grade fever. Confirmation is by a high erythrocyte sedimentation rate (ESR) and a normochromic anaemia. Alkaline phosphatase can also be elevated. Treat with steroids (15–20 mg day^{-1}) for a total of 2–4 years reducing the dose gradually over this time—titrate the dose according to symptoms and ESR. Relapses may occur.

POLYMYOSITIS: characterized by muscular wasting and weakness of the shoulder and pelvic girdle, neck and pharynx. It is more common in women with a peak age of 30–60 years. When accompanied by a rash it becomes dermatomyositis. It may be associated with carcinoma of the bronchus, breast and ovary. It can be acute in onset particularly in children. There is a chronic form with progressive muscular weakness. Muscular pain occurs in about half the cases as does arthralgia/arthritis affecting the small joints of the hand. Investigations show a high erythrocyte sedimentation rate, high creatine phosphokinase and aldolase. The electromyogram shows short polyphasic motor potentials with spontaneous fibrillation and high-frequency repetitive discharges. Muscle biopsy reveals necrosis of the muscle fibres with swelling of the muscle cells and inflammatory changes. Treatment is with high-dose steroids (occasionally need azathioprine) and physiotherapy.

PORPHYRIA: a metabolic disorder chemically characterized by the overproduction of porphyrins or their precursors (delta amino levulinic acid and porphobilinogen) and clinically by neurological and/or cutaneous manifestations (bullous lesions on the light-exposed parts). There are several different forms of porphyria of which acute intermittent porphyria (hepatic) is one of the commonest. It causes abdominal pain, dark urine and neuropsychiatric symptoms. There is a constitutional (genetic) predisposition to the condition which may be precipitated by certain drugs such as sulphonamides. Porphyria cutanea tarda is relatively commoner and characterized by mechanical fragility and bullous lesions on sun-exposed areas. Acute neurological attacks do not occur.

POSTMYOCARDIAL INFARCTION SYNDROME: see Dressler's syndrome.

PRIMARY PULMONARY HYPERTENSION: an idiopathic variety of pulmonary hypertension diagnosed by exclusion of other causes (e.g. thromboembolic disease) and predominantly occurring in females between the ages of 10 and 40 years.

PROGRESSIVE MASSIVE FIBROSIS: an advanced form of coal worker's pneumoconiosis with large, round fibrotic lesions affecting mainly the upper lobes. Pathogenesis is unknown but is thought to involve immune complexes. Lung function tests show a mixed obstructive and restrictive pattern with loss of lung volume and a reduced gas transfer. Can lead to respiratory failure and can progress even after stopping contact with coal dust.

PSEUDOXANTHOMA ELASTICUM: an inherited disorder of elastic tissue. The most obvious cutaneous features are over the flexural surfaces and the neck with lax skin hanging in folds together with the characteristic 'plucked-chicken' skin appearance. There is little elastic recoil on stretching the skin (cf. Ehlers–Danlos syndrome). There are widespread vascular changes including fibrous proliferation and deposition of calcium in the media of the arteries. Intermittent claudication and angina pectoris are common early symptoms. Gastrointestinal bleeding can be troublesome and angioid streaks can be seen in the retina.

PULMONARY HYPERTENSION: increased blood pressure in the pulmonary arteries secondary to lung diseases such as fibrosis and bronchitis, thromboembolic and veno-occlusive diseases, or to mitral valve disease.

PYODERMA GANGRENOSUM: ulcers often on the lower leg, usually large and necrotic with bluish-red overhanging edges. The patient often has ulcerative colitis, Crohn's, rheumatoid arthritis or a myeloproliferative disease.

RAMSAY HUNT SYNDROME: otic herpes zoster involving the geniculate and VIIth nerve ganglia causing ipsilateral lower motor neurone facial nerve palsy with a loss of taste on the anterior two-thirds of the affected side of the tongue. There can be pain in the ear as herpetic vesicles involve the tympanic membrane.

RAYNAUD'S PHENOMENON: it usually occurs in cold weather in young women. Fingers and (occasionally) toes become white. It is relieved by warmth. It is due to vasospasm of the arteries to the fingers and toes which produce the first stage of the phenomenon — whiteness. This is followed by blue discoloration due to sludging of the blood in the fingers and the final stage is redness due to hyperaemia as the digits warm up. This latter stage can be very painful. When it occurs with no underlying disease it is known as Raynaud's disease. Causes of Raynaud's phenomenon include the connective tissue disorders (especially systemic sclerosis) and cryoglobulinaemia.

REFSUM'S DISEASE: a rare, autosomal recessive disorder caused by the absence of phytanic acid hydroxylase. Clinical features include retinitis pigmentosa, demyelinating polyneuropathy, deafness, nystagmus and cerebellar signs. The cerebrospinal fluid protein is elevated and there may be cardiac conduction defects.

RENAL TUBULAR ACIDOSIS: an uncommon disorder leading to systemic acidosis caused by impairment of the renal tubules to maintain the body's acid–base balance. It can be of primary, drug-induced, immunological or inherited aetiology. Features include acidosis, hypokalaemia and an inability to reduce the urinary pH to below 5.5 after an acid load.

RETINAL VEIN THROMBOSIS: may be secondary to a hyperviscosity syndrome such as Waldenström's macroglobulinaemia or myeloma, but it also occurs in association with hypertension, chronic simple glaucoma and diabetes mellitus. Characterized by tortuous and engorged veins with haemorrhages scattered all over the retina with the appearance of 'bundles of straw'. It is a major cause of blindness in the elderly.

RHEUMATIC FEVER: a delayed inflammatory sequel of an upper respiratory infection with group A streptococci affecting the joints, heart, brain and skin. Now rare in the UK. Major criteria include carditis, polyarthritis, chorea, erythema marginatum and subcutaneous nodules. Minor criteria are fever, arthralgia, previous rheumatic fever, high erythrocyte sedimentation rate/C-reactive protein, leucocytosis, and prolonged PR interval on electrocardiography. Treat with bed rest and benzylpenicillin to eradicate the streptococci. Corticosteroids are needed for patients who have severe carditis.

RIEDEL'S LOBE: common congenital abnormality affecting the right lobe of the liver with extra liver tissue projecting downwards.

ROTH'S SPOTS: round, oval or elliptical retinal haemorrhages with a white centre (caused by a collection of lymphocytes) originally associated with bacterial endocarditis but can be seen in any of the collagen diseases, haemolytic anaemias and leukaemias.

SARCOIDOSIS: a multisystem granulomatous disorder. Usually a subacute syndrome in young adults, especially females, with fever, malaise, polyarthralgia, erythema nodosum and bilateral hilar lymphadenopathy (sometimes with pulmonary infiltrates) on chest X-ray. This form is usually benign and self-limiting. Less commonly it can present as a chronic insidious disease with progressive dyspnoea due to pulmonary fibrosis. There may be lupus pernio of the skin. Other manifestations of sarcoidosis include hypercalcaemia due to hypersensitivity to vitamin D, eye lesions (usually anterior uveitis), hepatosplenomegaly, generalized lymphadenopathy, parotid enlargement which may be bilateral, bone cysts, mononeuritis multiplex and peripheral neuropathy.

SCHISTOSOMIASIS: bilharziasis; a disease endemic in some tropical areas and caused by infection of the venous channels with trematode parasitic flukes which are transmitted through freshwater snails. The condition commonly affects the skin, and intestinal and urinary tracts.

SCLEROMALACIA: this is one of the ocular complications of rheumatoid disease. It presents as a bluish discoloration of the sclera mainly around the iris. The blueness is thought to be due to the choroid showing through the thin sclera. Perforation may (rarely) occur—scleromalacia perforans.

SCURVY: vitamin C (ascorbic acid) deficiency caused by an inadequate intake of citrus fruits, leafy vegetables and tomatoes. Usually seen in socially and economically deprived elderly people and in those who have bizarre food fads. In adults the symptoms are often non-specific (muscle pains and weakness). In infants there is irritability, anaemia, leg pains and subperiosteal haemorrhages especially at the ends of the long bones. Other features include spontaneous haemorrhages, corkscrew hairs and poor wound healing.

SENSORY ATAXIA: incoordination due to defective sensory input usually from the posterior column of the spinal cord (e.g. tabes dorsalis). Unlike cerebellar ataxia, incoordination is only revealed when the eyes are closed thereby eliminating visual correction (hence Romberg's test).

SHY—DRAGER SYNDROME: an example of the rare multisystem atrophies where parkinsonism is associated with primary autonomic failure.

SICKLE CELL ANAEMIA: can vary from a very mild, asymptomatic disorder to severe haemolytic anaemia with recurrent, severe and painful crises. Presents in childhood with anaemia and mild jaundice. Infarcts of the small bones of the hands and feet are common. In adults it presents with vaso-occlusive problems due to 'sickling' in the small vessels of any organ. It can present with bone pain, pleuritic chest pain, splenic infarcts, hemiparesis and fits, papillary necrosis of the kidneys and haematuria. Long-term problems include increased susceptibility to infection, chronic leg ulcers, gallstones, aseptic necrosis of bones and chronic renal disease. Haemoglobin can be low (6–8 g) with a high reticulocyte count. Sickling of the red cells can be seen on blood film. Treatment is supportive with fluids, oxygen, analgesics and antibiotics.

SILICOSIS: uncommon condition but can still be seen in workers in foundries, sand blasting, stone masonry, pottery and ceramics. Due to inhalation of silica, a dust that is very fibrogenic. The chest X-ray and clinical features are similar to progressive massive fibrosis though the chest X-ray has the distinctive appearance of 'egg shell' calcification (thin lines of calcium seen around the hilar lymph nodes).

SJÖGREN'S SYNDROME: dry eyes (keratoconjunctivitis sicca), dry mouth, telangiectasiae on the face, Raynaud's phenomenon and bilateral parotid enlargement, usually associated with rheumatoid arthritis.

STEELE—RICHARDSON—OLSZEWSKI SYNDROME: a rare, progressive neurological disorder of unknown cause which occurs mostly in middle-aged men. It is characterized by ophthalmoplegia (loss of upward gaze), ataxia, rigidity, pseudobulbar palsy and parkinsonian facies.

STILL'S DISEASE (JUVENILE CHRONIC ARTHRITIS): occurs in childhood either in infancy or early adolescence. Characterized by three subtypes—the systemic form (about 20%) with high fever, rash, lymphadenopathy, splenomegaly and pericarditis with arthralgia being a main feature; the oligoarticular form (40% of cases) affecting up to four large joints and associated with iritis; and the polyarticular form (40%; female preponderance) presenting similar to rheumatoid arthritis with systemic features. Treat with non-steroidals and avoid steroids because of their effect on growth. Spontaneous remissions occur in about 85% of patients before the age of 20.

STURGE—WEBER SYNDROME: congenital abnormality. Port wine stain on one side of the face associated with a vascular abnormality in the meninges with tramline calcification on the same side on skull X-ray. Can cause ipsilateral glaucoma, strabismus and optic atrophy and contralateral hemiparesis, hemismallness and epilepsy.

SUPERIOR VENA CAVA OBSTRUCTION: commonly secondary to a bronchial carcinoma involving the superior vena cava. Symptoms include early morning headache, facial congestion and oedema including the upper limbs. The jugular veins are distended as are the superficial veins on the chest due to the formation of a collateral circulation. Treat with urgent radiotherapy.

SYRINGOMYELIA: a progressive neurological condition due to fluid-filled cavities (syrinxes) within the spinal cord, often associated with bony anomalies at the foramen magnum. Clinical features include pain in the arms, dissociated sensory loss (intact touch and proprioception and impaired temperature and pain sensations), wasting, spastic paraparesis and loss of upper limb reflexes. Charcot's joints at the elbow may occur.

TABES DORSALIS: a syphilitic involvement of the dorsal column of the spinal cord causing sensory ataxia with loss of joint position sense. The patient may also have Argyll Robertson pupils (small irregular pupils less responsive to light than accommodation), ptosis with overaction of frontalis and Charcot's joints.

TABOPARESIS: neurosyphilis in which there are both features of tabes dorsalis and involvement of the pyramidal tracts (extensor plantar responses) leading to features of spastic paraparesis. There may be 'general paresis of the insane'.

TEMPORAL ARTERITIS: a condition of older age groups associated with headache and tenderness over the temporal arteries with loss of pulsation. The erythrocyte sedimentation rate is usually >100. Treat urgently with high-dose steroids to prevent the irreversible blindness that can occur early. See also polymyalgia rheumatica.

TESTICULAR FEMINIZATION SYNDROME (ANDROGEN-INSENSITIVITY SYNDROME, AIS): a disorder in which a genetic male with XY chromosomes appears to be a phenotypic female because of the inability of the body to respond to normal amounts of androgens. The external sexual appearance is normal for a female but there is a paucity of pubic and axillary hair. The vagina ends in a blind pouch and there is no uterus. The testes may be in the abdomen, inguinal canal or in the labia. These should be removed because of the high incidence of neoplastic disease.

TETANUS: an infective condition due to the toxins of *Clostridium tetani* entering the body usually through a skin wound. Characterized by both spasms of the masseters and generalized spasms; can be fatal. Treat with antitoxin and penicillin. Occasionally there may be need for ventilatory support.

THROMBOPHLEBITIS MIGRANS (TROUSSEAU'S SYNDROME): may occur in as many as 10% of cancer patients in some series. There is thrombophlebitis in multiple sites at different times and it is often associated with carcinoma of the gastrointestinal tract.

THYROID ACROPACHY: may occur in Graves' disease but is very rare. Clinically resembles clubbing and is characterized by curved nails, swollen fingertips and periosteal new bone formation.

TROISIER'S SIGN: enlargement of the supraclavicular lymph nodes, associated with either gastric carcinoma (when on the left) or an intrathoracic tumour (when on the right). Troisier diagnosed his own gastric cancer from a supraclavicular mass.

TROUSSEAU'S SIGN: important sign in hypocalcaemia. Inflation of the sphygmomanometer cuff above the diastolic blood pressure for 3 min induces tetanic spasm of the fingers and wrist. The patient may also have Chvostek's sign.

TUBEROUS SCLEROSIS: a rare inherited (autosomal dominant) disease characterized in its fully developed form by mental retardation, epilepsy and adenoma sebaceum (red and white papules mostly in the nasolabial folds) of the face. Sclerotic patches occur in the brain and benign tumours may be found in other organs. Shagreen patches (flesh-coloured lumpy plaques which resemble studded leather) may be seen over the back.

ULCERATIVE COLITIS: a severe ulcerative inflammation of the colon with abdominal pain, diarrhoea with loss of blood, mucus and pus from the bowel and anaemia. Can be mild, moderate or severe and is often associated with malaise and anorexia. The disease usually runs a course over many years with relapses and remissions. Acute episodes are characterized by severe diarrhoea, fever, tachycardia, high erythrocyte sedimentation rate, anaemia and low albumin. Sigmoidoscopy reveals an inflamed, friable and bleeding mucosa. Treatment may be medical with high-dose steroids or surgical with resection of the colon.

VASCULITIS: inflammation of a blood vessel presenting usually as purpura, bruises, nodules or ulceration. Can be seen as part of several systemic disorders, e.g. collagen vascular diseases or meningococcal septicaemia.

VIRCHOW'S NODE: left supraclavicular adenopathy associated with carcinoma of the stomach.

VON WILLEBRAND'S DISEASE: an autosomal dominant disorder due to deficiency of a plasma protein, von Willebrand factor, which is required for the stabilization of factor VIII in the circulation and for the normal adherence of platelets to sites of vascular injury. The condition is characterized by a low factor VIII level, prolonged bleeding time, haemorrhages after minor trauma, frequent epistaxis and menorrhagia. Haemarthrosis is rare.

WALDENSTROM'S MACROGLOBULINAEMA: see paraproteinaemia.

WALLENBERG'S SYNDROME: lateral medullary syndrome due to thrombosis of the posterior inferior cerebellar artery—commonest of the brainstem infarctions. Presents with sudden vertigo, vomiting, ipsilateral Horner's syndrome, palatal palsy, decreased perception of pain on the face, and ataxia, with contralateral loss of pain and temperature on the trunk.

WEBER'S SYNDROME: midbrain lesion characterized by ipsilateral oculomotor nerve paresis and contralateral hemiplegia.

WEGENER'S GRANULOMATOSIS: a disease of unknown cause involving the upper respiratory tract, lungs and kidneys. Can start with nasal granulomata and ulceration, cough, haemoptysis and pleuritic pain. The chest X-ray shows single or multiple nodules. There can be a necrotizing glomerulonephritis and vasculitis.

WEIL'S DISEASE (LEPTOSPIROSIS ICTEROHAEMORRHAGICA): infection by *Leptospira* is usually acquired through cuts in the skin from dirty water in canals and sewers. The condition is characterized by fever, headache, myalgia, conjunctival suffusion, abdominal pain, hepatomegaly, jaundice and gastrointestinal haemorrhage.

WERDNIG–HOFFMANN DISEASE: a rare, genetic disorder of the motor neurones which causes a slowly progressive, symmetrical (usually) muscle weakness and wasting. Occurs in infants and is usually quite acute in onset. Can be confused with the muscular dystrophies.

WICKHAM'S STRIAE: these are thin, lacy white lines that occur on the surface of the flat-topped papules of lichen planus. The striae may be radial or trabecular in character and are probably due to thickening of the epidermis.

WILSON'S DISEASE: hepatolenticular degeneration. Due to an inborn error of metabolism causing an accumulation of copper. It is a progressive and often familial disease. Starts in early life and is characterized by tremor, muscular rigidity, involuntary movements and hepatic dysfunction. There may be Kayser–Fleischer rings in the eyes.

YELLOW NAIL SYNDROME: complete or partial cessation of all nail growth with thickening and yellowish discoloration, excessive increase in convexity and loss of cuticles. Often associated with pulmonary disease (pleural effusion, bronchiectasis or a malignancy) and lymphatic abnormalities (e.g. aplasia, lymphangitis, lymphoedema).

ZOLLINGER–ELLISON SYNDROME (GASTRINOMA): a malignant tumour arising from the G cells of the pancreas secreting large amounts of gastrin. It stimulates maximum gastric acid secretion causing peptic ulcers in the usual areas of the stomach and duodenum but also in the jejunum. They can be large, deep and multiple. Haemorrhage and perforation can occur. Diagnosis is by finding high serum gastrin levels. Treat medically with omeprazole; surgery is reserved for the removal of the primary tumor.

4 / Pocket Snellen's chart

This pocket Snellen's chart held 2 m from the patient's eyes (i.e. just beyond the end of the bed) can be used to gain some bedside information about the visual acuity. It gives only an approximation because 6 m is the least distance at which the effects of accommodation can be ignored (hence visual acuity is normally tested at 6 m

with a Snellen's chart three times as big as this). Remember that the commonest cause of diminished visual acuity is a refractive error so that to gain information about other pathology in the eye (e.g. diabetic maculopathy), the corrected visual acuity needs to be assessed (with glasses on or through a pinhole).

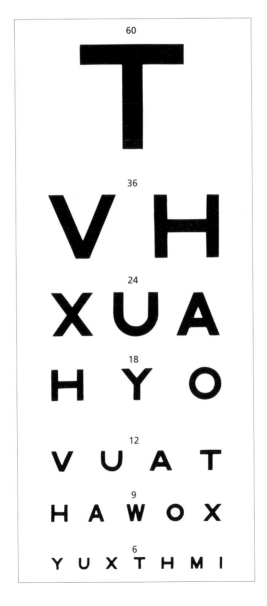

Index